P9-DSW-208

Born to Talk
An Introduction to Speech and Language Development
SECOND EDITION

Lloyd M. Hulit
Illinois State University

Merle R. Howard
Illinois State University

Allyn and Bacon
Boston • London • Toronto • Sydney • Tokyo • Singapore

Executive Editor: Stephen D. Dragin
Series Editorial Assistant: Christine Svitila
Editorial-Production Administrator: Rosalie Briand
Editorial-Production Service: Matrix Productions Inc.
Composition and Prepress Buyer: Linda Cox
Manufacturing Buyer: Suzanne Lareau
Cover Administrator: Linda Knowles

Copyright © 1997 by Allyn & Bacon
A Viacom Company
160 Gould Street
Needham Heights, MA 02194

Internet: www.abacon.com
America Online: keyword: College Online

All rights reserved. No part of the material protected by this copyright notice may be reproduced or uti-
lized in any form or by any means, electronic or mechanical, including photocopying, recording, or by
any information storage and retrieval system, without written permission from the copyright owner.

Library of Congress Cataloging-in-Publication Data
Hulit, Lloyd.
    Born to talk : an introduction to speech and language development
/ Lloyd M. Hulit, Merle R. Howard. — 2nd ed.
        p.   cm.
    Includes bibliographical references and index.
    ISBN 0-205-19411-7
    1. Language and languages.   2. Language acquisition.   3. Speech.
I. Howard, Merle R.   II. Title.
P106.H78   1996
401'.93—dc20
                                                      96-23772
                                                      CIP

Printed in the United States of America

10 9 8 7 6 5   01 00 99 98

To the most important people in our lives,
with immeasurable love and gratitude

Pamela, Yvonne, Carmen, Scot, John, Christopher, and Lance
Bonita and Lane

Photo Credits: Pages xiv, 160, 368 © Robert Finken/The Picture Cube. Page 14 © Larry Kolvoord/The Image Works. Pages 21, 39, 46, 148, 245, 300, 315 © Will Faller. Page 54 © D. Ogust/The Image Works. Page 65 © Tony Loreti/ The Picture Cube. Page 71 © George W. Gardner/The Image Works. Page 76 © Elizabeth Crews/The Image Works. Page 79 © Michael Ciluk/The Image Works. Page 108 © John Coletti/The Picture Cube. Page 116 © Julie O'Neil/ The Picture Cube. Page 132 © Robert V. Eckert Jr./The Picture Cube. Pages 171, 218 © Carol Palmer/The Picture Cube. Page 174 © Steve Takatsuno/The Picture Cube. Page 198 © CLEO Photography/The Picture Cube. Pages 224, 311 © Will Hart. Page 272 © Topham-OB/The Image Works. Page 306 © Eric Roth/The Picture Cube. Page 323 © Patricia Beringer/The Image Works. Page 334 © Stephen Marks.

Contents

Preface

This book is about one of the greatest natural wonders in the human experience—language. Despite having studied speech and language development and disorders for many years and our teaching of a wide range of courses on these topics to thousands of students, we retain the same curiosity and awe about speech and language that we had when we began. In fact, the more we learn about speech and language, the more convinced we are that the whole process by which language is generated and then transmitted by speech may never be fully understood. In the pages that follow, we hope to share our enthusiasm for this subject with our readers, to stimulate the same passion that has driven us to appreciate the complexity, power, and enormous creative potential of language in all its expressive forms.

Although this book is grounded in relevant research literature, it was not our intention to write a scholarly treatise. All university professors must serve in many roles, but we view ourselves first and foremost as teachers. The purpose of this book is to teach, and the style clearly represents the manner in which we each approach teaching in the classroom. When we teach, we do not merely present information. We explain and provide examples. We ask questions and try to anticipate questions that will or should be asked by our students. When we introduce new concepts, we thoroughly explain the terminology. We review information already discussed to provide a foundation for new information. We reach forward to help students understand where we are headed and to sense what the final outcome will be. We prefer to err on the side of providing too much information rather than on the side of assuming too much knowledge. Above all, we believe that learning should be stimulating and enjoyable, and we have tried to write a stimulating and enjoyable book.

Many books written by professors are heavy on jargon. This book is not. It was impossible to avoid the jargon entirely, of course—jargon is the language of the discipline—but when we use specialized terms, we do not assume familiarity.

One of the difficulties involved in writing a textbook is meeting the needs of instructors who teach certain targeted courses, yet at the same time creating an effective teaching tool addressed to the student. We have tried to walk the line between the instructor's needs and students' needs carefully. We will gladly admit, however, that when these needs appeared to collide, we chose to communicate as clearly and directly as possible to the students who will read the book. In doing so, we have created what we believe is an exceptionally reader-friendly introduction to speech and language development.

The first edition of this book was used in courses representing a number of disciplines and was read by students with widely varying academic backgrounds. We kept this wide audience in mind as we prepared the second edition. Some readers, for example, will be less familiar than others with information pertaining to the anatomy and physiology of speech, language, and hearing. We have included this information in Appendix A (*The Anatomical and Physiological Bases of Speech, Language, and Hearing*). Majors in speech–language pathology and audiology may want to consult this material for purposes of review, but it is strictly introductory in nature and is not intended to include all one needs to know about the structural and functional bases of human communication.

Two chapters of the book have been written as independent units: Chapter Eight (*Language Diversity: Regional, Social/Cultural, and Gender Differences*) and Chapter Nine (*Speech and Language Disorders*). These two chapters can be included or deleted without affecting the book's integrity.

Chapter Seven (*The Building Blocks of Speech*) presented a different problem. Any book on speech and language development must address the development of the sound system of speech, but there is always the question about where this information should be included. We chose to keep the language chapters together, make references to phonological issues in these chapters as necessary, and insert a separate, more comprehensive chapter on phonology following our discussion of speech and language development. It should be noted, however, that Chapter Seven, too, has been written so that it can be moved to the beginning or the end without affecting understanding of the material in any other part of the book.

The primary focus of this book is language. Chapters One through Six are devoted to language development. Whereas other books divide language development according to the various components of language (i.e., syntax, morphology, semantics, pragmatics, etc.), ours is a real-time presentation of development, divided by stages. We have integrated our discussion of the components within each stage. This will allow the reader to sense what the child is receiving and producing at each developmental level, and will facilitate an understanding about how one aspect of language affects all other aspects.

It is important that instructors and students alike clearly understand the purpose of Chapter One (*A Connection of Brains*). This chapter is not designed as much to present information as it is to pique the reader's interest. We understand that some students who read this book will already have some background in speech and language, but others will not. Students with little or no background in speech–language pathology or linguistics have probably not given much thought to the process of human communication. The sole, but important, purpose of Chapter One is to prod the reader into thinking about language as a unique human experience and appreciating speech as an incredible means by which messages encoded in language forms can be transmitted from one human brain to another. We believe that students cannot truly appreciate what we now understand and believe about language and language development without understanding the historical context from which our present knowledge originated. Chapter One provides that context.

Although every chapter has been touched by the revision process, the most important changes have been made in Chapters Two, Three, Seven, and Nine. Chapter Two (*Language Acquisition: A Theoretical Journey*) has been renamed to more accurately reflect the purpose of our presentation. Instead of concentrating just on the extremes of the nature-versus-nurture debate about how children acquire language, the revised chapter focuses on a range of theoretical perspectives representing a number of junctures on the nature-versus-nurture continuum.

In the first edition, Chapter Three (*Get Ready . . . Get Set . . . Talk!*) was devoted almost exclusively to a discussion of Jean Piaget's theory of cognitive development. That discussion remains in the second edition, but we now also include a section summarizing research findings that have challenged some of Piaget's assertions, and we have included a reasonably thorough discussion of Lev Vygotsky's theory of cognitive development.

In the first edition, Chapter Seven (*The Building Blocks of Speech*) included detailed discussions of the three approaches used to describe speech sounds: Traditional Phonetics, Distinctive Features, and Phonological Processes. These discussions have been retained, but significantly reduced in detail. The portion of the chapter devoted to theories of phonological development has been greatly expanded. As in Chapter Two, an effort was made to sample a range of theories, not just extreme perspectives.

The changes in Chapter Nine (*Speech and Language Disorders*) focus on phonological and language disorders. These sections have been completely rewritten to reflect current terminology and to represent current views about etiological and classification issues.

Before we get to our acknowledgments, I want to address the gender strategy we used in writing this book. As a husband and the father of two daughters, and member of a profession that is more than 80 percent female, I am sensitive to the gender problem in communication. As a writer, I am also frustrated by the limitations of American English pronouns. In order to gain a perspective on this issue beyond my own, I polled my undergraduate and graduate students, the overwhelming majority of whom were female, about the use of *he* and *she* in textbooks. They were unanimous in saying that they understand *he,* when used in this kind of writing, to be gender neutral, and that they find alternating between *he* and *she* by chapter distracting. For this reason, we decided to use *he, him, his,* with the understanding that these pronouns are intended to be gender neutral. We also decided that referring to the child in one gender would be consistent with our intention to create an image of *one* child whose speech and language development we trace through the pages of this book.

We want to acknowledge the invaluable contributions of several people. Howard Davis created the anatomical figures in Appendix A. Pamela Hulit provided computer assistance in creating a number of tables included in the book. We appreciate the special talents of these people and are grateful for their efforts on our behalf.

We also want to acknowledge Dr. David L. Tucker for his contributions to Chapter Six. Dr. Tucker, whose primary scholarly and teaching focus is reading, is a Professor in Illinois State University's Department of Specialized Educational Development. The material in the section of Chapter Six entitled, *Reading and Writing: New Applications of Language,* was contributed by Dr. Tucker and edited by the senior author.

We want to express a special gratitude to our students, a group of young women and men who have enriched our professional lives by their presence in our classrooms. Our students never allow us to be complacent. They constantly challenge us to know more and understand better, just as we try to challenge them to learn, integrate, and apply knowledge to the solution of real-life problems. They ask penetrating questions that require us to continue the process of learning. Their curiosity becomes our curiosity, and that is what makes teaching one of the most satisfying of human endeavors. We thank all Illinois State University students who have shared time with us in our collective effort to understand more about communication development and disorders.

Finally, we want to thank the following people who reviewed the second edition of this book: Delores E. Battle, Buffalo State College; Rhea Paul, Portland State University; and Sara Elizabeth Runyan, James Madison University..

Lloyd M. Hulit, Ph.D.
Merle R. Howard, Ph.D.

Born to Talk

ONE

A Connection of Brains

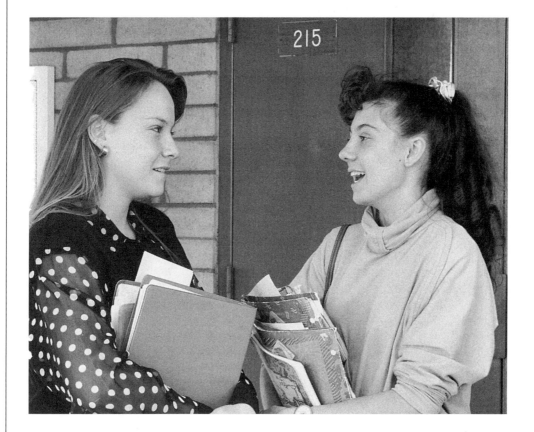

Chapter Objectives

This first chapter is designed to pique your interest in speech and language as processes within the broader process we call communication. We define and describe these processes, and we consider how speech and language interact to produce a form of communication unique to humans. We also consider how a speaker's thoughts are conveyed to a listener's brain through a series of communication transformations known collectively as the *speech chain*. Specifically, this chapter is designed to facilitate understanding of the following topics:

- Definitions of *communication, language,* and *speech.*
- Speech and language as separate but related processes.
- Design features of the human communication system.
- The speech chain that connects the speaker's thoughts to the listener's understanding of those thoughts.

Have you ever wished you could read someone's mind or ever wished or worried that someone could read your mind? I think all of us at one time or another have at least wondered about mental telepathy, and perhaps some of you reading this page believe you have that gift. I would like to suggest that every person reading this page who is able to speak is capable of a form of mental telepathy, because human speech allows one human brain to communicate with another human brain in a wondrous and almost magical manner.

Most people give very little thought to the magic of speech because it is acquired so naturally and used by humans so effortlessly. It is the purpose of this book to explore the miracles of speech and language, to examine the marvelous anatomic structures and physiological processes we humans have adapted for speech, to unravel the layers of language from sounds to words to elaborate sentence structure that together make up speech, to investigate the dialectal differences in our own language, and to consider the problems that occur when speech and language do not develop properly or when something goes wrong after communication skills have been normal for a time. By the time you have turned the final page in your journey through this book, I believe you will be convinced that words like *magic* and *wondrous* and *miraculous* in reference to speech and language are accurately descriptive, but before we go any further, we need to address some basic terminology.

Separate But Related Processes

In the preceding paragraphs I have used the words *speech* and *language* in a manner implying they are not the same thing, and that is correct. They are separate but related processes in the larger process we call communication. To understand any of these processes, you must understand all of them, and how they are interconnected.

Communication is the sending and receiving of information, ideas, feelings, or messages. In order to appreciate the breadth of communication, consider just some of the methods by which human beings communicate. We transmit messages of all kinds by speech, the written word, Morse code, semaphore flags, Braille, facial expressions, gestures, art, music, dance, the distances we maintain when we interact, vocal variations, the clothes we wear, hairstyles, our natural and purchased odors, and the list goes on. We communicate hundreds, perhaps thousands, of messages every day. Some of our communications are intended, but many are not. We hope that most of what we send is received according to our intent, but unfortunately this is not always the case. The fact is, we humans cannot stop communicating even when we want to. You may decide to say nothing, but your saying nothing may be saying more than your saying something. Even when you are asleep you may be sending messages. You may talk in your sleep, of course, but even in the silence of unconsciousness, you may communicate restlessness by the way you thrash around in your bed, or you may communicate a basic insecurity by the way you curl into the fetal position or you may transmit a message of utter tranquility by the relaxed and peaceful expression on your sleeping face. Do you get the point? Communication is so much a part of the human experience that we are constantly sending and receiving messages.

Language is an infinitely more difficult phenomenon to describe, so we will build a definition by first looking at some of the characteristics of language and then trying to piece them together. Most people think of language as "words strung together by grammar," but that captures only a part of language and only what appears on the surface of what we read or hear.

Language is an expression of an ability that is innate in all humans. We are born with the capacity to use language in the same way a spider is born with the ability to weave webs, and a bird is born with the ability to make a nest. To use language is instinctive in humans, but the capacity is realized differently in people according to the specific languages to which they are exposed. A child reared in a family of English-speaking adults, who hears only English during the language acquisition period, *will* speak English. You might be surprised that the logic of that observation escapes some people. My youngest sister, abandoned by her natural Korean parents, was adopted by the Hulit family when we lived in Korea. When we returned to a small town in rural Ohio 2 years later, some people were amazed that she spoke English without a Korean accent. Children do not know they are German, French, Russian, or Japanese when they are born. They speak the language they hear, but the innate capacity for that language is the same, no matter where they are born.

It is important to understand that language and the expression of language are two very different things. Language exists in the mind, and it exists whether it is expressed or not. It is useful to understand language as a system of abstract symbols organized according to basic rules that seem to be common to all the languages known to humankind. In other words, at the deepest, most basic level, all languages share common structural rules.

The fact that we do not all speak the same language suggests that some aspects of language are learned. Languages are different in many ways. They use different words. They have different rules for organizing words into grammatical sentences. English, for example, stresses word order in its grammar system, but other languages, like Latin, place greater emphasis on word endings than on order to indicate grammatical relationships. That is, all languages have rules for making sentences grammatically correct, but the means by which correctness is achieved vary. We can conclude, therefore, that although the capacity for language is innate and although certain very basic rules are shared by all languages, the specific conventions of any given language are learned. The child who will speak English, for example, must learn the sounds of English as well as its vocabulary and grammar.

Now let us put some of these pieces together into a definition. **Language** is a system of abstract symbols and rule-governed structures, the specific conventions of which are learned. The symbols of language may be sounds that are combined into spoken words, or letters that are combined into written words, or even the elements of sign language that are combined into larger units. It is important to note that whatever the symbols, they are arbitrarily established by the conventional usage of a given people. Furthermore, the symbols or their combinations will change over time because language is a constantly evolving phenomenon. Much more needs to be added to this definition (and will be in the chapters that follow), but this will serve as a starting point.

We can now define speech, a relatively simple task if we understand communication and language. Very simply, **speech** is the oral expression of language. Sometimes people use the terms "language" and "speech" as though they are interchangeable, but they are clearly not. If they were interchangeable, one could not exist without the other because they would be one and the same thing. In fact, speech can and does exist in the absence of language, and language exists in the absence of speech. Consider the parrot or mynah, birds that can mimic human speech, often with remarkable clarity. These birds produce speech, but they do not have language. That is, they can produce strings of sounds with the acoustic characteristics of human speech, and human listeners recognize the sequences of sounds as words, but the speech of these birds is devoid of meaning, and therefore, is not the oral expression of language. They have speech but no language. Some human beings, most notably severely mentally retarded individuals, may have the ability to imitate speech perfectly even if they do not fully understand the language underlying the speech. They have speech that reflects language abilities they do not have. Even normal children, between the ages of 18 to 24 months, often produce a form of speech known as **echolalia,** which is an imitation of words, phrases, or even whole sentences in the absence of an understanding of what they are saying.

Language can also exist independently of speech. Children who are born deaf, for example, may never learn to speak, but their deafness does not preclude language. If there are no other problems and if these children receive proper stimulation and appropriate educational opportunities, they can develop language abilities just as sophisticated and complete as the hearing child who speaks. The deaf child who does not have speech must learn a different way to express language, most likely through signs and gestures. In addition, of course, the deaf child can receive and express language through the written word.

We can best understand speech as a highly complex physiological process requiring the coordination of respiration, phonation, resonation, and articulation. Some of the movements involved in producing even the simplest of utterances are simultaneous and others are successive, but the synchronization of these movements is critical.

Consider just some of what happens in the production of the single word *statistics.* The tip of the tongue is lifted from a resting position to an area on the roof of the mouth just behind the upper teeth called the **alveolar ridge** to produce the "s" sound. The tongue is pressed against the alveolar ridge hard enough to produce constriction, but not so hard as to stop the airflow altogether. As the speaker slowly contracts the muscles of exhalation under precise control, air is forced between the tip of the tongue and the alveolar ridge. Leaving the tongue in the same area, the speaker now presses a little harder to stop the air flow and then quickly releases the contact for the production of the "t" sound. The tongue drops to a neutral position and the vocal folds in the larynx vibrate to produce the vowel "a." The speaker turns off the larynx and lifts the tongue to the alveolar ridge for the next "t," then vibrates the vocal folds for the vowel "i" while the tongue stays in a forward but slightly lowered position. The speaker turns the larynx off again and moves the tongue to the alveolar ridge yet again to produce the controlled constriction for the next "s," followed by increased pressure to stop the air flow and release it for the "t." The larynx is turned on one more time and the tongue lowered to a neutral position for the "i," and then turned off as the tongue arches to the back of the mouth where it contacts the velum, or fleshy part of the roof of the mouth, for the "k." Finally, the tongue tip darts to the alveolar ridge for the production of the final "s" sound.

All of this occurs in the production of *one* word! Imagine what occurs in the production of a long sentence produced at an average rate of speed. When you consider how many intricate adjustments are made so quickly in the speech mechanism, it is difficult to imagine that anyone learns to speak at all! But we do learn to speak, and we do it easily and naturally over a very brief period of time.

Speech and Language Rejoined

Now that we have established that speech and language are separate, although related, parts of the communication process, we will reconnect them for the remainder of our analysis. For practical purposes, in people with normal communicative abilities, they are not separate. Speech is commonly understood as oral language, and that understanding will serve our purposes well. It is certainly clear to anyone who has studied the development of communication in children that speech and language develop together, but we should always remember that they do not develop at the same pace. Most of what a child will ever know about language is acquired before entering school, but some speech sounds are not mastered until age seven or eight. Even within language itself, not all dimensions are acquired according to the same schedule. Rules pertaining to the structure of language are acquired early and most of the basic vocabulary of a language is learned early, but we may continue to add vocabulary as long as we live, and most of us are developing our knowledge about how to use language, a dimension called **pragmatics,** well into adulthood.

From this point on, however, we will consider speech and language as integrated parts of the same process in the same way that pictures and sounds are integrated parts of television. You can certainly have television without pictures: It's called radio. And you can have television without sound: That's called network difficulty. But television as we expect it includes not only pictures but also sound. Speech as we expect it in normal human beings combines phonated and articulated noises and the rule-governed structures of language.

The Unique Characteristics of Human Speech

To appreciate the powers of oral language, we can compare it to the communication systems of other animals. Other animals do communicate, of course, but there is much we do not understand about their systems. Some animals seem to communicate very general messages in simple ways. The beaver, for example, slaps his tail when he senses danger. Dogs bark when they are frightened or excited. Other animals are able to communicate more elaborate messages. Bees dance to tell their fellow bees where the flowers are. Other insects use their antennae to instruct or inform. There is a great deal of interest in the communication systems of dolphins and singing whales because they seem to be much more elaborate than the systems of most other animals (Herman & Forestell, 1985; Schusterman, 1986). No matter how much we discover about the abilities of other animals to communicate, however, we remain convinced that no animal has a communication system as powerful as human speech.

One of the first linguists to take a detailed, analytical look at the characteristics of human speech in comparison to the communication systems of other animals was Charles F. Hockett (1960), who wrote a classic essay entitled "The Origin of Speech," in which he describes what he calls "thirteen design-features" of language. Although many animals share some of these features in their communication systems, Hockett believed that when his thirteen features are taken together, they effectively separate human speech from other forms of animal communication. Since Hockett wrote this essay, many of his assumptions and conclusions have been dismissed as the result of research data and new theoretical interpretations. Nevertheless, "The Origin of Speech" remains an important part of the literature on human language, because it challenged linguists to think about language and those who use language in revolutionary ways.

From Mouths to Ears

Hockett's first design-feature is the **vocal-auditory channel.** That is, human beings communicate by forcing air through the vocal folds of the larynx and breaking the vibrating air stream into sounds of speech, which are organized into words and sentences. These sounds are received by the listener's ears. This feature is so obvious that we may need to note that other channels can be used in communication and are used by other animals. Bees, for example, communicate by dancing and that can be described as the visual channel. In fact, human beings who cannot hear use the visual channel when they produce and receive sign language. Still other animals communicate by touch or by odor. The primary advantage of the vocal-auditory channel for humans is that it leaves our hands free to do other things while we are communicating. We can build or repair, for example, while giving or receiving instructions. Imagine what it would be like for a construction crew building a house if everyone had to put down their tools every time one person needed to communicate with another through the gesture-visual channel. There is no question that vocal-auditory communication is convenient and allows us to be efficient in all tasks that involve communication in conjunction with other physical activities.

Sending and Receiving Signals

The second design-feature is **broadcast transmission and directional reception,** which is obviously related to the first feature. Two characteristics of speech are involved in this feature. When speech is produced, it radiates in all directions and can be received by any listener who is in range. In addition, a listener with two good ears can compare the loudness and timing of the signals reaching each ear, and can determine the direction from which the sound is coming. If communication is visual, reception is much more limited. Deaf sign language, for example, can be received only by someone who is close enough to the sender to see the details of the gestures, some of which are quite subtle, and the receiver must directly face the sender.

Hear Today, Gone Immediately

Rapid fading means that speech signals are transitory. They do not linger. Humans have developed writing to put language information into a more permanent form, but writing is a relatively new ability for human beings in comparison to speech. We have also developed electronic means for preserving speech, but each time a sample of speech is produced live or on tape, the signals are broadcast and rapidly fade. We cannot freeze-frame speech and study it in the same way we can read and study the written word or primitive paintings on the cave walls of prehistoric people.

If You Can Say It, I Can Say It

One feature of human speech that we may take for granted is **interchangeability**. This means that any human being can say anything that is said by any other human being. Children can and do imitate the speech of adults. Female humans can produce the same speech forms as are produced by males. Among other animals, this feature is rare. In courtship rituals, for example, the male of many species produces gender-limited communications, and the female produces gender-limited responses. Interchangeability removes communication barriers and is largely responsible for the unlimited exchange of information that characterizes human speech for both sexes and all ages.

Did I Say That?. . . Did I *Mean* That?

Total feedback means that human speakers have the capacity to monitor what we say and how we say it. We hear ourselves, of course, but we also receive information from the musculature of speech about what we feel as the articulators move and contact one another. This feedback component allows the speaker to make constant adjustments so that output is as finely tuned as possible in terms of conveying thoughts accurately. Feedback also provides controls for the mechanics of speech in the sense that speech errors are caught and corrected or even anticipated and avoided. The fact that the feedback system includes information from several sensory sources also protects the speaker from communicative disaster if part of the system fails. Adults who lose hearing, for example, can maintain reasonably good speech by attending more closely to how speech feels. If we lose some of our ability to monitor the motor aspects of speech, we can concentrate more intently on what our speech sounds like.

Speech Is for Talking—What Else?

The feature, **specialization**, suggests that speech is specifically designed for communication and serves no other purpose. In Appendix A, we will discover that the physical processes of speech are actually the secondary functions served by the structures involved. That is, human beings have adapted structures that serve more basic biological purposes for speech. Nevertheless, it is true that speech itself is a specialized human function. We speak to communicate and for no other purpose, although we may speak when no one is listening, and sometimes when we speak, we do not successfully communicate.

Sending Messages Loud and *Clear*

Most other animals communicate fairly general messages whereas humans can convey very specific messages with words having relatively stable relationships with the people, things, events, and concepts they represent. This feature of human speech is called **semanticity.** When the beaver slaps his tail against the water, and his fellow beavers scurry in fear, they do so because they have heard the message "Danger!" The danger could be a fire, an approaching bear, or a human hunter. Humans not only can warn that danger is present, we can name the danger.

Because We *Say* So!

One of the reasons languages differ so broadly across groups of people on earth is that the words we use to refer to the people, things, events, and concepts in our human experiences do not directly reflect their referents. There is an **arbitrariness** about language. That is, there is nothing inherent in a spoken word to account for its meaning. We call the piece of furniture upon which I now sit, a *chair*, not because it screams out to be called a chair, not because there is a connection between the nature of chairness and the word, but because someone at some time, for reasons of no interest to most of us living today, arbitrarily decided to call it a *chair*. The obvious advantage of arbitrariness is that there is absolutely no limit to how we can use language to describe anything and everything. Languages have different vocabularies because the arbitrary naming of the bits and pieces of the world has been done by different people at different places at different times.

The Limits on Speech

Discreteness is a feature that can be applied to human speech in at least two ways. Although the speech mechanism can produce an incredibly wide range of noises, each language is limited to a finite or discrete number of sounds. Furthermore, each sound used in one or more human languages has very specific characteristics so that each sound is discrete. Adult speakers adapt so completely to the specific sounds of a given language that they often have great difficulty breaking out of these patterns to produce sounds found in other languages but foreign to their own. Speakers whose native languages do not contain *l* or *r,* for example, struggle to produce these sounds when they are learning to speak English, and many of us who speak American English almost choke trying to produce some French vowels. The flexibility we have as infants to produce virtually all sounds known to all languages is quickly lost when we begin to narrow our range to the discrete sounds of our own language.

Back to the Future

One of the most intriguing features of human speech is **displacement.** That is, humans can talk about things that are distant in time and/or space. We can talk about what is going on in places across vast oceans or even across the infinite expanses of space. We can talk about events that occurred hundreds or thousands of years ago, and we can talk about things that have not yet happened. Although this feature may not be absolutely unique to human speech, we have no evidence that other animals have communication systems with this feature as fully developed as it is in speech.

The Creativity of the Mind and Mouth

According to Hockett, **productivity** is one of the most important design-features of human speech. Humans have the amazing ability to be creative in their communication efforts. We can say things that have never been said before, or we can put old messages in brand new language forms. We use words in speech in much the same way the sculptor uses clay. The sculptor can take one mass of clay and make everything from an ashtray to a bowl or a bust. We can use a finite collection of sounds and words to shape an infinite variety of messages, some simple, some profound, some old, some new. No matter what the message is, however, if we obey the rules of our language, the message will be understood by anyone who shares the language we speak. Just imagine that on this very day you may say something that no one has ever said before and perhaps no one will ever say again in exactly the same way. The productivity or creativity of language gives human speakers a communicative power that is not shared by any other animal.

Many Wholes from a Few Parts

Part of the creativity that is characteristic of human speech is made possible by another design-feature, **duality of patterning.** Although a given language is restricted in the number of sounds it uses, these sounds can be combined in an infinite number of ways to produce an infinite variety of words, and the words of a language can be combined into an infinite variety of sentences. Every year of your life you will be witness to the creation of new words that are the product of this duality of patterning. Many of these new words reflect neverending advances in science and technology. Before there were telephones, there was no word, "telephone," but the sounds making up the word have existed for as long as human language as we know it has existed. It remained for someone to arrange this particular collection of sounds into this specific word to refer to that object. Just think for a moment about all the words that have been invented over the past 40 years as a result of the technology supporting the exploration of space. The patterning of sounds into words and words into sentences will end only when humankind ceases to communicate, and that is likely to happen only when humankind ceases to exist.

Born to Talk

The final design-feature Hockett describes is **traditional transmission.** Hockett was on the leading edge of a new view of human speech and language, which will be described in more detail in the next chapter. The suggestion in this feature is that speech is instinctive in humans. We have a genetic or biological capacity for language so powerful that few environmental factors can stop the acquisition of speech, although they may affect the rate at which it is acquired and they may affect the quality of the language we use. Although the capacity for language is genetic, the details of a language, including vocabulary and structural rules, are learned.

Not All Features Are Created Equal

It should be obvious that not all of these features, even as originally described by Hockett, are of equal importance in describing human language and in separating human from animal communication. Of the thirteen features, four might be described as most important or differentiating: semanticity, displacement, productivity, and traditional transmission. That is, human beings have a communication system that allows us to communicate very specific messages. We are not limited by time and space in what we say, and we can say things that have never been said or heard before and be understood. In the next chapter, we will examine attempts to teach apes to use human language. The results of these attempts suggest that some other animals can be taught to communicate in ways that approximate human language, but it still seems reasonable to conclude that only humans are born with a capacity for language as we know and understand it. Only humans, it seems, have such a strong biological drive to acquire language, that they often talk even when the environmental odds are against them.

Speech: The Tale of Two Brains

We are now ready to return to the query that opened this chapter, or more specifically to a more complete response to that question. All human beings who are able to speak are capable of using a kind of mental telepathy because speech allows two human brains to connect.

This connection is described in another portrait of human speech contained in a book entitled *The Speech Chain* (Denes & Pinson, 1993, pp. 1–9). A summary of this description will show how the brains of a speaker and a listener connect in a communicative sense.

There are six steps or links in the speech chain. In the first step, the speaker sorts through his or her thoughts, decides which of these thoughts to express, and makes some decisions about how to express them. Although this process occurs very quickly, within seconds or fractions of a second, it is actually a very complex process. If, for example, a friend wearing the most atrocious dress you have ever seen, asks you, "What do you think of my new dress?", you have some serious decisions to make. Your brain is filled with conflicting thoughts as you consider your response. You know that this article of clothing is an affront to anything resembling good taste. You must also consider that your friend must have liked it because she did, in fact, actually give someone real, government-green money for it. You want to be honest, but you do not want to hurt her feelings. What do you do? What do you say? Well, you sort through all your thoughts. You make a decision about the relative merits of honesty and compassion, and you finally decide what to say. Incidentally, this step is much easier for very young children who typically spend very little time arranging and editing their thoughts. The three-year-old is likely to say the first thing that comes to mind, which may be tactless and unintentionally hurtful. One of the aspects of communication acquired most slowly is the ability to make good decisions in the first step of the speech chain.

Regardless of how the decisions are made in the first step or whether or not they are appropriate decisions, the second step remains the same. You as speaker put your message into language form by leafing through your mental dictionary to pick out the right words and by selecting the appropriate rules of grammar to create the correct word forms and place them into the right order. This step also occurs so quickly that you cannot monitor yourself doing it, unless you cannot think of the right word. Only when the process is interrupted by this kind of failure do we begin to appreciate just how easily and naturally we translate thoughts into language. Notice that the first two steps are confined to the brain. We may think of speech as flapping lips and a wagging tongue, but the beginning of even the simplest utterance begins in the gray matter of the brain.

In the third step, the brain sends instructions, in the form of neural impulses, to the muscles of speech, and keep in mind that these are not just the muscles of the structures in the mouth. The brain must send instructions to the muscles of respiration, the muscles of the larynx and pharynx, as well as to the muscles of the face that support speech with nonverbal expressions, and even to the muscles of the arms, hands, fingers, perhaps even the legs and torso, which provide additional nonverbal support to the speaker's words. The complexity of this operation is unbelievable and becomes even more amazing when you consider the speed at which all the parts are made operative.

In the fourth step, the movements of the structures of speech interrupt and constrict the flow of vibrating air from the larynx, setting up minute pressure changes in the air surrounding the speaker's mouth. These patterns of air pressure changes are called **sound waves.** Sound waves cause air particles to bump into each other, creating compression between some particles and spaces or rarefactions between others. The bumping, compression, and rarefaction of air particles continue until the sound waves reach the listener's ears.

As the air particles bump into the listener's eardrums in the fifth step, the listener's hearing mechanism is activated. As you will discover in more detail in Appendix A, the ear has the capacity to transform the mechanical energy of vibrating air particles into hydraulic energy in the fluids of the inner ear, and eventually into neural energy that travels along the acoustic nerve to the brain.

Finally, in the listener's brain, the neural impulses are analyzed and interpreted so that the listener recognizes the speaker's message. Consider what has happened in the speech chain. Thoughts have been transformed into language forms, which have been transformed into neural signals, which trigger the structures of speech, which by means of their movements disturb air particles into sound waves, which bombard the listener's ears, which transform the sound waves into neural patterns, which are received and decoded by the listener's brain. Incredibly, the message is not lost or changed. I may not always successfully understand what you intended to communicate, but if I am within hearing range and if you speak clearly, I will receive precisely the same pattern you sent.

Speech does indeed give us the power of mental telepathy. It allows brains to connect. Speech is so much a part of the human experience that we truly take it for granted, but it is a wondrous human gift. The next time you engage in a conversation with one or more people, consider the speech chains that connect speakers and listeners. Marvel at the speed involved in the sending and receiving of messages. Notice how quickly speakers become listeners and listeners become speakers in a ballistic communication give-and-take that almost defies understanding. Now consider that human beings know much of what they will ever know about language and have the basic skills involved in speech by the time they are just four or five years old! How does this happen?

In the remainder of this book, we will take a closer look at many of the elements in the speech chain. We will consider what the child must know to be a competent language user, and we will explore the acquisition process along all important dimensions of speech and language. You will learn that there is much we still do not know about human language. The experts argue about almost every major topic, but we know much more about speech and language today than we did just 30 years ago. It is the purpose of this book to help you understand what we know, to recognize what we do not know, and most importantly to appreciate the almost mystical nature of this uniquely human talent.

Review Questions

1. Define *communication, language,* and *speech.*

2. How are speech and language "separate but related" aspects of communication?

3. Which of Hockett's design-features most effectively separate human communication from animal communication, and why?

4. Trace the six steps in the speech chain that transforms the speaker's thoughts into the listener's understanding.

References and Suggested Readings

Bohannon, J. (1982). Close encounters of the primate kind. *American Journal of Primatology, 3*, 353–358.

Denes, P., & Pinson, E. (1993). *The speech chain* (2nd ed.), New York: W. H. Freeman and Co.

Fillmore, C., Kempler, D., & Wang, S. (Eds.) (1979). *Individual differences in language ability and language behavior*. New York: Academic Press.

Gardner, R., & Gardner, B. (1980). Two comparative psychologists look at language acquisition. In K. Nelson (Ed.), *Children's language* (Vol. 2). New York: Gardner Press.

Geschwind, N. (1982). Specializations of the brain. In W. Wang (Ed.), *Human communication: Language and its psycho-biological bases* (pp. 110–119). San Francisco: W. H. Freeman.

Herman, L. (1981). Cognitive characteristics of dolphins. In L. Herman (Ed.), *Cetacean behavior* (pp. 363–429). New York: Wiley.

Herman, L., & Forestell, P. (1985). Reporting presence or absence of named objects by a language-trained dolphin. *Neuroscience and Biobehavioral Reviews, 9*, 667–681.

Herman, L., Hovancik, J., Gory, J., & Bradshaw, G. (1989). Generalization of visual matching by a bottlenosed dolphin (tursiops truncatus): Evidence for invariance of cognitive performance with visual and auditory materials. *Journal of Experimental Psychology Animal Behavior Processes, 15*, 124–136.

Hockett, C. (1960). The origin of speech. *Scientific American, 203*, 89–97.

Lane, H. (1979). *The wild boy of Aveyron*. Cambridge, MA: Harvard University Press.

Nelson, K. (1981). Individual differences in language development: Implications for development and language. *Developmental Psychology, 17*, 170–187.

Quigley, S., & King, C. (1982). The language of deaf children and youth. In S. Rosenberg, (Ed.), *Handbook of applied psycholinguistics: Major thrusts of research and theory* (pp. 429–475). Hillsdale, NJ: Erlbaum.

Schusterman, R. (1986). Cognition and intelligence of dolphins. In R. Schusterman, J. Thomas, & F. Wood (Eds.) *Dolphin cognition and behavior: A comparative approach* (pp. 137–139). Hillsdale, NJ: Erlbaum.

Slobin, D. (Ed.). (1985). *A cross-linguistic study of language acquisition*. Hillsdale, NJ: Erlbaum.

Von Frisch, K. (1967). *The dance language and orientation of bees* (L. E. Chadwick, Trans.). Cambridge, MA: Belknap Press.

TWO

Language Acquisition: A Theoretical Journey

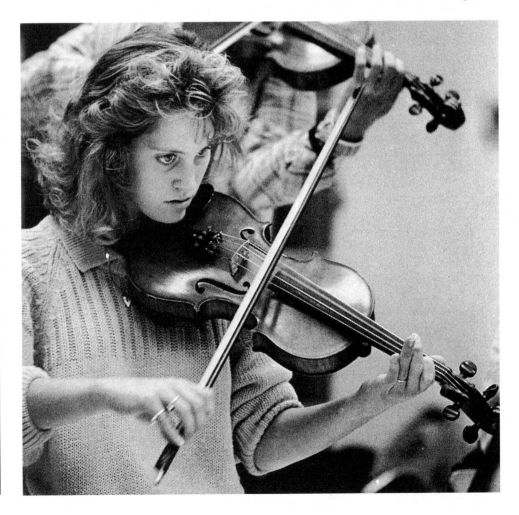

Chapter Objectives

One can only guess when the first nature-versus-nurture argument occurred. We do know, however, that whenever human behaviors are discussed, this argument is sure to arise. It is not surprising then that language experts have debated the relative influences of genetics and the environment on speech and language development. Is the child genetically predisposed to talk, or taught to talk? In this chapter, we consider the implications of this question and some of the answers experts have suggested. The answers, as you will discover, cover the entire nature-nurture continuum.

This chapter is designed to facilitate comprehension of the evolutionary changes that have occurred over the past four decades in the theories of language acquisition. It will consider the contributions made by each major theoretical view along the evolutionary continuum to furthering our understanding about how the various components of language emerge. Specifically, this chapter will address the following topics:

- The general character of the nature-versus-nurture argument and its potential impact on our understanding of speech and language development.
- The *behaviorist,* or nurture, interpretation.
- The *nativist,* or nature, interpretation.
- The *generative semantic* and *cognitivist* interpretations.
- The *information processing* interpretation.
- The *pragmatics* view and the *social interactionist* interpretation.

People probably have argued about how human talents are acquired from the earliest days of our species. Is an artist born or made? Does the musician inherit talent, or is it shaped by hours of rehearsal? Is the great athlete destined to become a physiological virtuoso because of genes, or is athletic skill the product of teaching and practice? Even the casual observer must understand that in most nature-versus-nurture arguments, the truth does not come down on only one side. The master artist must surely be born with the ability to paint or sculpt, but it is only through study, training, and practice that an artist's skills are developed and refined. The child born with the genetic makeup to become a gifted athlete will realize that potential only when provided the opportunity to learn and perfect the skills of the game he chooses. In other words, most human talents are both born and made.

Even human traits we would consider to be purely genetic can be influenced by the environment. A child might be smaller than his genetically determined size because he is malnourished. A child born with great intellectual capacity might function at a normal or below normal level because he has not been provided adequate opportunities for learning. Sadly, if the poor diet continues long enough, the small child will remain undersized, and if the educational opportunities are withheld long enough, the intellectually gifted child will lose his gift. Sometimes, of course, environment can affect nature's outcomes in less dramatic and less permanent ways. A child born brown-eyed can have blue eyes by wearing tinted contact lenses. A short child can wear elevator shoes. The adult with naturally brown hair can have blonde hair by using peroxide. The list of environmental manipulations of natural conditions becomes longer with each generation of humans.

Theories designed to explain how language develops address the nature-versus-nurture debate at various points along the continuum, and the reader will note that each theoretical view addresses certain aspects of language more directly than others. Some theories, for example, focus primarily on the function of language. Others are more concerned with the structure of language. Others consider the connections between cognition and language, and still others attend to environmental factors as facilitators in the acquisition process.

Choosing Sides

Until about 1960, most people who studied the development of speech and language in children assumed that oral communication skills are learned. During the first half of this century, much emphasis was placed on parents teaching their children to talk, even though there was concern that parents were not very good teachers. Van Riper, as late as 1964 (p. 92), observed that "children learn to talk. Their parents do the teaching, and it is usually very poor." Many experts during this era believed that children learn to talk not because of their parents, but in spite of them.

The nature-versus-nurture argument in speech and language became heated during the 1960s and early 1970s when theorists called *nativists* or *biological-nativists* suggested that children are genetically predisposed to talk. That is, oral language is instinctive in humans, and like instincts in other animals, speech is a behavior the child produces with minimal environmental involvement. It is a genetically coded behavior and is as natural for the child as walking.

What is sometimes lost in discussions about this debate is that neither side completely discounts the other. Those who believe language is learned recognize that the child must have the right anatomic equipment, and must be ready to acquire language in terms of cognitive, perceptual, and neuromuscular maturation. Their emphasis, however, is on environmental influences. They argue, for example, that a child reared in a stable home with parents who provide good language models has a distinct advantage over one reared in an economically, culturally, and socially impoverished home by parents who provide few and inadequate language models. The nativists accept the fact that environment plays some role in the acquisition of speech and language. That is, the child must be exposed to language models, but the nativists view these models as mere triggers for a natural, biological acquisition process. They argue that the innate drive for the development of language in humans is so powerful that even a poor environment will not prevent the child from talking.

As the debate has continued, the extreme views have moderated, and there is a general understanding that what the child brings to language development genetically is important, but so is the environment into which he is born. There are still differences among theorists relative to the importance they place on the nature or the nurture, and given the history of this ongoing debate in all aspects of human development, it is unlikely the experts will ever agree.

With the general nature-versus-nurture debate as a backdrop, we will take a closer look at a number of theoretical interpretations reflecting the evolutionary changes in thinking about language acquisition over the past half century. These include behaviorism, nativism and the government-binding theory, generative semantics and cognitivism, information processing theory, and the pragmatics revolution that gave birth to the social interactionist view.

The Behaviorist Interpretation

Several basic assumptions underlie the **behaviorist** or **empiricist** interpretation of language development.

It is assumed, for example, that attention should be focused on observable and measurable behaviors. Behaviorists do not emphasize mental constructs or internal mechanisms that generate language structures. The problem from this perspective is that since mental activities cannot be seen, they cannot be defined or measured. Behaviorists do not deny the existence of these mental processes. They acknowledge that observable behaviors are connected to internal or physiological mechanisms, but, they argue, we cannot study what we cannot observe. Behaviorists, therefore, look for the overt behaviors that occur together in language performance. On the basis of their observations and measurements, they draw conclusions about the relationships among co-occurring stimuli and make predictions about future behaviors based on these relationships (Bohannon & Warren-Leubecker, 1989, pp. 171–172).

Using Watson (1924) and Skinner (1957) as examples, Bohannon and Warren-Luebecker (1989, p. 173), make the point that behaviorists believe language is learned because they do not believe language is unique among human behaviors. Watson (1924), in fact, says that in its early stages, language is "a very simple type of behavior . . . a manipulative habit." Behaviorists argue that language is something humans *do,* not something they *have,* and it should be understood, therefore, in the same context of learning as other behaviors humans do like brushing their teeth or tying their shoes. They contend that language is learned according to the same principles used in training animals, and that like trained animal behaviors, language behaviors are learned by imitation, reinforcement, and successive approximations toward adult language behaviors.

One of the more controversial aspects of the behaviorist view is that the child is passive during the process of learning language (Bryen, 1982). That is, the child begins life with his "language tank" on empty. He becomes a language user as his tank is filled by the experiences provided by the language models in his environment. This is not to say that the child is totally inactive, of course. He is active in the sense that he imitates language forms, but he does not initiate these behaviors on his own, and the shape of his emerging language is determined not by self-discovery or creative experimentation, but by the selective reinforcements received from his speech and language models.

This leads us to the key assumption underlying behaviorist views of language development. Although behaviorists have differing opinions about exactly how the process of learning occurs, they all agree that environment is the critical and most important factor in the acquisition formula. While nativists stress the *similarities* that occur in the language development of children, the behaviorists stress the *differences* that are explained by the widely varying environments of children during the language acquisition period. The behaviorists focus on the external forces that shape the child's verbal behaviors into language. They see the child simply as a reactor to these forces (Bryen, 1982).

Speech and Language as Operant Behaviors

The theorist most closely associated with the behaviorist interpretation of speech and language development is B. F. Skinner. It is not surprising that Skinner (1957) viewed speech as learned behavior because he viewed virtually all behaviors as learned according to operant conditioning principles. To understand Skinner's explanation of speech and language development, therefore, one must understand the basic principles of operant conditioning.

An *operant* is any behavior whose frequency can be affected by the responses that follow it. If a target behavior's frequency of occurrence increases as a consequence of the response that follows it, **reinforcement** has occurred. If the frequency decreases, the target behavior has been **punished.** Very often people try to understand operant punishment in terms of aversiveness or unpleasantness, but these judgments may interfere with an understanding of the principle involved. If a target behavior's frequency of occurrence decreases as a consequence of the response that follows it, punishment has occurred whether or not the organism being conditioned perceives the response as unpleasant or aversive. In other words, reinforcement and punishment are defined on the basis of their effects.

In operant conditioning, the events that follow target behaviors are critical to learning, but the events preceding the target behaviors are also important, because they can come to control whether or not these target behaviors will be produced. Assume, for example, that a parent has conditioned a child to say "thank you" whenever he receives a gift by praising him (reinforcement) each time he remembers to say the words. If the "thank you" behavior increases as a result of the praise, we can conclude that reinforcement and learning have occurred. During the learning period, the parent may, consciously or not, give the child a certain look as he is receiving the gift, a look that reminds the child that he should say "thank you." We call this look a **discriminative stimulus.** Now notice the sequence. The child receives the gift. The parent gives the "look." The child says "thank you," and the parent praises him for his gratitude. Over time, the "look" or discriminative stimulus comes to control the frequency with which the child says "thank you." There are other preceding events. The **delta stimulus** is a signal indicating that reinforcement will not follow a particular response, and an **aversive stimulus** warns that there will be an unpleasant consequence for a particular behavior. It is very important to remember, however, that these preceding events have only as much power to control behaviors as provided by the strength and consistency of the events that follow targeted behaviors. A parent might try to use an aversive stimulus by threatening to spank a child if he produces a certain behavior, but if that behavior is never followed by a spanking, the preceding event will have no power to control. This is why parents are counseled not to make empty threats. Behavior in children and all organisms can be managed by operant principles only if preceding events are connected to following events, at least part of the time. In other words, behavior management is effective only if efforts to manage are consistent and if the manager follows through on the promises or threats inherent in the preceding events.

Sometimes the behavior we want must be **shaped** in small steps that gradually approximate the target behavior. When the child is learning to say "water," he might begin by saying "wawa." The adult accepts this production as a step toward the target behavior and reinforces it, perhaps by giving the child a drink when he says "wawa." As the child gets older and expectations for his speech rise, he might be reinforced for saying "wada" but is no longer reinforced for saying "wawa." The next approximation might be "wata" and finally "water." In each step of the shaping process, what is reinforced is closer to the target. Productions that are not advanced or are perceived as regressions are ignored.

Many behaviors, including speech behaviors, occur in sequences. These sequences are learned through a procedure known as **chaining.** An example from Holland and Skinner (1961, pp. 161–162) makes the process more understandable than a definition: "At the same time sight of food is a discriminative stimulus for seizing food, it is a reinforcer for bending down to the food magazine and looking in. This sequence forms a chain: bending down, seeing food, seizing food. . . ." This same procedure can be used to explain a sequence of behaviors involving language. A child sees his mother getting ready to go out and thinks she looks pretty. He says, "You sure look pretty, Mommy." The mother, flattered, responds, "Well, thank you! That was a nice thing to say." The child says, "You're welcome." Seeing his mother looking pretty is the discriminative stimulus for the child's initial comment, which is followed by the mother's response and the child's response to her response, each reinforcing the preceding utterance.

It is not too difficult to understand how Skinner and others have applied these basic principles to speech and language development. In general, the child acquires language as a result of selective reinforcements provided by his caregivers. The caregivers provide models. The child imitates the models. Imitations most closely resembling the models are reinforced by the caregivers when they give the child what he wants, when they respond with another comment, or when they give the child adoring attention. Over time, the child will cease to use productions that have not been reinforced and will continue to use those that have been reinforced. Stringing words together into sentences occurs as the result of chaining. Imitation, important throughout the learning process, undergoes a change as the child moves from single words to sentences. Staats (1971) suggests that this new version of imitation is introduced by the child's parents as their expectations for his speech increase. The child produces a single-word utterance. One of the parents, believing he can produce a longer utterance, expands this single word into a sentence and withholds reinforcement until the child imitates the expanded form.

Remember that behaviorists stress the idea that language is a doing or performing phenomenon more than a knowing phenomenon. Skinner (1957), for example, argues that verbal behaviors serve one of five specific functions defined according to what they do: echoic, tact, mand, intraverbal, and autoclitic. (1) Perhaps the simplest of these behaviors is **echoic,** the imitation of a model in the presence of a nonverbal stimulus to which the word refers. For example, as a parent hands the child a dessert, she says "cookie." The child takes the treat and imitates the model, "cookie." Eventually the child will associate the word with the object and will use the word to refer to or request a cookie, but in the beginning his production is simple, meaningless imitation. (2) After the child has established an association between an object and its corresponding word, an echoic becomes a tact. A **tact** is a verbal behavior used to name or label something, typically in response to things or events the speaker is discussing. (3) The next term sounds and looks something like the word "demand," and that is not a coincidence. A

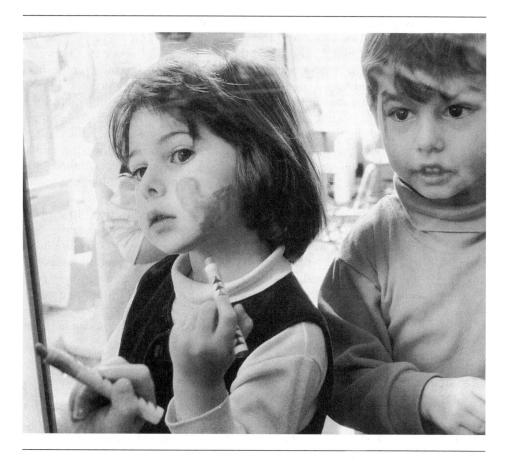

The chaining of behaviors.

mand is a verbal behavior used to request, command, or make a demand, and it identifies its own reinforcer. An utterance like "me want drink" indicates a request. If the request is granted, the drink becomes the reinforcement for the utterance. (4) An **intraverbal** is a production that often seems to have no direct connection to the utterance that precipitated it. A mother might say "Daddy went to work" and the child might reply "Go outside and play now?" Although there might seem to be no direct link between these two utterances, the child might be conditioned to go outside to play only after his father goes to work. In this context, the child's response makes sense. Intraverbals are used in the free association characteristic of conversation. In conversation, what one person says may not dictate the response received. In some cases, a person responds even when there is no request for a response. The free-associated and nonrequested responses in conversation and social gesture talk are intraverbals. (5) **Autoclitic** responses can be understood in two important ways. First, these responses influence and are influenced by the speaker's behaviors. Second, autoclitic responses account for the linking of words into sentences. Using operant terminology, each word serves as a discriminative stimulus for the following word. Another way to understand the linking of words into autoclitic responses is to consider how the child is combining isolated ideas. The child, for example, might be watching her brother, Billy, playing baseball, and she wants to comment on this observation. She knows the names for "Billy" and "ball," and she knows that striking the ball with a bat is called "hitting." She links the three ideas together to create the utterance "Billy hitting the ball." This is an autoclitic response.

As language structures become more complex, it is more difficult to explain them on the basis of learning alone. In reference to autoclitics, for example, Fey (1986) says there is the implication that only strings of words which have been specifically reinforced can be produced. We know, however, that all speakers, including young children, produce strings of words that have never been produced or heard before. In other words, operant principles cannot adequately account for the creativity that is a dominant characteristic of language. Additionally, operant principles alone fail to account for the acquisition of meaning in novel utterances.

Classical Conditioning in Meaning Acquisition

Staats (1971) believes we must include classical conditioning principles to explain language acquisition, especially the meaning component. In classical conditioning, an originally neutral stimulus is paired with an unconditioned stimulus that elicits an unconditioned response. In the famous Pavlovian experiment, the dog hears a bell just before seeing food, which elicits the unconditioned response, salivation. After a number of trials, the bell alone, now a conditioned stimulus, will elicit salivation, now a conditioned response. That is, the dog has learned or been conditioned to salivate upon hearing the bell. Staats argues that a word is, in the beginning, a neutral stimulus that acquires meaning only as responses are classically conditioned to it. The word *sit* develops meaning as it comes to represent the physical act associated with it through the process of conditioning. At first, when the child hears his parent say "Sit!" there is no reaction, but if the word is paired with the physical act of being placed on a chair, the word alone, after enough trials, will elicit the act of sitting and will be understood to represent the act.

The Behaviorist Perspective in Review

The behaviorists stress the importance of environment. The child is viewed as an empty vessel to be filled by the experiences provided by the important people in his life. The child is typically viewed as having no knowledge about the rules of language. His parents and other speakers are credited for "teaching" language by providing models that the child imitates. By selective reinforcement, the parents shape the child's utterances into adult forms.

Obviously, the behaviorist perspective of language acquisition has not gone unchallenged. James (1990) provides an excellent and succinct summary of some of the problems and criticisms. The role of imitation has been questioned, for example. As noted earlier, children produce sentences they have never heard before. This may mean they produce sentences that are more creative and elaborate than their models, but it also means they produce utterances that are simply not produced by adults because such utterances are infantile. The child will typically say things like "Daddy goed work" and "That mine milk," productions that are clearly not imitations of sentences produced by parents. Perhaps more importantly, the frequency of imitation decreases dramatically after the second birthday, but there is still a lot of language to be acquired beyond age two. Some children, even from the beginning, imitate very little. If imitation is as important as the behaviorists argue, we would expect to see imitations more consistent with the models provided, and we certainly would expect to see imitation play a major role in acquisition throughout the learning period. James also notes that since parents are more likely to correct a child for the content of his utterances than for the grammatical accuracy of his sentences, syntactic development cannot be explained solely on the basis of selective parental reinforcement.

Whatever the problems with the behaviorist perspective, there seems little doubt that learning explains some aspects of language acquisition. We know that language changes over the course of a person's lifetime, well beyond the age range identified by the nativists as the critical acquisition period. These changes are best explained by general learning principles. An innate capacity for language, for example, cannot account for how humans learn the crazy nuances of language, like when to use "who" and when to use "whom," and environmental influences seem to be very important in changing a person from an adequate user of language into an exceptional user of language.

The Nativist Interpretation

If the behaviorist view represents the extreme nurture end of the nature-nurture continuum, the nativist perspective is the extreme nature end of the same continuum. As the name of this view suggests, nativists stress the idea that language is innate or biologically based. They argue that human beings are born with a species-specific capacity for language, a capacity that is realized with minimal assistance from the environment. While behaviorists seem solely concerned with performance, nativists stress competence or knowledge that leads to performance.

The theorist most closely associated with the nativist view is Noam Chomsky, a linguist. Chomsky (1968, p. 59) expresses one of the basic assumptions of nativism in this declaration: "Anyone concerned with the study of human nature and capabilities must somehow come to grips with the fact that all humans acquire language." The idea that language is universal among humans and unique to humans is the foundation of the nativistic interpretation of language acquisition. These theorists point out that unless there are severe physical or mental limitations, human beings will acquire language, and that the innate drive to acquire language is so powerful that many humans talk in spite of what may seem to be insurmountable limitations. They also argue that only human beings are capable of acquiring and using language as we know and understand it.

One of the questions embedded in the larger issue of the relative influences of genetics and environment in language acquisition centers on whether or not animals can be taught to communicate using something comparable to human language. Among the strongest voices in the nativist movement of the 1960s was Eric Lenneberg, who was so convinced that language is unique to humans that he asserted "there is no evidence that any nonhuman form has the capacity to acquire even the most primitive stages of language development" (1964, p. 67). Although this seemed a reasonable conclusion at the time, some research conducted in the late 1960s and throughout the 1970s raised doubts about what other animals can and cannot do as users of language.

The earliest attempts to teach chimpanzees to speak failed, but when Gardner and Gardner (1969, 1971, 1975) began their research with Washoe, a ten-month-old female chimpanzee, they tried a different language avenue. They taught Washoe how to use American Sign Language, the manual communication system used by deaf people. Washoe eventually learned more than 100 signs, and according to the Gardners, spontaneously produced combinations of signs to express basic requests such as "Listen dog" and "Give me food". The fact that Washoe brought her hands to a resting position only after a series of signs was produced was interpreted to mean that she intended to combine these signs. There is no question that what Washoe accomplished was beyond what Lenneberg would have imagined possible when he talked about language as a uniquely human ability, but even those most excited about attempts to teach apes to use language have recognized some important limitations. There is no evidence, for example, that Washoe learned any rules of grammar as reflected by consistent or meaningful word order. Some have suggested that this failure to acquire grammatical rules may be a function of American Sign Language, which is not bound by the strict word order rules used in spoken and written language. On the other hand, it may simply be that chimpanzees do not have the ability to learn syntax, a conclusion that seems to be supported by the findings of another researcher, Terrace (1980), who specifically analyzed his chimpanzee's signed utterances to determine if there were any word order consistencies. He found none.

More recently, efforts have been made to teach language to pygmy chimpanzees (Savage-Rumbaugh, MacDonald, Sevcik, Hopkins, & Rubert, 1986). Pygmy chimpanzees are reportedly more intelligent and social than those used in earlier experiments, and the preliminary evidence suggests they have a greater capacity for language-based communication skills. According to their trainers, these chimpanzees have acquired symbols simply by observing their human trainers, and they have used these symbols spontaneously in apparent attempts to communicate with humans. There is also evidence that they can combine these symbols to create more complex utterances, and they seem to understand some spoken words. Chimpanzees, including the pygmy variety, have so far not shown the ability to acquire adult-like syntax, but some researchers feel comfortable in concluding that chimpanzees are capable of acquiring and using the kind of language we expect of very young human children (Greenfield & Savage-Rumbaugh, 1984; Savage-Rumbaugh et al., 1986; Savage-Rumbaugh, 1990).

All the research conducted with apes must be understood in the context of the criticisms raised about the general methods used. Skeptics have noted that whatever "language" is learned is the result of extraordinary efforts to teach on the part of human trainers—the kind of constant and powerful teaching that is not necessary for humans to acquire language. Critics also suggest that the successes noted are more the result of imitation and prompting than any natural capacity for language (Terrance, Pettito, Saunder, & Bever, 1979).

Based on all the data now available, we have no reason to believe that nonhumans are capable of acquiring and using language, at least not a language directly and completely comparable to human language. Even if we accept that apes can acquire symbols and combine them, and that they can understand some spoken words, we have no evidence that they can acquire the rules for combining words into grammatical structures, engage in conversation, or use language creatively. If we believe that language goes beyond vocabulary to include structure, the layering of meanings, the transformations of word forms to indicate things like plurality, possession, and tense changes, the use of language as a pragmatic tool, and the creativity that allows even young children to formulate utterances never produced or heard before, we must conclude that Lenneberg (1964) was more right than wrong—at least so far.

Another basic assumption of the nativist perspective is that since language is acquired so quickly and so early in the child's life, learning alone cannot adequately account for acquisition. Nativists argue that caregivers do not provide language models that are designed to "teach" progressive understanding of language forms. In fact, the nativist would question whether caregivers teach language at all. The child is exposed to language forms of enormous complexity, variety, and inconsistency, and he is never given specific feedback about whether or not his utterances are correct or incorrect (Wexler & Culicover, 1980; Pinker, 1984, 1987). If language is learned, the nativist argues, we would expect the teacher to provide models that allow the child to develop progressively more sophisticated hypotheses about the rules and forms he is learning, and we would certainly expect the teacher to clearly indicate when the child's productions are right or wrong.

One of the most compelling arguments for the nativistic perspective is that language is essentially the same experience for all human beings no matter what language they speak, where they live, or how they interact with their language models. As listeners and speakers of languages, we may be most impressed by their differences, but when languages are studied carefully, we discover many common-alities. All languages, for example, have rules for organizing words into grammatical sentence forms. They do not all use the same rules, of course. Some languages, like English, stress word order in developing grammatical sentences. Latin, on the other hand, allows more freedom in word order but stresses word endings to indicate the relationships among words. A given Latin noun, for example, has a different ending when it is the subject of a sentence than when it is a direct object.

Nativists stress the common ground, however. That is, all languages have rules to indicate the structural relationships among words in sentences. All languages distinguish between subjects and predicates and allow the embedding of one sentence structure into another to create an elaborated sentence representing both original structures. All languages have rules to indicate changes in tense and plurality, and draw sets of speech sounds from a common pool of sounds, and the list goes on. These commonalities or *linguistic universals* are evidence, say the nativists, that language is an ability humans possess, not by virtue of specific learning or teaching, but by virtue of their humanness. Spiders weave webs. Birds build nests. Humans speak. Enough said. Well, more needs to be said, of course, but you should be able to appreciate the form of this argument. If language were truly and solely learned, we would expect great differences among the languages spoken by people from different parts of the world. No matter which side of the debate you ultimately take, you must admit that language is a universal human experience and that there are startling similarities in the way people from widely varying cultures acquire and use language.

All of these assumptions led to the creation of a concept that underlies the nativist's understanding of language development. The concept is called the **language acquisition device** or **LAD** (Chomsky, 1965; Lenneberg, 1967). The LAD is an innate language reservoir filled with information about the rules of language structure. Nativists contend that it should be understood as a real part of the brain, that part specifically designed to process language. The LAD takes the syntactic information provided by the child's models and generates the grammar of that child's native language. Since no child is predetermined to speak any specific language, the LAD is driven by knowledge common to all languages. As you might imagine, the existence and certainly the nature of the LAD have been widely debated (Bohannon & Warren-Leubecker, 1989).

As you may have sensed in this discussion, nativists believe that the structure of language is somehow independent of its use. In fact, they view structure as being independent of meaning and almost every other aspect of the total language package. The rules for structuring sentences determine, for any given language, that some forms are grammatical and allowable and others are not. There is a finite, or specifically limited, number of rules for a given language. These rules allow the speaker to create an infinite number of grammatically acceptable sentences. The rules should not be understood in a prescriptive sense but in a descriptive sense. In other words, these rules do not tell the speaker what he should do but what he does do. They are rules that describe the regularities of a language. Once the speaker knows what these rules are, he can create an unlimited number of grammatical sentences, including the possibility of sentences that have never been produced by any other human. Language acquisition, therefore, is a matter of discovering and applying the rules or regularities of one's native language.

Transformational Generative Grammar

Chomsky (1957) devised **Transformational Generative Grammar** to account for the production of an unlimited number of grammatically acceptable sentences. This grammar suggests that language is processed at two levels, and there are two kinds of rules to describe what is occurring at each level. **Phrase structure rules** describe the underlying relationships of words and phrases, the level of structure referred to as **deep.** These rules are universal and operate in all languages. **Transformations** are rules that describe the rearrangement of deep structures as they are moved to the next level of structure, referred to as **surface.** These rules are not universal. Each language has its own set of transformations, although the basic principles that operate in transformations are much the same in all languages. A complete description of Transformational Generative Grammar is beyond the scope of this book, but the reader should understand how the grammar works to appreciate Chomsky's point of view about language.

If we take a simple sentence like "The little boy hit the white ball," we can identify three basic phrase structure rules that operate to create this kind of sentence:

1. *Sentence = Noun Phrase + Verb Phrase.* Our sample sentence consists of the noun phrase ("The little boy") and the verb phrase ("hit the white ball").
2. *Verb Phrase = Verb + Noun Phrase.* The verb phrase in our sentence consists of the verb ("hit") and the noun phrase ("the white ball").
3. *Noun Phrase = Modifier(s) + Noun.* There are two noun phrases in our sentence. In the first noun phrase, there are two modifiers ("The" and "little") and the noun ("boy"). In the second noun phrase, there are also two modifiers ("the" and "white") and the noun ("ball").

Keep in mind that Chomsky was devising a grammar to account for the production of an infinite number of grammatical sentences with a finite number of rules. By using just these three rules, it is possible to create an unlimited number of sentences. The example here is an English sentence, but these same rules can be used to describe the deep structure of similar sentences in any language.

Think of deep structures as the origins of a sentence in the brain before it is spoken or written. Phrase structure rules describe the relationships of the most basic elements of sentences while they are thoughts, before they become spoken or written sentences. In order to move these deep structures to the surface, we need transformations (rules that determine how words are shaped and organized to make sentences grammatical). Each language has its own set of transformations.

In English, for example, we can understand the creation of a grammatically correct question by understanding what happens as we move from the deep structure of a particular sentence to the surface. Let's assume that I want to know if Billy is going to the library. At the deep structure level, the origin of the question is something like this:

"Billy is going to the library."—Question?

The rule in English for transforming this deep structure into a grammatically correct interrogative form is fairly simple. I rearrange the words. I reverse "Billy" and "is" to create the surface structure, "Is Billy going to the library?" The rule for rearranging the words to create a question is a transformation. If I am thinking:

"Billy is going to the library."—No!,

I can use a negative transformation to express that idea on the surface. In this case, I insert the word "not" between "is" and "going" to create the grammatically acceptable sentence "Billy is not going to the library." The transformation describes what I do on the surface to express what I have thought at the deep level.

It is also important to understand that every sentence has a deep structure and a surface structure. Notice, for example, that "The boy hit the ball" and "The ball was hit by the boy" mean the same thing. That is, they have the same deep structure. They differ only on the surface. The transformation used to change the first sentence into the second is called the **passive transformation.** Notice the reordering of words necessary to transform the active sentence into the passive sentence. Once you understand the rule, you can transform any active sentence into its correct passive version. Try it on sentences like "The beautiful woman rode the aging horse" or "The vicious cat chased the frightened dog under the porch." If several people try the same transformation, assuming basic competence in English, the resulting sentences will be the same:

The aging horse was ridden by the beautiful woman.

The frightened dog was chased under the porch by the vicious cat.

How did you do? You have just demonstrated something many nativists believe supports their view. That is, you know what you know about language even if you do not know what you know. Think about that for a few seconds. The point is, you might not have known what the term passive transformation means, and if asked how to make a sentence passive, you might not have been able to explain it, but by changing active sentences that you have never seen before into passive versions, you have demonstrated your knowledge of not only the deep structures of these sentences but the rules for surface structure as well. The nativists would argue that if language were purely learned, you would have a more conscious understanding of what you are doing when you create sentences at the deep level and as you move them to the surface. Instead, they contend, your Language Acquisition Device provides you with innate knowledge of deep structures and the ability to easily acquire the rules for surface structures for your native language, an acquisition that comes by exposure to models, not direct teaching.

Chomsky (1981) has significantly expanded and extended his theoretical views regarding the acquisition of grammar with what is called the **government-binding theory.** One of the problems with previous theories of transformational grammar is that they were so powerful they could account not only for language patterns that are possible and realistic, but also for language patterns that are outlandish. One of the primary emphases of the government-binding theory is "learnability." Chomsky suggests that there are limits on the possible hypotheses about language structure the learner can formulate. According to Leonard and Loeb (1988), the "government-binding theory is currently the dominant (though by no means the only) theory in linguistics."

While still allowing the language learner considerable latitude in terms of how language knowledge is processed and organized, the government-binding theory asserts that the learner's language knowledge must be consistent with the knowledge inherent in the grammars of presently existing and possible languages, and it must be possible to develop this knowledge from limited evidence. The internalized complex of rules and principles by which language knowledge meets these parameters is called *Universal Grammar*. Universal Grammar operates at four levels of representation: (1) Deep structures, (2) Surface structures, (3) Phonetic form rules, and (4) Logical form rules. In addition to these levels of representation, Universal Grammar also includes several subtheories.

Deep structures include the speaker's personal dictionary as well as rules for formulating sentences (rules comparable to those in Chomsky's earlier versions of phrase structure grammar). The personal dictionary specifies the meanings of words, but also specifies how words are to be treated syntactically. The sentence formulation rules are complex and versatile enough to explain how alternative sentences, such as question forms, are created from a basic form.

The **surface structures** of the Universal Grammar are similar to Chomsky's earlier versions. They differ in the sense that they come closer to spoken forms than the earlier versions, but they are still quite abstract and they are still derived from deep structures. **Phonetic form** and **logical form** rules operate at the same level of representation, but add differentiated information. Phonetic form rules are abstractions of the sound system and include the rules that govern the phonological shaping of words. Logical form rules are concerned with interpretation. If, for example, relationships between pronouns and antecedents in sentences are not clear based on structure alone, these rules, by the application of abstract logical interpretation, help clarify which pronouns are associated with which antecedents.

The subtheories of the government-binding theory are designed to explain the constraints and principles that allow language to be quickly acquired. According to the **bounding theory,** the movement of a grammatical constituent or component is limited. That is, no constituent can be moved out of a noun phrase and a sentence or clause by application of a single rule. *Noun phrase* and *sentence* are considered *bounding nodes* because they determine the extent to which constituents can move. **Government theory** is concerned with the "privileged relations" among certain syntactic constituents. For example, in prepositional phrases prepositions "govern," or exert influence over, the noun phrases that follow them. In a sense, the prepositions dominate and control their noun phrases. **Case theory** is concerned with the rules by which meaning category or semantic case is assigned to noun phrases. Consider the assignment of nominative or objective case to noun phrases. For example, the active verb, *hit,* determines that the following noun phrase, *the ball,* will be objective case, whereas the preceding noun phrase, *The little girl,* will be nominative case. Even though case theory is a distinct subtheory, one can easily see government theory principles in operation. **Binding theory** addresses the issue of "coreference," the idea that a given noun phrase may or may not refer to the same entity as one or more other noun phrases. For example, a reflexive clearly refers to the preceding noun phrase. In the sentence, *John made himself sick,* the reflexive pronoun *himself* unambiguously refers to *John.* A pronominal such as *I, he,* or *she* may make an independent reference (as in the sentence, *John thinks she is pretty,* in which the reference for *she* is not specified), or it may refer to a noun phrase (as in the sentence, *Mary thinks she is pretty,* in which *she* refers to *Mary.*) **Thematic theory** addresses the designation of roles such as *agent-of-action* and *goal-of-action.* The purposes of thematic theory and case theory are somewhat parallel. While case theory assigns grammatical case roles, thematic theory assigns semantic roles. In the sentence, *Paul planted the tree,* the grammatical case assigned to *Paul* is nominative, and the thematic role assigned to *Paul* is agent-of-action. The last of the subtheories, **control theory,** is concerned with determining the possible references for pronouns or words used like pronouns when the references are not clear. The subject of an embedded infinitive phrase, for example, may be controlled by a noun phrase or it may make an independent reference. The sentence, *Coach Smith considered what to do with the bases loaded,* suggests that *Coach Smith* is the subject of the infinitive phrase. The subject of the embedded infinitive phrase is controlled by the noun phrase of the sentence. In the sentence, *It is difficult to know what to do with the bases loaded,* the reference is not controlled by the noun phrase and is not so clear. It is an independent reference to some unidentified *one,* as in a paraphrased version of the sentence, *It is difficult for one to know what to do with the bases loaded.*

The speaker who has acquired language presumably uses all of these components to decipher language and to create language forms. In the process, the Universal Grammar which forms the foundation for the acquisition of language is shaped to fit the specific and idiosyncratic characteristics of the speaker's native language. In closing this section on Chomsky's view of language acquisition, it must be emphasized that while Chomsky is certainly interested in the entire breadth of language, his primary focus has always been on language form or structure. He believes that the Universal Grammar is innate and that the child masters his native language by using the various components of the Universal Grammar to make sense of the language to which he is exposed.

The Nativist Perspective in Review

Nativists are clearly at the nature end of the nature-versus-nurture continuum. They believe human beings are born with a capacity for language—that given exposure to language, the human child will talk, even if environmental conditions are not favorable. Nativists contend that the universality of language among all human beings, the striking commonalities in how language is acquired, and the schedule by which it is acquired, regardless of cultural or other environmental variations, are evidence of the innateness of language. They believe children are born with a Language Acquisition Device, a neurophysiological entity filled with language knowledge. The LAD provides the child the knowledge he needs to understand any language at the deep structure level and provides him the ability to acquire easily and quickly the surface structure rules specific to the language he will speak.

James (1990, pp. 169–171) notes that it is difficult to either confirm or refute the nativist perspective, although several of its basic assumptions have been challenged. The assumption that language is unique to humans has been challenged, however inconclusively, by attempts to teach apes to use language. The assumption that language acquisition is essentially complete by the time the child is four or five appears to be overstated. There is evidence that significant language acquisition occurs well beyond five years and that some complex language forms are not mastered until adolescence. The argument that language must be innate because parents and others provide models that are too complex and ambiguous for progressive learning also appears to be incorrect. Although it is true that adults talk to other adults in language that is often confused, incomplete, and grammatically ambiguous, there is evidence that adults use a different kind of language with children. That is, adults tend to use short, simple, and grammatically correct sentences when they talk to young children, the kind of models that could very well allow for approximations toward adult forms. Do not lose sight, however, based on the evidence gathered so far, that we have not ruled out the nativists' basic contention, which is that human beings are born with an innate capacity for language. What remains in the debate is to determine the relative importance of this innate capacity in comparison to the influence of environmental factors.

The Generative Semantics Interpretation

Not surprisingly, not all linguists accept Chomsky's views on language and language development. There are specific objections to his emphasis on syntax and his cursory attention to the meaning system of language. Chomsky does, of course, acknowledge the meaning level of language reflected in what he calls *deep structure,* but his primary focus is always on syntax and on how speakers generate syntax. Those who take the semantics view argue that in order for a language to be truly generative, it must generate meaning as well as structure, and that meaning in language is expressed not only in words but through the syntactic relationships among words. If we are to understand the acquisition of language, we must account for the expression of meaning.

One of the earliest and most often-cited generative semantics theories was developed by Fillmore (1968). Fillmore's **case grammar** is designed to explain the importance and influence of semantics on the form of language. Fillmore suggested that there is a deeper level of deep structure than that proposed by Chomsky. Beneath deep structure is a level comprised of universal concepts that determine how nouns and verbs are related to one another. These are semantic concepts, not syntactic relations, and they are independent of surface structure. Even though these semantic concepts are universal, they are not necessarily innate. According to generative semantics theorists, these concepts are either genetic or environmental phenomena (Chafe, 1970).

Fillmore suggests that sentences have two components: modality and proposition. **Modality** is concerned with sentence characteristics such as verb tense, or the expression of negation or interrogation. The second component, proposition, is more critical to the semantic theory. **Proposition** is concerned with the relationship between nouns and verbs in sentences. The relationship between the noun and verb in a given sentence determines the meaning underlying that sentence. Each proposition represents a type of sentence that includes a verb in combination with a *case* or a set of nouns. In the context of this view of language, certain categories of verbs require certain cases. Case refers to a specific semantic role or function that can be filled by a particular type of noun phrase.

Fillmore identifies seven universal cases. An **agentive** case noun phrase is the initiator of an action, and as you would expect, is usually animate. A **dative** case is a person, animal, or other animate being that is affected by the action or by the state of being ascribed by the verb. An **experiencer** is a person, animal, or other animate being that experiences an action or a mental or emotional state. A **factitive** is an object or a being that is the product of an action or state ascribed by a verb. An **instrumental** is an inanimate object that is not the instigator of an action but the means by which the action occurs. A **locative** is the place or location where the action or state ascribed by the verb occurs. An **objective,** considered the most neutral of the cases, is a noun phrase whose role in the action or state ascribed by the verb is determined by the specific meaning of the verb. A summary of these cases with sample sentences is displayed in Table 2-1.

It should be noted that there are not exclusive sets of nouns for each case. A given noun may be used in any case if it meets the definition and requirements of that case. The word *boy* is agentive in the sentence, *The boy broke the window.* It is dative in the sentence, *The woman gave a generous tip to the boy.* It is experiencer in the sentence, *The boy dreamed about owning his car,* and it is objective in the sentence, *The homecoming queen kissed the embarrassed little boy.* In each case, the verb determines the case of the noun phrase, which means that structure can be explained on the basis of the semantic functions of nouns as determined by verbs. In short, structure is a product of semantic relations.

TABLE 2-1 Fillmore's (1968) Seven Universal Cases

Case	Definition	Example
Agentive	The initiator of an action.	*Tom* hid the present.
Dative	A being affected by the action or state of being ascribed by the verb.	Sally gave *him* a generous tip.
Experiencer	A being who experiences an action or a mental or emotional state.	*Jerry* enjoyed the concert.
Factitive	An object or being that is the product of an action or state ascribed by the verb.	They built the *house*.
Instrumental	An inanimate object that is the means by which an action occurs.	He made the fire with *charcoal*.
Locative	The place where the action or state ascribed by the verb occurs.	He went camping in the *forest*.
Objective	A noun phrase whose role in the action or state ascribed by the verb is determined by the specific meaning of the verb.	Dad kicked *the ball* to me.

Chomsky and Fillmore share an important viewpoint relative to language production. Each believes that language production is a generative process and that any theory of language acquisition must account for how language is generated. The essential difference between Chomsky and Fillmore should be clear, however. Chomsky devised a theory to account for the generation of structure. Fillmore devised a theory to account for the generation of semantic relationships, which underlie and provide a foundation for structure.

Chomsky's ideas about generative transformational grammar led many linguists during the late 1960s to analyze children's emerging language from a syntactic point of view. Lois Bloom joined this movement. She discovered that syntactic analysis provided valuable information about the early utterances of children, but she also concluded that it did not provide adequate information about the meaning system underlying early language production. Based on her experiences in analyzing the meanings of early utterances using contextual information, Bloom (1970) asserted that transformational generative grammar is more useful in explaining children's language if the analysis includes semantic information that can be used to help analysts draw conclusions about underlying structure. This shift from syntactic analysis to semantic analysis was the beginning of what has been called the *semantic revolution*, a point of view about children's language that suggests that we should study the structure of early language within the context of the speakers intended message. This context must necessarily take into account linguistic and nonlinguistic information because the communications of children are not words—only events. This kind of analysis is described as a *richer* form of analysis than the transformational generative analysis precisely because it goes beyond the speakers words to take into account environmental and other nonverbal factors that contribute to the total message.

Other linguists, including Schlesinger (1971) and Brown (1973), reached essentially the same conclusions as Bloom about the importance of semantics in the analysis of early language. Schlesinger went a step further when he concluded that the grammar of early language is semantic, not syntactic, and that early productions are best understood in terms of the semantic relationships expressed in these productions rather than in terms of abstract syntactic categories such as *subject, verb, object.*

The Cognitive Interpretation

At about the same time as the semantic revolution was underway, there was renewed interest in Piaget's cognitive theory and its relationship to language acquisition. Theorists considered specific connections between Piaget's stages of cognitive development and stages of speech and language development, with special emphasis on Piaget's sensorimotor period. This stage of cognitive development extends from birth through two years, the period of time which, not coincidentally, is critical for early speech and language development. In other words, it is easy to understand why linguists would be intrigued by possible, and highly plausible, connections between cognitive development and language acquisition.

It should be noted that all theorists accept that there is a relationship between cognitive development and language development. What separates cognitive theorists from others is their belief that language does not hold an absolutely unique position in overall development. They believe that language itself is not innate, even though the cognitive precursors for language *are* innate. They also believe that language is not learned as behaviorists suggest it is learned. Language emerges, in the cognitive view, not because children are specifically genetically predisposed to produce language and not because language is shaped by learning principles. Language emerges as a product of cognitive organization and development. Language is one of several abilities the child develops for the purpose of conceptual representation and manipulation. All of these abilities emerge as a consequence of cognitive maturation. They emerge when there is imbalance between the child's existing cognitive structures and new information he is receiving from his environment. These theorists agree that the child's cognitive abilities differ from the adult's in terms of how much information is processed and how effectively it is processed. But no matter where a person is in cognitive development, he adds new information into existing cognitive categories, or if the new information does not fit, he extends, combines, or creates new categories. The process of language acquisition, according to this view, is not separate from but related to cognitive development; it is one part of, and fully integrated into, cognitive development.

Cognitive theorists have noted a number of correlations between language and other cognitive behaviors, correlations that may help us understand how language is acquired. There certainly seems to be a relationship, for example, between the child's understanding that words represent people, places, things, and ideas and the cognitive behavior known as *symbolic play*. There seems to be a connection between understanding that language can be used to get things done and the cognitive behaviors involved in solving problems with tools. Imitation is an important behavior in overall cognitive development, and imitation is clearly an important behavior in speech and language acquisition.

The Information Processing Interpretation

In order to appreciate the **information processing theory,** one must first understand how it relates to other theoretical perspectives, and how these other perspectives relate to one another. By way of a brief review of where we have been so far, the reader should understand that the behaviorist view stresses language function. Linguistic views, best represented by Chomsky's transformational generative grammar and government-binding theory, emphasize language structure. The cognitivist view stresses logical structure. Into this context, we bring the information processing theory. This theory shares with the behaviorist perspective a greater emphasis on *how* language is learned than on the abstract rule system that presumably underlies language, but it goes a step further by making a concerted effort to relate structure and function.

The information processing view is represented well in the *competition model* developed by Bates and MacWhinney (1987). The basic assertion of this theoretical view is that function, not abstract grammar, generates language structure. This view suggests that a human being processes information in much the same way a computer does. That is, a human being has an information processing system that gathers information from the environment and puts that information into symbolic codes, codes that include but are not limited to words and numbers. This internal information processing system interprets these symbolic codes, holds them in memory, and allows for the retrieval of stored information. Language acquisition occurs when a child experiences and gathers language evidence in the productions of his speech and language models and uses that evidence to make fundamental changes within his personal information processing system. The system is constantly adjusted to make its functions consistent with the language evidence the child is gathering.

According to this view, the child is not born with an internally wired system for language. Rather, he is born with a potential for all kinds of connections between symbols and the things and ideas symbols can represent. Based on his experiences, some connections are firmly established because they are repeated over and over again. Other possible connections eventually fade away because the child does not experience the evidence to activate them. The child internalizes language and the connections between language symbols and the things and ideas they represent because there is a constant inpouring of language evidence.

The information processing theory suggests that the processing patterns responsible for the acquisition of language are *parallel* rather than *serial*. Parallel patterns occur at many levels at the same time. By contrast, serial patterns, which are suggested by Chomsky's linguistic view, occur in a kind of vertical sequence. That is, deep structures are generated and are then transformed in a highly predictable sequence into surface structures. Information processing theory suggests that the order in which language forms are acquired is determined by what these forms accomplish. Those language forms that show up most often in the child's language models and that tend to serve the same purpose are acquired first. If, for example, the child's earliest language evidence is filled with examples of structures that make requests, language structures that fill the requesting function will emerge early.

Those who take the information processing view try to explain what occurs in the child's mind when he acquires language. They suggest, as already mentioned, that the child processes language information at a number of levels at the same time, a form of processing known as *parallel distributed processing* or *PDP*. The competition model of Bates and MacWhinney (1987) is an example of a PDP system. A basic premise of this model is that the child is not born with an innate understanding of language, but he is born with a powerful PDP device that has the capacity to process many different forms of information, including language information. In the earliest stages of language development, the PDP device does not differentiate among words, phonological patterns, and language forms in terms of their ability to represent communicative functions or meanings. This changes, however, as the child's experiences with language increase and become more differentiated. Words, phonological patterns, and language forms that are experienced repeatedly activate and strengthen connections in the PDP device. Other connections weaken. As the name of the model suggests, the patterns or connections that are most consistent with the language evidence the child is gathering win the *competition*. They are retained within the child's communication system. Patterns that do not match the evidence lose the competition and are discarded.

So, is the information processing view (and therefore the competition model) a nature or a nurture view of language acquisition? The reader has probably already surmised, correctly so, that this view includes elements of both extremes. Bates, Bretherton, and Snyder (1988) suggest the child is innately predisposed to acquire language just as he is innately predisposed to acquire other behaviors. In this sense, they believe that there is a biological, or innate, basis for language acquisition, though they do not believe that it necessarily accounts for language universals. In terms of nurture, they assert that each child uses his biologically based abilities to learn language creatively. They point out, for example, that there are significant individual variations in language acquisition among children within the same culture as well as across cultures. Within the context of the competition model, these differences are the result of varying experiences resulting in differentiated connections within the PDP system.

The Pragmatics Revolution

The semantic revolution that was a reaction to Chomsky's narrow emphasis on structure eventually led to a focus on *pragmatics,* the study of the functions served by communication. Researchers became concerned with how the context of language influences meaning and how language serves different functions for speakers under varying circumstances. The pragmatics revolution of the 1980s and 1990s had its origins many years earlier in work completed by Austin (1962) and Searle (1969). Austin's primary assertion was that when speakers produce utterances, they are doing more than saying words organized by conventional language rules. They are also using these words to get things done. They are ". . . performing acts with their words." Searle, a student of Austin's, suggested that every speech act consists of three separate acts: (1) the locutionary act, (2) the illocutionary act, and (3) the perlocutionary act.

The **locutionary act** is the most obvious part of the utterance because it is the part that strikes our ears. It is the expression of the words. If I say to a friend, "You've lost some weight," the locutionary act is limited to the utterance itself. It is the sentence the speaker speaks and the hearer hears. The locutionary act, because it is a sentence, consists of a subject, or *referring expression,* and a predicate, or *predicating expression.* Beyond the words, however, consider the possible reasons for my making this observation and you will get some sense that there may be more to my utterance than meets the listener's ears.

The **illocutionary act,** or **illocutionary force** (Searle, 1976) is concerned with the motive or purpose underlying an utterance. When someone says, "I know what you said, but I want to know what you meant," he is asking the speaker to identify his illocutionary act. Using the example above, if I say to my friend, "You've lost some weight," I could be telling him that he looks good, but I could also be saying that he looks sickly. My motive might be even more contrived. I might believe that my friend should be losing a lot of weight, and hope by saying that I have noticed some weight loss to motivate him to lose more. Consider the purpose that might be served by what Searle (1975) calls an *indirect speech act.* If my wife says to me, "It's a little drafty in here," it is not likely she is simply making an observation about the wind currents and the temperature level in the room. It is more likely that her comment is an indirect way of saying to me, "Close the window!".

The **perlocutionary act** takes the listener into account. It is concerned with the effect the locutionary act might have on the listener, an effect that may or may not be consistent with the speaker's communicative intention. If I intend to compliment my friend by saying, "You've lost some weight," but my friend knows that he has, in fact, gained a few pounds, he might be offended by my comment, believing I am being sarcastic. Communication works best, of course, when the listener's reactions match the speaker's intentions in terms of communicative content (locutionary act) and purpose (illocutionary act). When this happens, the speaker and listener agree that they are "on the same page," communicatively speaking. When they are not on the same page, communication can be very frustrating. The speaker may be frustrated because he knows what he is trying to say, but no matter how he tries to say it, the listener does not seem to get it. The listener may be frustrated by a sense of communicative paranoia that may or not be justified. The disconnection between speaker and listener, relative to communicative purpose, is not pleasant for either party, and it causes the process of communication to break down.

The Social Interactionist Interpretation

The evolution in theoretical interpretations relative to language acquisition eventually led theorists to explore a middle ground. This is what usually happens in nature-versus-nurture arguments, so the emergence of a compromise view was probably inevitable, although it has emerged later than some might have expected. This middle ground view is known as **social interactionism.**

According to the social interactionist interpretation of speech and language development, both biological and environmental factors are important in the acquisition process, although not necessarily equally. Some interactionist theorists are closer to the nature end of the continuum in that they understand language development as a product of general cognitive development (Bates & MacWhinney, 1982). Others place more emphasis on the contributions of the environment, but all agree that the interaction of biological abilities with environmental influences accounts for language acquisition, and they note the importance of the interaction of the child with his parents or other caregivers. This basic assumption about the importance of both biology and environment has led to other basic interactionist assumptions about language development.

For example, these theories assume that language acquisition is a product of the child's early social interactions with the important people in his life. They point out that the child communicates and interacts socially with other people before he is able to produce language forms. They believe that language develops as a natural consequence of these interactions. That is, the child's attempts to communicate and socialize prompt his parents and other caregivers to provide the language appropriate for these exchanges. As the child develops language, his communicative and social skills increase, allowing more mature and sophisticated interactions. These more mature interactions prompt more complex language forms from the parents, and the cycle continues until the child's language system and corresponding social skills reach adult levels. James (1990) provides an excellent example of this progression. She suggests that a nine-month-old child requests a cookie by reaching for it and vocalizing with an utterance like "Uh, uh, uh," while making eye contact with his mother. The mother, recognizing the communicative

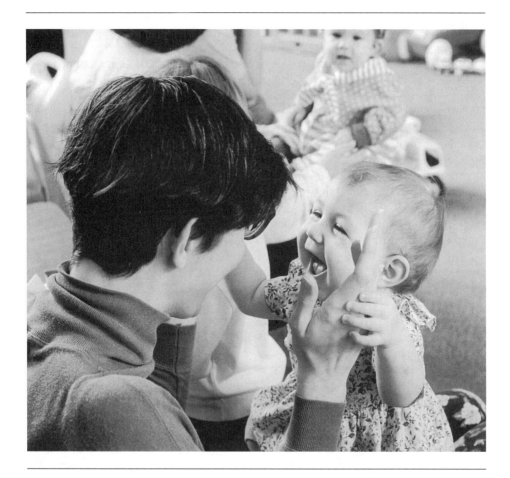

Language development is facilitated by social interaction.

intent, might provide a language form as she gives the child a cookie: "Do you want a cookie? Say cookie . . . cookie." By the time the child is two years old, he might make the same request by saying, "Mommy, want cookie," an utterance met with a cookie and an expanded language form modeled by mother: "Say 'Mommy, I want a cookie.' " By the time the child is four, he will have learned, on the basis of his social and communication experiences, to ask for the cookie by hinting. He might say, "You know, Mommy, I haven't had a cookie for long time." Notice what happens in this progression. The child is able to make a request from the beginning, before he has any language, and he certainly is able to interact with other people before he can speak. As he acquires language, however, his communicative and interactive abilities improve, and he is able to make his request known in more socially appropriate, more adult-like ways.

James's (1990) example illustrates another emphasis in the interactionist perspective. Unlike the nativists who stress structure independent of communicative function or intent, interactionists focus on language use. The intent to communicate leads the child to interact with people who can respond to his intent. The intent shapes his initial attempts to communicate, no matter how crude or unsophisticated these attempts may be. The recognition of the child's intent and associated communicative attempt prompts the caregiver to not only meet the intent, but provide an appropriate language model to support the intent. It may be that the model is given only to provide the child an opportunity to confirm or deny the intent, but the model is provided nonetheless. Over time, even though a given intent remains constant, the child acquires more sophisticated language forms by which he can make the intent more immediately and clearly known to his caregivers.

Interactionists, like the behaviorists, emphasize the importance of parents or caregivers in the language acquisition process. Behaviorists, however, view the child as a passive recipient of language shaped by selective reinforcement. Interactionists believe the child is an active participant in language acquisition by virtue of his bidirectional involvement with his parents. That is, the child initiates communicative and social efforts, perhaps as often as he receives them.

In comparison to the nativists, the interactionists would concede that the child comes to the language acquisition process with innate cognitive and linguistic abilities, but they do not believe these innate abilities are of greatest importance in language development. The child's interactions, socially and communicatively, with the important people in his environment are the most important factors in the acquisition of language.

Interactionists do not ignore structure or grammar in their understanding of language development. In fact, like the nativists, they try to discover common forms of structure in a variety of languages and cultures (DePaulo & Bonvillian, 1978). They believe, however, that these forms are fairly simple imitations of models to which children are exposed in social interactions (Moerk, 1975, 1983). It can be concluded, therefore, that although interactionists look for and try to explain structure, they are not as focused on structure as nativists. Since their emphasis, as already noted, is on the function of language within social-interactive contexts, they are concerned with how structure contributes to the use of language in getting things done.

Whereas nativists see structure or grammar as almost an end unto itself, interactionists view structure as a means to the end of accomplishing intent. This has led them to study language structure within the child–parent or child–caregiver interaction. In the beginning, these studies focused on the language forms of the caregiver (James, 1990), but more recent studies have examined the child's role and responses in these exchanges.

James (1990) notes that studies of caregivers' speech have revealed that the language forms adults use with young children are very different from the forms they use with other adults or even older children. According to James's review of the relevant research, when caregivers talk to young children, they:

1. Use short, simple sentences.
2. Talk about objects that the child is attending to or actions being engaged in.
3. Repeat their own utterances.
4. Repeat the child's utterances.
5. Use a slightly higher pitch and an exaggerated intonation pattern.
6. Introduce significant pauses between utterances.
7. Use a lot of questions and commands. (James, 1990, p. 179).

This style of speech has been given several names, but perhaps the most popular and descriptive is **motherese.** It should be noted, of course, that this general style is used by all adults when they talk to young children, although there may be some gender differences. Ratner (1988) has found, for example, that although mothers and fathers use the same vocabulary in talking with young children, fathers are more likely than mothers to include the less commonly used words in that vocabulary.

Although there are no empirical data to confirm the efficacy of any of the elements of motherese in facilitating language development, interactionists believe that motherese is ideally designed to help children in language acquisition. It can be argued that repetition, for example, provides multiple models and, depending on the nature of the communicative exchange, several opportunities for the child to practice a particular language form. The use of short, simple sentences seems to provide the child with models he can reasonably expect to imitate. The use of pauses may help him recognize where utterances begin and end. The use of emphatic prosodic patterns might direct the child to those words or structures that are most important. Talking about what is present and readily observable helps keep the communicative process concrete, which in turn probably helps hold the child's attention. The use of questions and commands seems to have the effect of keeping the child active in the communicative process.

On the basis of some research (Cross, 1978; Barnes, Gutfreund, Satterly, & Wells, 1983), one facet of motherese that seems to be related to language acquisition is the use of a technique known as **expansion.** Expansion occurs when the adult repeats what a child has said but adds additional words and/or structure. For example, the child might point to a passing vehicle and say, "Truck!" The parent might respond with "That's a fire truck." Parents and other caregivers frequently use expansions when they talk to young children, and they seem to do it naturally, without instruction. Because expansions are more frequently used by the caregivers of linguistically advanced children, and because the use of this technique seems to be associated with an increase in the mean length of children's utterances, it is reasonable to conclude that expansion probably facilitates language development. We must be careful, however, not to take the conclusion too far. We do not have evidence suggesting that this technique is essential for normal language development.

Remember that the interactionist view emphasizes the importance of the interaction between the child and his caregiver(s). What do we know about the nature of this interaction, especially as it might be related to communication and language development? We know that many adults treat the child as a communicator from the time he is born and begins to cry. That is, when the infant cries, his caregivers try to figure out why. They want to know what he is communicating. His caregivers also try to understand what the infant's cooing and babbling sounds mean and even what his facial grimaces and body movements mean. Even though the infant's vocalizations, grimaces, and body movements may be random and accidental, his caregivers assume that they have meaning and respond as though they are intentional communications. What we have here is a bidirectional communicative exchange in which the child is treated as an active participant.

As the child grows older, the interactions become a little more elaborate. Many parents, for example, read aloud to their children long before the children are producing language. Why do parents read to speechless children? They may assume that the child is receiving something of linguistic value in the exercise even if he cannot express anything in language form. They may assume that the interaction itself

TABLE 2-2 Motherese in Action

In your mind's eye, imagine a toddler walking through a zoo with her mother. She is seeing animals she has never seen before, and she is very curious about these new and different creatures. Imagine in your mind's ear the rate, pitch, and intonational patterns of the child's speech as well as the mother's speech. In the following exchange, notice some of the typical characteristics of motherese: a topic selected by the child's attention; short, simple sentences; repetition of key elements of the child's utterances; the use of questions to prompt additional responses; and expansion of the child's utterances into more complete, adult-like productions.

CHILD (pointing to a monkey):	Mommy, what's that?
MOTHER:	That's a monkey. Can you say 'monkey'?
CHILD:	Monkey!
MOTHER:	Yes, 'monkey.' What's the monkey doing?
CHILD:	Him eating.
MOTHER:	What's he eating?
CHILD:	Him eating banana.
MOTHER:	Do you eat bananas?
CHILD:	I like bananas!
MOTHER:	The monkey likes bananas too. . . . What's he doing now?
CHILD:	Him swinging by his tail.
MOTHER:	Can you swing by your tail?
CHILD:	No. I don't gots a tail.
MOTHER:	No, you don't have a tail like the monkey.

is valuable because it is establishing a bond that will facilitate more meaningful learning when the child is old enough to talk. Parents and other caregivers also play speech-related social games, such as peekaboo, with children. This kind of routine is highly structured, allows the child to participate by predicting what is going to happen (Bruner, 1978), and is a simple but comfortable communication activity. It is, after all, a game. It is nonthreatening and fun, but it provides the child an opportunity to experience all aspects of oral and nonverbal communication, and it gives him a chance to experiment with some of the components of language he is acquiring.

When a young child interacts with a caregiver, his nonverbal communications contribute to the fun and pleasure of the activity, but his nonverbal signals may also be helpful to the caregiver. When the adult uses a language form that the child cannot understand because it contains unfamiliar words or because it is too long or syntactically complex, the child will very likely send some kind of signal, perhaps verbal, but more often nonverbal to indicate that he is confused and needs help. He might simply look puzzled, or he might shrug his shoulders. When the adult receives this kind of signal, he offers another utterance, which he adjusts toward what he believes is necessary to facilitate the child's understanding. In this way, the verbal and nonverbal interaction allows the adult to simplify and reformulate language forms in ways that certainly facilitate improved communication and may facilitate language development.

Once again we must be careful not to read too much into what is happening in these interactions. If, as has been suggested, adults adjust their language to facilitate child–adult communication, it is probably not because adults are making conscious efforts to "teach" their children how to talk. Keep in mind that when adults talk to other adults, and there is an obvious failure to communicate, the listener lets the speaker know that the message has not been received, and the speaker tries again by creating a new version of the original message that is more carefully crafted, in terms of vocabulary and/or structure. When adults talk to children, they make exactly the same kinds of adjustments, and interestingly, when children talk to adults, they sometimes have to adjust in ways that help us understand. Are these adjustments essential in helping children acquire language? As tempting as it may be to let common sense answer "yes," we do not have the data to draw that conclusion.

Let's consider a specific example of the social interactionist view. One of the most recent formulations of this interpretation of early language acquisition is the **Child Talk** model proposed by Chapman, Streim, Crais, Salmon, Strand, and Negri (1992). Chapman and her colleagues have developed a model that purports to address the diversity of everyday conversational experiences we observe in young children during the language acquisition period. This model fully incorporates the most recent evidence researchers have gathered demonstrating the essential contributions of *context* and *world knowledge* to language understanding and production. *Context* includes the physical characteristics associated with a communication experience: the nature of events the child is experiencing at the time of the communication, the child's social relationships with other people involved in the communication experience, and all utterances previously produced during the communication. *World knowledge* includes the speaker's past and present knowledge about those aspects of context that might be used to facilitate understanding of or to formulate an utterance. The Child Talk model suggests that language develops as the child becomes increasingly expert in using context and world knowledge.

According to Chapman and her colleagues, "classical accounts" of language acquisition make a number of assertions that need to be challenged. Specifically, these accounts claim that early language formulation is creative, that early productions consist of linguistic units, that language development essentially involves learning rules for how to combine linguistic units, and that language development involves the generation and application of hypotheses about linguistic rules. Each of these assertions, according to Chapman and her colleagues, is problematic.

To argue, for example, that an utterance such as, *He runned fast,* is evidence that a child is creative in his language production is not wrong, but too simplistic. Nelson (1986) and Peters (1984), among others, have shown that while children are sometimes creative in their language productions, they often repeat what they have heard others say in a given circumstance, or they say what they themselves have said in the same or similar situation. The Child Talk model suggests that children sometimes do create utterances, but they also sometimes reproduce utterances. A child needs to have a history of being exposed to conversations associated with a variety of interactions in order to create a kind of language reservoir. The history he develops will result in a compilation of the utterances the child has heard and understood in all these conversational situations. It constitutes what is called a *lexical script*, a kind of linguistic background the child uses in the process of formulating his own utterances.

The classical accounts of language development suggesting that children learn linguistic units arrived at this conclusion based on two observations: (1) that when children learn to talk, they acquire one word at a time and that their single-word productions are devoid of prosody, and (2) that the measure of average length of utterances, using morphemes as the basic linguistic unit, is a reliable indicator of grammatical complexity and early language competence. The problem with this view, according to Child Talk proponents, is that it oversimplifies what actually occurs in early productions. During the early stages of language acquisition, children produce phrases as whole units, with no apparent understanding of the constituent parts. Children typically include utterances such as *Night-night, Allgone, Wannago,* and *Sobig* among their first meaningful productions. These are single-unit productions, not adult-like combinations of morphemes. Even adults, Chapman and her colleagues note, do not always formulate sentences by drawing linguistic units from a morpheme-restricted well. The adult, when producing idioms, proverbs, or other common expressions, probably gives no attention to the individual morphemes in these utterances. The adult says, *The more you know the more you know you don't know,* or *You can lead a horse to water, but you can't make it drink,* without paying attention to the morphemes in these words. In fact, the adult probably gives little attention to the individual words or their meanings in these productions. The focus, whether linguistic or semantic, is on the whole unit, not on its parts. Child Talk people argue that units of language production can range from syllables to sentences. The only criterion that must be met for a unit to be considered a unit is that it must be connected, in a general sense, to meaning.

The third assumption derived from classical structural models is that when children acquire language, they acquire rules by which they formulate sentences. The Child Talk people note, however, that over the past three decades, theorists have revised the nature of these rules. Early models, including pivot grammar, focused on syntactic category rules. These models gave way to case grammar models that describe rules based on the semantic roles or functions of noun phrases, and then to models that identify rules based on semantics and pragmatics. We have progressed, therefore, from views of language development that narrowly focused on rules based on linguistic structure to views that take into account how words are used in reference to one another, what they mean, and for what communicative purposes they are used. Slobin (1986) and Nelson (1986), for example, suggest that rules for selecting and structuring words and their morphemes into productive utterances are based on the roles of referents in events as children conceptualize these referents and events. In other words, you cannot separate children's language productions from children's real-life experiences and their understandings of these experiences. The idea that children organize language based on what they experience and on how they conceptualize the people, things, and events in their experiences suggests that language is organized, not by linguistic universals, but by conceptual universals. Conceptual universals refer to the shared views children have about what is happening around them, a phenomenon Nelson (1986) calls *event knowledge.*

Finally, there is the classical account assertion that during language acquisition, the child acquires rules by developing and testing hypotheses. The suggestion is that the child applies principles of scientific inquiry to the acquisition of language, an idea the Child Talk people believe challenges the limits of plausibility. Beyond the plausibility issue, however, is a more practical concern. The classical view suggests that the child develops and tests language hypotheses without getting specific affirmations or denials from his environment. In other words, the child operates independently in developing hypotheses and in either retaining or rejecting them. This assumption had its origins in the work of Brown and Hanlon (1970) who found very few specific and explicit reactions from parents in reference to the syntactic accuracy of their children's utterances. They found that parents reacted to the accuracy of their children's observations rather than the syntactic correctness of their utterances, and even these reactions were limited. The Child Talk people wonder how the child determines which hypotheses are valid and should be retained and which hypotheses are incorrect and disposable. Chapman and her colleagues acknowledge that other studies, utilizing a more liberal view

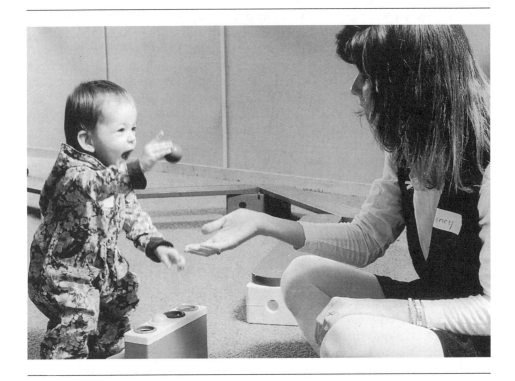

Language acquisition occurs within the child's total environment.

of negative feedback in reference to children's language errors, have generated evidence of more negative feedback from parents in their exchanges with their children than suggested by Brown and Hanlon. Even these studies, however, do not make clear how this kind of negative reaction leads the child to accept, modify, or reject his hypotheses about language production. Child Talk proponents further argue that even if children's productions can be described as analogous productions or as overextensions, we have still not explained why the child does not dispose of these forms when adults try to correct them.

To this point, we have identified the assumptions of the classical view that have been refuted by Child Talk theorists. But what assumptions underlly the Child Talk view of language acquisition? They assume that early language acquisition occurs as the child is introduced to his world, becomes acquainted with the social and physical characteristics of his environment, learns about the people and objects to be found in his environment, experiences the sounds, sights, and movements associated with all these things, and learns that he can make things happen by means of his own vocalizations and nonverbal actions. The basic assumption then that underlies the Child Talk model is that language acquisition occurs in context, broadly defined. The child's developing knowledge of everything in the life that swirls around him helps him establish goals for getting things done and develop strategies for successfully meeting these goals. According to the Child Talk view, the child formulates utterances because he has goals in mind that can best be met by using these utterances. Drawing upon the linguistic and nonlinguistic experiences of his own past, however brief that past is, the child uses his language knowledge in combination with his knowledge about other relevant aspects of his world to formulate utterances that will serve as means to today's ends. Consistent with other interactive models of language production, the Child Talk model suggests that a variety of language components, including semantics, syntax, and phonology, interact as the child formulates and interprets language.

TABLE 2-3 Tracing the Evolution of Language Acquisition Theories

Theory	Primary Architect/ Date(s)	Essential Idea	Primary Focus
Behaviorist	Skinner/1957	Language is learned by selective reinforcement.	General
Transformational Generative Grammar	Chomsky/1957	Language is processed by universal and innate rules governing deep and surface structure.	Syntax
Government-Binding Theory	Chomsky/1981	Extended version of GTG, but with emphasis on *learnability*.	Syntax
Case Grammar	Fillmore/1968	There is a level beneath deep structure comprised of universal semantic concepts that determines the relationships between nouns and verbs.	Semantics
Information Processing Theory	Bates & MacWhinney/ 1987	Function, not abstract grammar, generates language structure.	Structure by Function
Child Talk Model	Chapman et al./1992	Context and world knowledge drive language acquisition.	Interaction of all Language Components

And the Evolution Continues

Where does the evolution in theories of language acquisition stand as we approach the end of the twentieth century? It would be inaccurate to say that the experts have reached consensus about how children acquire language, but it would also be erroneous to conclude that we have not made progress in our considerations. Some are still convinced that language is a uniquely human and innate ability that only needs an environmental trigger to emerge, almost magically, according to a biologically predetermined schedule. Some still believe that language is almost entirely the product of environmental influences, and that the human child does not "develop" language as much as he "receives" language from his caregivers by virtue of their selective reinforcement and shaping of his initially random language-like behaviors. There seems to be growing support, however, for the middle ground in this nature-versus-nurture argument. As suggested in the opening of this chapter, this kind of compromise was almost inevitable. The interactionist perspective, therefore, is likely to have an increasingly greater voice in how theorists describe language acquisition and in formulating the questions researchers will attempt to answer about human language and its development.

Our three chapters tracing the development of language from the preparation stage through late childhood are written primarily from the interactionist point of view, with references to other explanations where appropriate. For people who are just beginning to explore language and its development in children, it is particularly important to take the broadest possible view. Humans are complex beings. We do not live in vacuums, and we certainly do not grow up in vacuums. To a large extent we are shaped by our environments and especially by our parents and other significant caregivers. At the same time, we should not lose sight of the enormous power of our genetic talents. We all marvel at world-class musicians and athletes. These people have worked hard to develop their considerable skills, but we must appreciate that without the right genetic stuff a man cannot high jump 7 feet, no matter how much he practices, and without the appropriate genetic gift, a pianist will never do justice to great music, no matter how many hours he spends at the keyboard. Language, like many other human abilities, is acquired by way of genetic gift shaped by environmental forces. Which is the greater factor, heredity or environment? Don't get me started!

Review Questions

1. What is the general nature-versus-nurture argument, and how does it apply to language development?

2. Summarize the behaviorist interpretation of speech and language development.

3. What do behaviorists mean when they describe language as a doing or performing phenomenon as opposed to a knowing phenomenon?

4. How can classical conditioning principles be used to explain the acquisition of meaning in language?

5. What have we learned about language development from experimental attempts to teach chimpanzees to use language?

6. What is the Language Acquisition Device (LAD), and what is its role in language development, according to the nativist interpretation?

7. In Transformational Generative Grammar, what is the difference between surface structure and deep structure?

8. How does the issue of "learnability" separate government-binding theory from Chomsky's earlier versions of transformational generative grammar?

9. Identify the four levels of representation at which Universal Grammar operates, and briefly explain what each level contributes to language production.

10. Briefly explain the following subtheories of the government-binding theory: bounding theory, government theory, case theory, binding theory, thematic theory, and control theory.

11. In the context of Fillmore's case grammar, what is meant by modality and proposition?

12. Briefly define and provide an example for each of Fillmore's seven universal cases.

13. What is the essence of the cognitive interpretation of language development?

14. What is meant by *parallel distributed processing* (PDP), and how does a model based on PDP, such as the competition model, explain language acquisition?

15. Compare and contrast the LAD and the PDP.

16. What are the three parts of the "speech act," according to Searle, and what does each part contribute to the whole speech act?

17. Discuss the objections of Child Talk proponents to the assumptions underlying the so-called "classical accounts" of language acquisition.

18. What assumptions underlie the Child Talk view? Explain why proponents of this view believe these assumptions are more valid than the assumptions underlying the classical interpretations of early language development.

19. How does the social interactionist interpretation fill the gap between the nativist interpretation at one end of the nature-versus-nurture continuum and the behaviorist interpretation at the other end of the continuum?

20. Based on your understanding of the twists and turns in the evolution of theories regarding language development over the past 50 years, what kinds of theoretical interpretations do you think language experts will be considering 50 years from now?

References and Suggested Readings

Austin, J. (1962). *How to do things with words.* London: Oxford University Press.

Barnes, S., Gutfreund, M., Satterly, D., & Wells, G. (1983). Characteristics of adult speech which predict children's language development. *Journal of Child Language, 10,* 65–84.

Bates, E., Bretherton, I., Beeghly-Smith, M., & McNew, S. (1983). Social basis of language development: a reassessment. In H. Reese & L. Lipsitt (Eds.), *Advances in child development and behavior* (Vol. 16, pp. 8–75). New York: Academic Press.

Bates, E., Bretherton, I., & Snyder, L. (1988). *From first words to grammar: Individual differences and dissociable mechanisms.* New York: Cambridge University Press.

Bates, E., & MacWhinney, B. (1982). Functionalist approaches to grammar. In E. Wanner & L. Gleitman (Eds.), *Language acquisition: The state of the art* (pp. 173–218). Cambridge, MA: Cambridge University Press.

Bates, E., & MacWhinney, B. (1987). Competition, variation, and language learning. In B. MacWhinney (Ed.), *Mechanisms of language acquisition.* Hillsdale, NJ: Lawrence Erlbaum.

Berko-Gleason, J. (Ed.) (1989). *The development of language* (2nd ed.). Columbus, OH: Merrill/Macmillan.

Bloom, L. (1970). *Language development: Form and function in emerging grammars.* Cambridge, MA: MIT Press.

Bloom, L., Hood, P., & Lightbown, P. (1974). Imitation in language development: If, when and why? *Cognitive Psychology, 6,* 380–420.

Bohannon, J., & Hirsch-Pasek, K. (1984). "Do children say as they're told? A new perspective on motherese." In L. Feagans, C. Garvey, & R. Golinkoff (Eds.), *The origins and growth of communication* (pp. 176–195). Norwood, NJ: Ablex.

Bohannon, J., & Warren-Leubecker, A. (1988). Recent developments in child-directed speech: You've come a long way, baby-talk. *Language Science, 10,* 89–110.

Bohannon, J., & Warren-Leubecker, A. (1989). Theoretical approaches to language acquisition. In J. Berko-Gleason (Ed.), *The development of language* (pp. 167–213). Columbus, OH: Merrill/Macmillan.

Brown, R., & Hanlon, C. (1970). Derivational complexity and order of acquisition in child speech. In J. Hayes (Ed.), *Cognition and the development of language.* New York: John Wiley & Sons.

Brown, R. (1973). *A first language: The early stages.* Cambridge, MA: Harvard University Press.

Bruner, J. (1978). Learning the mother tongue. *Human Nature, 1,* 42–49.

Bryen, D. (1982). *Inquiries into child language.* Boston: Allyn & Bacon, Inc.

Chafe, W. (1970). *Meaning and the structure of language.* Chicago: University of Chicago Press.

Chapman, R., Streim, N., Crais, E., Salmon, D., Strand, E., & Negri, N. (1992). Child talk: Assumptions of a developmental process model for early language learning. In R. Chapman (Ed.), *Processes in language acquisition and disorders.* St. Louis, MO: Mosby-Year Book, Inc.

Chomsky, C. (1969). *The acquisition of syntax in children from 5 to 10.* Cambridge, MA: MIT Press.

Chomsky, N. (1957). *Syntactic structures.* The Hague: Mouton.

Chomsky, N. (1965). *Aspects of a theory of syntax.* Cambridge, MA: MIT Press.

Chomsky, N. (1968). *Language and mind.* New York: Harcourt, Brace & World.

Chomsky, N. (1979). Human language and other semiotic systems. *Semiotica, 25,* 31–44.

Chomsky, N. (1981). *Lectures on government and binding.* Dordrecht, Holland: Foris.

Clark, E. (1977). Strategies and the mapping problem in first language acquisition. In J. MacNamara (Ed.), *Language Learning and thought* (pp. 147–168). New York: Academic Press.

Cross, T. (1977). Mother's speech adjustments: the contribution of selected child listener variables. In C. Snow & C. Ferguson (Eds.), *Talking to children: Language input and acquisition.* Cambridge, MA: Cambridge University Press.

Cross, T. (1978). Mother's speech and its association with rate of linguistic development in young children. In N. Waterson & C. Snow (Eds.), *The development of communication.* New York: Wiley.

DePaulo, B., & Bonvillian, J. (1978). The effect on language development of the special characteristics of speech addressed to children. *Journal of Psycholinguistic Research, 7,* 189–211.

Derwing, B. (1973). *Transformational grammar as a theory of language acquisition.* Cambridge, MA: Cambridge University Press.

Fey, M. (1986). *Language intervention with young children.* San Diego, CA: College-Hill Press.

Fillmore, C. (1968). The case for case. In E. Bach & R. Harmas (Eds.), *Universals in linguistic theory.* New York: Holt, Rinehart & Winston.

Gardner, R., & Gardner, B. (1969). Teaching sign language to a chimpanzee. *Science, 165,* 664–672.

Gardner, R., & Gardner, B. (1971). Two-way communication with a chimpanzee. In A. Schrier & F. Stollnitz (Eds.), *Behavior of nonhuman primates* (Vol. 4 pp. 117–184). New York: Academic Press.

Gardner, R., & Gardner, B. (1975). Early signs of language in child and chimpanzee. *Science, 187,* 752–753.

Gleitman, L., Newport, E., & Gleitman, H. (1984). The current status of the motherese hypothesis. *Journal of Child Language, 11,* 43–79.

Gleitman, L., & Wanner, E. (1982). Language acquisition: the state of the state of the art. In E. Wanner & L. Gleitman (Eds.), *Language acquisition: The state of the art* (pp. 3–48). Cambridge, MA: Cambridge University Press.

Greenfield, P., & Savage-Rumbaugh, S. (1984). Perceived variability and symbol use: A common language-cognition interface in children and chimpanzees (pan troglodytes). *Journal of Comparative Psychology, 2,* 201–218.

Hoff-Ginsberg, E. (1986). Function and structure in maternal speech: Their relation to the child's development of syntax. *Developmental Psychology, 22,* 155–163.

Hoff-Ginsberg, E., & Shatz, M. (1982). Linguistic input and the child's acquisition of language. *Psychological Bulletin, 92,* 3–26.

Holland, J., & Skinner, B. F. (1961). *The analysis of behavior.* New York: McGraw-Hill.

James, S. (1990). *Normal language acquisition.* Austin, TX: Pro-Ed.

Lenneberg, E. (1964). A biological perspective of language. In E. Lenneberg (Ed.), *New directions in the study of language.* Cambridge, MA: MIT Press.

Lenneberg, E. (1967). *Biological foundations of language.* New York: Wiley.

Leonard, L., & Loeb, D. (1988). Government-binding theory and some of its implications: A tutorial. *Journal of Speech and Hearing Research, 31,* 515–524.

Lovaas, O. (1977). *The autistic child: Language development through behavior modification.* New York: Irvington.

MacWhinney, B. (1987). *Mechanisms of language acquisition.* Hillsdale, NJ: Erlbaum.

Maratsos, M., & Chalkley, M. (1980). The internal language of children's syntax: the ontogenesis and representation of syntactic categories. In K. Nelson (Ed.), *Children's language* (Vol. 2). New York: Gardner Press.

Maratsos, M., Kuczaj, S., Fox, D., & Chalkley, M. (1979). Some empirical studies in the acquisition of transformation relations: Passives, negatives, and the past tense. In W. Collins (Ed.), *Children's language and communication.* Hillsdale, NJ: Erlbaum.

Menyuk, P. (1977). *Language and maturation.* Cambridge, MA: MIT Press.

Moerk, E. (1975). Verbal interactions between children and their mothers during the preschool years. *Developmental Psychology, 11,* 788–794.

Moerk, E. (1983). *The mother of Eve—As a first language teacher.* Norwood, NJ: Ablex Publishing Corporation.

Moerk, E. (1989). The LAD was a lady and the tasks were ill-defined. *Developmental Review, 9,* 21–57.

Nelson, K. (1986). *Event knowledge.* New York: Academic Press.

Newport, E. (1976). Motherese: the speech of mothers to young children. In N. Castellan, D. Pisoni, & G. Potts (Eds.), *Cognitive theory* (Vol. 2). Hillsdale, NJ: Erlbaum.

Owens, R. (1992). *Language development: An introduction* (3rd ed.). Columbus, OH: Merrill/Macmillan.

Palermo, D. (1978). *Psychology of language.* Glenview, IL: Scott, Foresman & Co.

Penner, S. (1987). Parental responses to grammatical and ungrammatical child utterances. *Child Development, 58,* 376–384.

Peters, A. (1984). *The units of language acquisition.* New York: Cambridge University Press.

Pinker, S. (1979). Formal models of language learning. *Cognition, 7,* 217–283.

Pinker, S. (1984). *Language, learnability and language development.* Cambridge, MA: Harvard University Press.

Pinker, S. (1987). The bootstrapping problem in language acquisition. In B. MacWhinney (Ed.), *Mechanisms of language acquisition* (pp. 399–439). Hillsdale, NJ: Erlbaum.

Ratner, N. (1988). Patterns of parental vocabulary selection in speech to very young children. *Journal of Child Language, 15,* 481–492.

Savage-Rumbaugh, E. (1987). A new look at ape language: Comprehension of vocal speech and syntax. In D. Leger (Ed.), *The Nebraska symposium on motivation.* Lincoln, NE: University of Nebraska.

Savage-Rumbaugh, E. (1990). Verbal communication in the chimpanzee. In N. Krasnegor, D. Rumbaugh, R. Schiefelbusch, & M. Studdert-Kennedy (Eds.), *Biobehavioral foundations of language development.* Hinsdale, NJ: Erlbaum.

Savage-Rumbaugh, E., MacDonald, K., Sevcik, R., Hopkins, W., & Rubert, E. (1986). Spontaneous symbol acquisition and communicative use by pygmy chimpanzees (pan paniscus). *Journal of Experimental Psychology: General, 115,* 211–235.

Savage-Rumbaugh, E., Sevcik, R., Brakke, K., & Rumbaugh, D. (1990). Symbols: Their communicative use, combination, and comprehension by bonobos (pan paniscus). In L. Lipsitt & C. Rovee-Collier (Eds.), *Advances in infancy research.* Norwood, NJ: Ablex Publishing Corporation.

Schlesinger, I. (1971). Production of utterances and language acquisition. In D. Slobin (Ed.) *The ontogenesis of grammar.* New York: Academic Press.

Searle, J. (1969). *Speech acts.* Cambridge, England: Cambridge University Press.

Searle, J. (1975). *Indirect speech acts.* In P. Cole & J. L. Morgan (Eds.), *Syntax and semantics 3: Speech acts.* New York: Academic Press.

Searle, J. (1976). The classification of illocutionary acts. *Language in Society, 5,* 1–24.

Shatz, M. (1982). On mechanisms of language acquisition: Can features of the communicative environment account for development? In E. Wanner & L. Gleitman (Eds.), *Language acquisition: The state of the art.* Cambridge, MA: Cambridge University Press.

Skinner, B. F. (1957). *Verbal behavior.* Englewood Cliffs, NJ: Prentice-Hall.

Slobin, D. (1986). Cross-linguistic evidence for the language-making capacity. In D. Slobin (Ed.), *The cross-linguistic study of language acquisition: Theoretical issues.* Hillsdale, NJ: Lawrence Erlbaum.

Snow, C. (1981a). Social interaction and language acquisition. In P. Dale & D. Ingram (Eds.), *Child language: An international perspective.* Baltimore: University Park Press.

Snow, C. (1981b). The uses of imitation. *Journal of Child Language, 8,* 205–208.

Staats, A. (1971). Linguistic-mentalistic theory versus an explanatory S-R learning theory of language development. In D. Slobin (Ed.), *The ontogenesis of grammar.* New York: Academic Press.

Staats, C., & Staats, A. (1957). Meaning established by classical conditioning. *Journal of Experimental Psychology, 54,* 74–80.

Stine, E., & Bohannon, J. (1983). Imitation, interactions and acquisition. *Journal of Child Language, 10,* 589–604.

Tager-Flusberg, H., & Calkins, S. (1990). Does imitation facilitate the acquisition of grammar? Evidence from a study of autistic, Down's syndrome, and normal children. *Journal of Child Language, 17,* 591–606.

Terrace, H. (1980). *Nim: A chimpanzee who learned sign language.* New York: Knopf.

Terrance, H., Pettito, L., Saunder, R., & Bever, J. (1979). Can an ape create a sentence? *Science, 206,* 891–902.

Van Riper, C. (1964). *Speech correction, principles and methods* (4th ed.). Englewood Cliffs, NJ: Prentice-Hall.

Watson, J. (1924). *Behaviorism.* Chicago: University of Chicago Press.

Wexler, K., & Culicover, P. (1980). *Formal principles of language acquisition.* Cambridge, MA: MIT Press.

Whitehurst, G., & Vasta, R. (1975). Is language acquired through imitation? *Journal of Psycholinguistic Research, 4,* 37–59.

Zimmerman, B., & Whitehurst, G. (1979). Structure and function: a comparison of two views of the development of language and cognition. In G. Whitehurst & B. Zimmerman (Eds.), *The functions of language and cognition.* New York: Academic Press.

THREE

Get Ready . . . Get Set . . . Talk!

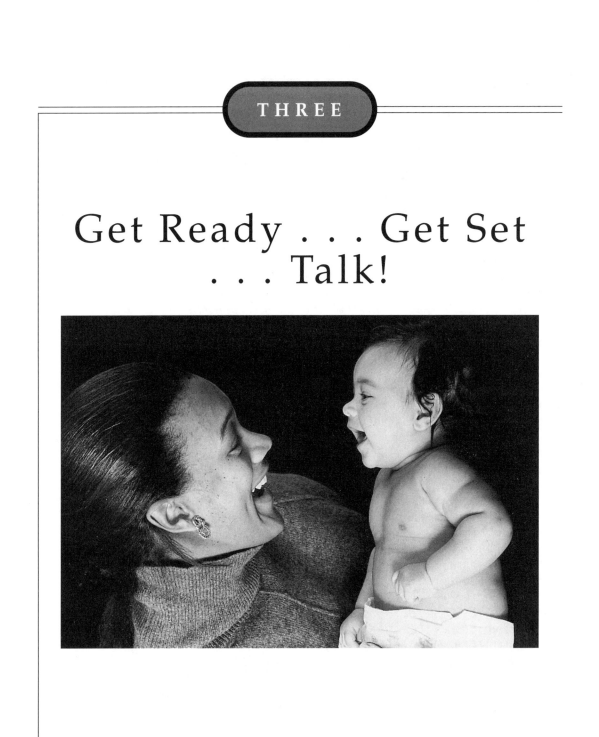

Chapter Objectives

What is the role of intellectual development in language development? This is one of the most interesting and challenging questions we must address in our study of human communication development. Since language is a means by which we express what we are thinking, the relationship between cognition and language is important, but does the development of one precede the development of the other? Do cognition and language develop in a parallel manner, and if they are connected, how are they connected? In this chapter, we address these and related questions, and in the process, discover that theorists hold widely varying views about whether language and thinking depend upon one another and how.

We then examine two major theoretical views of cognitive development, one proposed by Jean Piaget and the other by Lev Vygotsky. We consider how these two interpretations account for early intellectual development, with special attention to the implications relative to child language development. Finally, we consider the perceptual bases that underlie early cognitive and language development. Specifically, this chapter is designed to facilitate understanding of the following topics:

- Jean Piaget's theory of cognitive development, with emphasis on the first of the four stages of intellectual development he describes.

- *Distancing,* a basic perceptual principle critical to early intellectual development.

- Concepts and behaviors central to intellectual functioning and development, including *object permanence, causality, means-ends, play,* and *communication.*

- Challenges to Piaget's theory as the result of recent research.
- Lev Vygotsky's theory of cognitive development, which emphasizes the role of language in intellectual and social development.
- The perceptual preparation for communication development, focusing on visual perception, auditory perception, and the child's early interest in the human voice and speech.

In Chapter Two, we examined a number of theories of language development that can be arranged along a continuum representing the possible influences of nurture and nature on the language acquisition process. The basic question that has driven the writers of these theories can be framed as follows: "Is language genetically or environmentally determined?" The answer, as you discovered, is not to be found in any simple extreme, but the question provides an appropriate segue into this chapter.

Are you ready for another question about language for which there is no answer, or more accurately, no easy answer? Well, ready or not, here it is. Does thought shape language or does language shape thought? This is an important question in the context of our discussion because we need to know whether the development of thought, or *cognition,* precedes the emergence of language, follows the emergence of language, or develops concurrently with language.

Since language is used to express what we think, common sense would certainly suggest that thought shapes language, at least in the early stages of human development. Common sense would also suggest, however, that at some point in development, language begins to shape thought. In this case, common sense is probably correct on both counts. The point we need to make sure we do not miss is that, for many thought processes, it is not possible to separate thinking and language. As you read the words on this page, you are processing language to interpret the intended thoughts of the writer, and as you consider what the messages on this page mean, you are manipulating your thoughts in some kind of language form. You might not use complete sentences in your inner language, and your cognitive sentences may not always be grammatically correct, but they are in language form.

At the same time, we must be sensitive to the fact that human beings can and do think in ways that do not involve language. When Beethoven wrote his music, he *thought* music. When artists paint, they think in colors and forms and visual messages. When a football coach designs plays, he thinks in *Xs* and *Os*. Mathematicians think in numbers and formulas. Thinking takes many forms other than language. We all think emotions, and sometimes these emotions cannot even be expressed in language. We all think images and sounds and smells, and even though these sensory experiences can sometimes be described in words, words often fail to do them justice. If a picture is worth a thousand words, a thought, even a simple thought, has the potential to bankrupt the vocabulary.

What can we conclude, therefore, about the relationship between thought and language? We can conclude that thought does shape language because thought determines what we will say and how we will say it. We can conclude that language shapes thought because we often use language in our thought processes and manipulate our thoughts in language forms. And we can conclude that some thoughts are expressed in forms other than language, such as musical tones and chords, mental images, or even mathematic abstractions.

In order to facilitate an understanding of the critical relationship between cognition and language, we will examine two highly regarded theories of cognitive development. We will consider the research evidence that supports each view, the scholarly ponderings these theories have generated, and we will determine what each theory suggests about the role of language in cognitive development. Before we examine each of these theories in some detail, a few general observations are in order. First, it must be emphasized that Piaget did not specifically propose a theory of language development. He treated language as just one of a number of symbolic functions a child develops as he interacts with his environment. Piaget viewed cognitive development as an essential prerequisite for the development of all symbolic functions. It should also be noted that while Piaget's theoretical views are widely respected among those who study human intellectual development and language development, several aspects of his theory have been challenged. One aspect of particular interest to us is the theory's failure to adequately account for how the child assigns words to their referents (Owens, 1996, p. 148). Both Piaget and Vygotsky assert that the child is an active player in the process of acquiring knowledge about his world, but beyond this general agreement, there is a crucial difference. Piaget believed that the child is an independent operative in cognitive development. Vygotsky believed that during cognitive development, the child maintains a cooperative relationship with his environment and his culture. In his view, this cooperative relationship is a vitally important component in the process of achieving cognitive competence.

Piaget's Theory of Cognitive Development

Jean Piaget is well known by Americans, who usually think of him as a child psychologist. Although his work has certainly been applied to child psychology and education, Piaget was actually a genetic epistemologist. **Genetic epistemology** is the study of how knowledge is acquired, so Piaget devoted his life to understanding cognitive or intellectual development. This science has rather obvious applications to both education and psychology. Piaget moved easily in these disciplines, and his ideas have been influential in both.

Piaget's original passion was biology, a passion born and cultivated at a young age. By the time he was only ten years old, he had already published an article describing a partly albino sparrow. This intellectually gifted child earned his bachelor's degree at eighteen and his doctorate at twenty-one, by which time he had already published twenty-five professional papers. Piaget's early studies of mollusks caused him to believe that development was not just the product of biological maturation guided by genetics, but was also affected by environmental factors. Over the years of his professional career, this conclusion led him to understand that cognitive development is the result of biological maturation in interaction with the environment (Wadsworth, 1971, pp. 2–3).

This conclusion about the interaction of heredity and environment can be clearly observed in Piaget's stages of cognitive development. We will begin our examination of Piaget's theory by identifying and describing several basic concepts underlying the theory. Using this understanding as a foundation, we will consider the overall framework of the theory. We will briefly describe the four stages before examining the first stage, the **sensorimotor period,** in detail. This discussion will reflect Piaget's theory as he originally proposed it, but we will follow this discussion with a review of recent research evidence that calls some aspects of Piaget's theory into question.

The Elements and Processes of Cognitive Organization

It is important to remember what Piaget learned from his work as a biologist. He came to understand that many actions of living creatures are *adaptations* to their environments and that these actions help creatures *organize* their environments (Wadsworth, 1971, p. 9). He applied this understanding in explaining the cognitive development of a child by assuming that cognitive acts *organize* the child's environment and are the result of the child's *adaptation* to his environment. According to Piaget (1952), four basic concepts underlie cognitive organization: schema, assimilation, accommodation, and equilibrium. As you will discover, it is difficult to understand one of these concepts without considering the others because they are related. We will begin by defining and explaining schema, but your understanding of schema will not be complete until you understand how the other three concepts relate to schema and to one another.

A **schema** can be understood as a concept, mental category, or cognitive structure. The plural of schema is **schemata,** so as a child develops intellectually, he develops many schemata by which he organizes and adapts to his environment. Think of a schema as a computer file of the brain. A personal computer's memory bank might be filled with a number of specific files for things like business expenses, addresses, letters, appointments, checking account, etc. When you process new information on the computer, you save that information in the appropriate file. In much the same way, adults use many schemata to process, identify, and store information. Even if I see a dog unlike any dog I have ever seen before, I have no difficulty processing that stimulus as a dog. My dog schema is so well developed that I can put the smallest Chihuahua and the largest Great Dane in the same category. I know what dogness is. I may encounter a rat bigger than a Chihuahua or a horse smaller than a Great Dane, but I do not misfile these stimuli into my dog schema because I have a rat schema and a horse schema, and I know the differences among these three animals. If, however, I see an animal unlike any animal I have ever seen before, I will scan all my schemata and find no place to fit this new stimulus. I will either modify an existing schema to make the new stimulus fit, or I will create a new schema so that I can put this new creature into its proper file. This brings us to the next two concepts: assimilation and accommodation.

Let's return to the computer file analogy for a moment. If I have a letters file in my computer's memory, any letter I compose will be saved into that file. Other things I may write, such as recipes, memos to professional colleagues, lyrics for songs I am composing, or material for what I hope is the next great American novel, go in other files, but every letter I write is saved into my letters file. In much the same way, each time I encounter a new stimulus, I scan my schemata to decide where this stimulus fits. **Assimilation** is the cognitive process whereby a person includes a new stimulus into an existing schema. Until a few years ago, I had never seen a Sharpei, the cuddly and wrinkled Chinese dog that has become popular in America. I recognized this stimulus as a dog, however, and assimilated it into my existing dog schema, right there with Chihuahua, Great Dane, German Shepherd, Schnauzer, and all the other dog stimuli. As we experience life, our existing schemata are constantly being expanded by the inclusion of new stimuli that fit these categories.

What happens when some new stimulus just does not fit into an existing schema? Let us return once more to the computer file analogy. I may be a prolific letter writer, so after months or years of producing and saving letters, my letter file becomes very large. Because I write many different kinds of letters, it also becomes unmanageable and virtually meaningless. I may have family letters, letters to friends, business letters, and love letters in the same file, and it becomes clear they do not all belong in the same computer file. What do I do? I create new files, of course. I might develop a file for personal letters, another for business letters, and another for love letters. In other words, I accommodate the diversity of letters by creating separate categories for them in my computer's memory. When people develop new schemata to allow for the organization of stimuli that do not fit into existing schemata, we say that **accommodation** has occurred.

My dog schema may be well developed as an adult, but for the young child this schema presents some organizational problems. You have probably known a child who has pointed to a horse, cow, perhaps even an elephant or giraffe, and said, "Doggie!" What is going on here? The child is observing a stimulus he has never experienced before. He searches his schemata for a category into which to place this new stimulus. He sees a creature with four legs. His "doggie" schema includes animals with four legs. Eureka! This must be a doggie, he thinks, so he assimilates the horse, cow, elephant, or giraffe into his existing doggie schema.

Unlike a computer file, which has a size limit based on a computer's memory capacity, a schema has no size limits. No matter how many new dogs I may see in my lifetime, I will always have room for new varieties of dogs in my dog schema.

If, however, I assimilate stimuli into a schema that I gradually recognize as not fitting the shape of the schema, I must accommodate either by reshaping an existing schema or by developing new schemata. As a child, I might understand dogness as "any animal with four legs," but as I have more experiences with my environment, I begin to reshape my dog schema to include "any animal with four legs, fur, a wet nose, a wagging tail, within certain size limitations, which barks." As this understanding of dogness develops, I begin to separate dogs from other animals who might share some traits with dogs but who differ in other important ways. As a result of my experiences with my environment, I adapt and reorganize by developing new schemata to accommodate stimuli that do not belong in my reshaped dog schema. Eventually, I will have schemata for horses, cows, elephants, giraffes, and all other animals with whom I become acquainted in a cognitive sense.

The dog example illustrates an important difference between children's and adults' schemata. When the child is young, his schemata tend to be very large, and in comparison to adult schemata, imprecisely defined. As the child develops intellectually, his schemata become more adult-like in that they become more narrowly and more accurately defined. It should be noted here that some schemata, even for the most intelligent adults, are never completely accurate. An adult, for example, who has little interest in football, might have a schema for football player as incompletely formed as the young child's doggie schema that includes all four-legged animals. This adult might not understand the specialized responsibilities of the various players on offense and defense. He might not understand the difference between a nose guard and an outside linebacker, between a cornerback and a safety, or between a slot back and a wide receiver. He might not understand that the punter is considered a defensive player and the place kicker is considered an offensive player even though they both kick when their team possesses the football. To the person who knows little or nothing about football, these players all fit into one large, undifferentiated schema called "football player." The point is, we are all ignorant in our own ways, and our ignorance is reflected in how our schemata are shaped and cataloged.

We are now ready to consider the final basic concept, equilibrium. Think of **equilibrium** as a balance between assimilation and accommodation. Cognitive development can be understood as a process resulting from assimilation and accommodation, but if these cognitive strategies are not in balance, there are problems. If, for example, a person *assimilates* all new stimuli he experiences, he will have relatively few schemata—but these schemata will be so broadly defined that he will be unable to recognize important differences among the things he is trying to categorize. But if he *accommodates* all new stimuli, he will have many narrowly defined schema and will be unable to recognize the commonalities among the things he is trying to categorize. Too much of either strategy results in an inadequate understanding of the parts and wholes of life and life's experiences. Each person is constantly in the process of finding a balance between assimilation and accommodation to create a kind of cognitive peace.

Each time the child encounters a new stimulus, he either assimilates or he accommodates, but he places the stimulus somewhere. He might assimilate a new stimulus for a short time before he accommodates by creating a new schema more appropriate for that stimulus, but he does not leave his cognitive organization in disarray. Unlike the retailer who might be a few pennies short or a few pennies over at the end of the day, the child balances his cognitive account every day. It does not matter that his schemata are right or wrong in comparison to adult schemata. In fact, you should not understand assimilation and accommodation in cognitive development as right or wrong. The child places stimuli according to *his* understanding of the world at any given moment in his intellectual development. As he grows older, his schemata become more and more adultlike, but they are always right, within the context of his understanding. In other words, he always finds his **equilibrium,** his cognitive peace, even though his balance might represent **disequilibrium** in an adult's cognitive organization.

When does a person stop assimilating and accommodating? These processes cease only when a person no longer has new experiences or new understandings of old experiences. As long as the brain continues to function, existing schemata accept new stimuli, existing schemata are reshaped, and new schemata are created. One of the marvelous aspects of intellectual development is that it continues throughout life. You may reach your maximum height when you are nineteen or twenty, and you may reach your athletic peak in your late twenties or early thirties, but you can continue to grow intellectually by assimilating and accommodating into your eighth or ninth decade and beyond.

The Stage Concept of Cognitive Development

Throughout our discussion of language acquisition, we will encounter stages and substages of development. It is important to remember that these stages are *not* like stair steps, where moving from a lower step to the next higher step means leave the lower step behind. In language development, what is acquired in one stage is carried over and integrated into the next stage. The same is true in cognitive development. Piaget's stages of intellectual development are not discrete. Each stage builds on the preceding stage so that development is a continuing process of qualitative changes in a person's schemata. As the child grows intellectually, he does not discard schemata. He accommodates by reshaping a schema and by creating new schemata, but schemata are not disposable any more than stages of development are passed through and forgotten. Intellectual growth is a cumulative, integrative, expanding process. As the child comes to understand that not all four-legged animals are dogs, he does not throw away his dog schema. He accommodates this schema to make it more dog-like, and he acquires new schemata to allow for other four-legged animals. He might for a time put horses, cows, donkeys, and zebras in his horse schema, but he eventually sorts out all the four-legged animals into adult-like schemata.

Piaget compares the progression through the stages of cognitive development to the building of a pyramid, and that may be a helpful way to understand the progression of one stage to the next and the interdependence of the stages. Just as the structure of a pyramid is layered, each stage of cognitive development lays the foundation for the following stage, but what is acquired in each stage is not forgotten. The child's schemata are corrected and refined, and he continually adds schemata. Cognitive development should be understood as an improving and adding process like remodeling and adding on to an existing house as opposed to destroying it and building a new one.

The Big Picture

Piaget (1963) describes four stages of intellectual development from birth through late adolescence, briefly summarized here:

1. *Sensorimotor Intelligence* (Birth to 2 Years). Most of the child's behaviors during the sensorimotor intelligence stage are reflexive and motor. That is, he interacts with his environment in physical and mostly unlearned ways, especially early in the stage. He does not manipulate ideas in a conceptual sense, although cognitive development occurs in this stage, and it occurs rapidly. The child at two is a very different creature intellectually from the child in infancy.

2. *Preoperational Thought* (2 to 7 Years). The most rapid period of language development occurs during the stage of preoperational thought. The child begins to think conceptually, is able to categorize things in his environment, and is able to solve physical problems.

3. *Concrete Operations* (7 to 11 Years). The child develops the ability to think logically in dealing with concrete or physical problems. He is able to place stimuli into categories based on order and levels.

4. *Formal Operations* (11 to 15 Years). During the stage of formal operations cognitive abilities become fully developed. The child is able to think abstractly, to solve problems mentally, and to develop and test mental hypotheses. He reasons and thinks logically.

Remember, *these stages are not independent.* They are cumulative and are integrated into one another. The ages attached to these stages are not absolute. They simply represent the ages when most normal children are experiencing the cognitive developments indicated. One child might show signs of preoperational thought at fourteen months, but another child ten or eleven years old might still be demonstrating characteristics of preoperational thought, and both children could be normal. There is a great deal of variability among children in terms of when and how quickly they pass through each stage, but, as Piaget insists, each child must pass through the stages in the order listed, and a child will not skip a stage.

With this overview of cognitive development in mind, we will now direct our collective attention to the first stage, sensorimotor intelligence. During this stage, according to Piaget, the child develops those intellectual abilities that lay the foundation for symbolic behaviors such as dreaming, drawing, and language. Within the larger context of symbolic behaviors, therefore, this stage of cognitive development allows the child to get ready . . . get set . . . talk!

The Principle of Distancing in Sensorimotor Development

The primary focus of this chapter is on the intellectual and perceptual prerequisites experts assume are necessary for the development of early language. We must take care to note, however, that as important as these factors are to language development, the acquisition of language is an extraordinarily complex process that depends on factors other than cognition and perception. This complexity being established, we will consider how perception works with cognition in helping to establish a foundation for language. In order to understand this relationship, we must go back one step further to sensory input.

A person receives stimuli through his senses: touch, taste, smell, hearing, and vision. **Perception** refers to the processes by which the person selects, organizes, integrates, and interprets the sensory stimuli he is receiving. It should be obvious, therefore, that the child must be able to receive and perceptually process sensory stimuli to put this information into manipulable thought forms. Later in this chapter, we consider some of the child's earliest perceptual abilities, which appear to be related to his first attempts to communicate.

Before we can continue our explanation of the sensorimotor stage of cognitive development, however, we must identify and describe **distancing,** a basic perceptual principle affecting those cognitive changes that apparently precede and lay the foundation for language acquisition.

The infant relates to his environment in a very physical way. He grasps things with his hands and puts things into his mouth. In fact, parents often believe that everything goes into the infant's mouth. The infant is trying to understand his world primarily through touch, taste, and smell. Now consider how you relate to the world, especially to new stimuli. The first time you saw a computer or a CD player, you did not put these new things into your mouth. You looked at the computer. You looked at and listened to the CD player. You used senses that placed you at a greater distance from these new stimuli than if you had explored them by touch, taste, or smell. One can reasonably assume that you would eventually touch these items, but unless you are very strange, you probably would not taste or smell a computer during your first encounter. One thing that happens during perceptual development, therefore, is that the child relates to stimuli from a greater and greater distance. Moerk (1977) believes that the child's long-range visual and/or auditory images of new stimuli are the forerunners of representational meaning. That is, he first relates to an object by putting it into his mouth—immediate and maximal contact. As he develops, he creates a kind of mental picture of the object based on what he sees. The visual image represents the real thing, and the child recognizes the real thing based on that image.

Consider what happens as distancing progresses. A toy truck represents a real truck. A block of wood might be used by the child to represent a toy truck, which represents a real truck. The child will then recognize a truck in a picture. Eventually, the word truck represents the real thing. In each progression, the distance between the child and contact with the actual object becomes greater. Language represents the ultimate perceptual distance, and consider the advantages gained in the use of language. Linguistic symbols allow the child to mentally manipulate objects more quickly and easily than the objects themselves can be physically manipulated, and the mental manipulation of symbols representing things, people, places, and ideas is unfettered by time or space. Distancing moves the child's experiences with his environment from his hands and mouth to his brain. This is a short trip when measured in feet and inches, but when understood in the context of cognitive development, it is a journey spanning an intellectual universe.

Concepts and Behaviors Central to Early Cognitive Development

As we progress through the six substages of the sensorimotor phase of cognitive development, we will encounter three concepts (object permanence, causality, and means-ends) and three behaviors (imitation, play, and communication), which account for increasingly advanced intellectual functioning as they change. Consider these concepts and behaviors the principal players in the unfolding sensorimotor drama. Although the roles of these six characters in our cognitive drama change from scene to scene or substage to substage, these concepts and behaviors are the forces that together, in an interactive manner, shape the child's intellectual growth during this rapidly evolving first stage of cognitive development. And now, before the curtain goes up, let's meet the players.

A common bond shared by, all six players in our drama is **representation,** the idea that a stimulus can stand for or represent something else. A stop sign itself does not prevent me from driving my car through an intersection, but the sign represents the law, which says I must stop before proceeding. The whistle of an approaching train will not destroy my car, but the distinctive sound of the whistle causes me to approach the railroad crossing cautiously because I know the whistle represents the train, which can destroy my car and me if I put myself in its path. As I drive down the road, I watch the rear lights of the car in front of me. If the brake lights go on, I slow down because these lights represent the driver's intention to slow down or stop. If the right turn signal flashes, I assume the driver is about to turn right because that signal represents the driver's intention to turn. All day, every day, we are bombarded by stimuli representing ideas, people, things, and directions. An important and basic part of cognitive development is the evolutionary understanding of the concept of representation. Without this understanding, language is not possible because words are symbols that direct our thoughts to the things for which they stand.

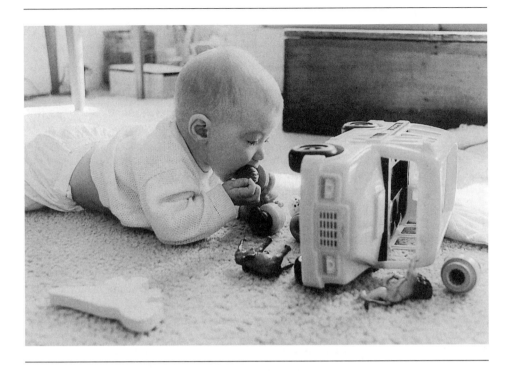

The child's first contacts with his world are physical and sensory.

The first player in our drama is a concept clearly related to representation, **object permanence.** It would not be accurate to say that the infant is not aware of objects, because even the youngest child will grasp or suck the things in his environment with which he has direct contact. When an object is removed, however, the infant pays no attention to its removal and does not look for it. When an object is out of sight, it is literally out of mind. As cognitive development proceeds, the child understands that objects exist even when they are not being touched, tasted, smelled, seen, or heard. Only when the child understands that things are permanent can he represent them cognitively, perhaps first in mental pictures, but eventually in words.

The next member of our cast is **causality.** In the beginning, the child has no concept of cause and effect. As he develops intellectually, he realizes that certain events cause other events, and he understands that he can produce behaviors that have predictable effects. According to Bates, Benigni, Bretherton, Camaioni, and Volterra (1979), the development of causality is a significant factor in the child's social and communicative maturation. Communication is a process driven by intentions. I do things or say things to produce desired and predictable results. An early understanding of causality might be reflected in the child's pushing a spoonful of strained carrots out of his mouth with his tongue. As he develops language, he might simply say "No!" He uses a word to represent his intention to cause the carrots to not be delivered to his stomach.

Means-ends can be understood as a concept that extends causality. As this concept develops, the child learns to use the cause-effect concept to solve problems. The young infant's first behaviors are random and unintentional. Perhaps he sees a cookie he would like to consume. He reaches out to grab it, but it is beyond his reach. His mother sees the child reaching, figures out what he wants, and gives him the cookie. Although the child got what he wanted, he stretched out his arms not to communicate intent, but to reach the cookie. As he becomes more cognitively sophisticated, he is able to establish goals and to figure out *means* by which to accomplish these goals or *ends*. He will eventually reach for an object he knows is beyond his reach because he is intentionally signalling by this gesture that he wants the targeted object. In terms of language development, means-ends is important because language is used to get things done. It becomes a means by which many ends are accomplished. The child must learn not only that language is a means-ends phenomenon, but that adjustments in language must be made depending on who the listener is and what kind of relationship the child has with the listener. If he wants a cookie from his younger brother, he might simply demand it. If he wants a cookie from his mother, he will likely ask for it—and say "Please!" In both cases, the end is thoughtfully targeted and the means is carefully created to maximize the possibility of success.

The fourth principal player is **imitation.** Anyone who observes young children will quickly and comfortably conclude that imitation is an important factor in cognitive development and in language development. Most of what children learn, and much of what adults learn, appears to be the result of attending to models and trying to duplicate them. The research data concerning the acquisition of communication skills support the conclusion that imitation is an important developmental factor (Rees, 1975; Moore & Meltzoff, 1978; Snyder, 1978). It is assumed that imitation facilitates the child's ability to internalize models of the behaviors of others, which he can then duplicate. Early imitations are crude, imprecise, and always immediate, but over the course of development, imitated behaviors become more accurate and sophisticated, and they occur in a delayed manner. **Delayed or deferred imitation** is important because it allows the child to produce a desired behavior even when the model is not present. Without deferred imitation, language would not progress beyond the kind of parroted productions accomplished by talking birds. Even before the child can imitate language forms, he imitates movements and gestures. Imitations of behaviors associated with objects seem to suggest some understanding of the objects themselves. For example, if the child, with or without a real comb in his hands, imitates a combing motion, we might reasonably assume he knows something about the function of the comb. Bates and Snyder (1987) suggest that imitation is a primitive kind of labeling. That is, the child labels a comb by imitating, immediately or on a deferred basis, the action of combing. In the sensorimotor drama, imitation is a major player, as you will see.

Our next player is **play** itself. Many adults think of playing as a frivolous activity, but play is viewed by professionals concerned with child development as fairly serious business. Play is certainly a fun and entertaining activity, but it also provides the child many opportunities for learning about the things and people in his world, as well as concepts ranging from colors, numbers, and simple prepositions such as *in* and *on,* to more complex things like sharing and social interactions. As the child grows older, language and other forms of communication become increasingly prominent and important components in play activities. Experts in cognitive and language development are especially interested in **symbolic play,** an activity in which one object represents another object. How many times, for example, have you watched children play for hours in a big box, pretending it was a house or a fort. A child might use a block as a truck. My youngest daughter, when she was about two years old, used rubber bands as bracelets and often had ten or twelve on her wrist at one time. All of these are examples of symbolic play. This kind of play has a rather obvious connection to language. In symbolic play, the child might use a stick to represent a nail-driving tool. In language, he can use the word *hammer* to refer to the same object. Both are representational activities. It is probably not a coincidence then that Bates, Bretherton, Snyder, Shore, and Volterra (1980) found that children who are able and willing to use objects to represent other objects progress more quickly in language development than children who are more rigid in their use of objects.

Sixth, **communication** is the leading character in our version of the sensorimotor drama, because speech and language are the focus of this book. The development of the concepts we have identified are reflected in the child's increasingly sophisticated communication system, and few would argue with the conclusion that imitation and play are important in helping the child acquire greater conceptual understandings and more advanced communicative skills by which to express his understandings. It is also reasonable to assume that, at some point, the child uses his communication abilities, especially language, to facilitate advances in his cognitive development. As we proceed through the substages of sensorimotor development, we will track changes in communication as well as changes in the other concepts and behaviors we have identified. For the sake of convenience and to allow for direct comparison of the substages, we discuss the players in the same order in each substage; however, keep in mind that the order signifies nothing about the importance of these players. The interactions among the players are more important than the individual players themselves. The further into cognitive development we proceed, the more inextricably connected the players become.

The cast is set. The curtain is rising. Let the play begin.

The Sensorimotor Period (Birth to 2 Years)

Scene One—Substage One (0 to 1 Month)

Piaget believes the understanding that objects are permanent is not innate. That is, the newborn infant reacts to objects as though they no longer exist when they are not in sight. The concept of object permanence develops in stages as the child gets to know the things in his environment (Piaget, 1954, p. 4). At birth, the child has no concept of objects. He gives no indication that he understands the difference between himself and the things around him. He reacts to objects only by looking, grasping, and sucking them, and even these reactions are reflexive, or unlearned, and they are undifferentiated. That is, he does not demonstrate preferences for some objects over others based on an understanding of meaningful differences. The world, to the newborn, consists of unexplored and relatively uninteresting things that pass, with little notice, in and out of his sensory fields.

At birth and through the first three substages of the sensorimotor period, the child is egocentric. As Piaget uses the term, **egocentrism** means that the child sees and understands the world only as an extension of himself. He has no other point of view. He does not understand that he is one thing among many other things in the environment. This means that the newborn infant has no concept of causality. He is so far removed from this concept, in fact, that he does not understand that there is a difference between himself and other objects. It will be some months before we glimpse even the beginning of cause-effect understanding. From the newborn's perspective, there are not even parts to act upon one another. Everything in the newborn's world is a member of a whole, and the whole is **him!**

If the newborn sees the world as one undifferentiated mass of himness, it should not be surprising that he shows no understanding of means-ends. One cannot identify an objective and plot a strategy to obtain it if the world is ensconced in one tightly bound, leakproof package. Imagine what it would be like to have no goals, no tasks to be done, no chores to complete, no responsibilities to fill. Since there are no identifiable ends, the newborn does not need to devise any means.

The Substage One infant is not capable of imitation, but does produce behaviors that seem to be imitative. McCormick (1990) refers to one example of this behavior as "vocal contagion." That is, when one newborn begins to cry, other newborns in the same room are likely to cry, too. Piaget believes that what happens in this case is not imitation but the stimulation of an already established response by an external stimulus. In other words, the newborn has already established the ability to cry. His crying is usually triggered by pain or hunger, but in the case of vocal contagion his crying is triggered by another newborn's cries.

The newborn infant does not play. He exists. He sees, hears, grasps, sucks, eats, sleeps, and relieves himself—often, but he does not play. Playing must wait until the time when he knows there are other people and other things in the world.

There is not much communication during the first substage. There is certainly nothing we can call language. The newborn child produces reflexive cries, usually in response to stimuli of discomfiture, and fairly early in his life he makes sounds of pleasure, sounds we might interpret as sighs, but the communicative effects of these behaviors are limited. Parents quickly learn to identify the conditions under which cries and sighs are produced, and in that sense, there is communication, but there is no communicative intent on the part of the child in Substage One.

As dramas go, this has not been the most exciting opening scene one might imagine. What do we have here? We have a living organism with enormous cognitive and communicative potential, but he is just sitting on the stage crying, grasping, and sucking. He pays little or no attention to the audience, and is constantly falling asleep. This drama builds in excitement, so hang in there. It gets better.

Scene Two—Substage Two (1 to 4 Months)

During this substage, the child begins to show some awareness of objects, but the awareness is sensory rather than conceptual. He reacts to objects visually and auditorially, and more significantly, he is able to coordinate his visual and auditory contacts with objects. That is, when he hears a noise, he searches for the source with his eyes, and if the sound source moves within his field of vision, he follows its movement. Piaget (1954, pp. 10–11) reports that one of his daughters during this substage not only visually located objects but was also able to look away from an object and then locate it again. Whether or not a child reacts to this visual and auditory hide-and-seek activity with disappointment and expectation as Piaget suggests, it is reasonable to conclude that the child is developing an interest in objects and is using his senses to make and maintain contact with them.

Even though there is sensory interest in objects during this substage, the child still does not demonstrate an understanding that objects are separate from him. He makes few, if any, meaningful differentiations among objects, and he does not differentiate objects from himself, even when the objects move in and out of his sensory fields. In other words, he is still very much egocentric. As was true in the first substage, there are no parts, and therefore, there is no possibility for a demonstration of causality.

Since the child has not yet developed the concept of causality, we should not be surprised that there is no evidence of means-ends in the second substage. Even though we see sensorimotor behaviors in this substage that we did not see earlier, such as visually locating and following a moving object or grasping and looking at an object, we should not conclude that these behaviors reflect intentionality. These are still essentially reflexive behaviors even though they can be modified by other people who cause objects to move or make noise. Piaget (1952, p. 143) contends that "Even when the child grasps an object in order to look at it, one cannot infer that there is a conscious purpose." In this example, it might be tempting to think of looking as the end and the grasping as the means, but since grasping is a reflexive behavior, we cannot conclude that the sequence of behaviors from grasping to look-ing is intentional. It just happens, and the looking is part of the reflexive sequence.

We see the beginning of imitation in this substage, although it is a specialized kind of imitation. The child produces a behavior that someone, perhaps a parent, imitates. The child then repeats the behavior. What we have then is the child imi-tating a behavior which he produced, but only after someone else imitated him. Got it? These behaviors might be gestural but are usually vocal. In a common example, the child says "goo-goo." The parent mimics the child saying, "goo-goo." The child, terribly excited by this insightful communicative exchange, repeats his original production, "goo-goo." Piaget calls this behavior "pre-imitation," sug-gesting it is behavior that sets the stage for true imitation. McCormick (1990) calls the same behavior "mutual imitation," which describes the nature of the exchange.

It would be a real stretch to call anything the child does in the second substage play, but he is engaging in sensorimotor behaviors that are preliminary to play. He is not only grasping objects, but holding them for brief periods of time and looking at them, and is showing some interest in the sensory characteristics of objects. Even the primitive imitative responses we see in this substage are preparing the child for play activities seen in later substages. Early play activities involve very basic motor and sensory behaviors, and they often involve imitation, so the child is getting ready for play.

During the early weeks of this substage, most of the child's communications are still in the form of reflexive cries, but as the substage progresses, the child cries less frequently and develops distinctly different types of cries. According to D'Odorico (1984), at about four months the child produces three differentiated cries to signal discomfort, to call, and to request. Noncrying vocalizations sig-nalling pleasure develop during this substage. The child begins to coo, especially when interacting with someone else. These productions are described as vowel-like to indicate that there are no consonant approximations and to suggest that the sounds produced are not true vowels. They are random, undifferentiated produc-tions of sounds with vowel characteristics. Toward the end of this substage, at about four months, the child is also laughing (Stark, 1979), a delightful develop-ment for child and parents. The child may not be receptive to political humor or satire at this point, but he does laugh. It is, in fact, often difficult to figure out what makes a four-month-old child laugh, but if gentle pokes in the belly accompanied by funny faces and silly vocal noises make him laugh, parents will enjoy it! They have made communicative contact with their child about subjects other than hunger and soiled diapers.

Scene Three—Substage Three (4 to 8 Months)

In the third substage, the child begins to develop the concept of object permanence, the idea that objects exist even when they are not in view or in physical contact with the child. The concept at this point is limited, however. The child watching an object move will anticipate its future position. If he is sitting in a high chair, he might drop food and watch it fall onto the floor, and he will react to the general

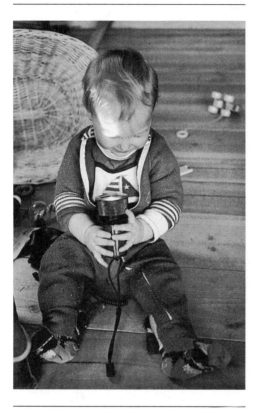

Where did this light
come from and where is
it going?

direction of the fall, anticipating the food's final resting position on Mom's newly
scrubbed vinyl floor. As in the previous stage, he will grasp an object and look at
it, but now he seems to examine it with greater interest. If a toy is partially hidden
by a piece of paper, he might reach for it, but if the same toy is out of sight, he will
not search for it. This is what Flavell (1977, p. 43) calls the "essential limitation" of
Substage Three. That is, the child will briefly look for an object that is hidden, but
will not conduct a physical search for it. Even though the child in this substage has
not yet developed the concept of object permanence, he is rapidly moving toward
this understanding.

To appreciate what this child understands about causality, one must remember
that he is still very much egocentric. The child will repeat actions he finds interesting or pleasurable, and in that sense, he knows he is causing the action that precip-
itates the pleasure. There are two important limitations, however. First, the child
pays little attention to the effects of his behaviors, especially in a cognitive sense. For
the concept of causality to be truly developed, the child must understand cause *and*

effect. Second, the child in this substage behaves as though he is the cause of all actions. He does not recognize that other people or objects cause actions. If, while holding the child, I ring a bell, he might throw his arms up or push my face to cause the bell to ring again. He does not understand that it is my hand, moving in a specific manner, which causes the bell to ring. The child believes it is *his* action that causes bell ringing and all other events because he is still the master of his universe.

The sophistication of means-ends in this stage matches the child's understanding of causality, as we would reasonably expect. In the first two substages, we saw no evidence of intentionality. In the third substage, there is a limited but important progression in means-ends development. The child might pick up a new rattle, for example. In the course of examining the rattle, he shakes it and it makes a noise he finds interesting. He continues to shake the rattle. This can certainly be construed as intentional or goal-oriented behavior, but the goals in this substage are established only after the activity has begun (Wadsworth, 1971, p. 46). Behavior based on a complete understanding of means-ends is initiated in an intentional manner after a goal has been identified and a strategy for reaching that goal has been developed. At this point, the child is engaging in intentional behaviors, but is not yet a planner.

Interesting changes in imitation occur in the third substage, but as with the other concepts we have described in this substage, it is important to stress the limitations as we identify the progressions. McCormick (1990) refers to Substage Three imitation as "systematic imitation." The most significant progressions are that the child imitates a wider range of behaviors, and he will imitate the behaviors of others. Most imitations are of sounds and physical actions, but the child will not imitate an action he himself has not performed spontaneously at an earlier time. He will imitate only complete sequences of behaviors, not isolated parts of a sequence. The child must be able to see himself perform the activity he is imitating, and if it involves sound, he must be able to hear himself. If we put these limitations together, they mean the child will imitate making and releasing a fist if he has previously done this on his own. If, in releasing his fist, the child spontaneously spreads his fingers, he will spread his fingers when he imitates the fist making/fist releasing sequence, but he will not imitate only the spreading of his fingers. He will imitate fist making/fist releasing if he can watch himself, but he will not imitate this sequence of behaviors while holding his hand behind his back.

In the third substage, we see the child engaging in activities that more closely resemble play. The child is interacting with other people. Even though his imitations are limited to his repertoire of behaviors, he does respond to models of physical and vocal activity. He is finding toys more interesting and repeats actions on toys that may or may not be appropriate. That is, he might shake a rattle, but he might also bang it on the floor or on Mom's forehead. He is still very much a sensory creature. He grasps toys, ears, nostrils, and dog's paws, and he still tries to put all objects, including the coffee table leg, into his mouth. The child is deriving pleasure from his play activities, and they provide him opportunities for developing concepts and elaborating behaviors important for later cognitive and communicative development.

There are few dramatic changes in communication in this substage. The child continues to produce vowel-like utterances, but we do notice the emergence of consonant-like sounds. Keep in mind that the "-like" qualification affixed to "vowel" and "consonant" means that these productions are random and not meaningful, but they are sounds that have characteristics of true sounds. Toward the end of this substage, at about six to eight months, the child begins to produce productions referred to as **babbling.** These are combinations of vowel-like and consonant-like sounds, resulting in utterances like "gagaga" or "mamama." As you might imagine, parents often interpret these babbled productions as "words," but until a production is used in a consistent, intentional, and meaningful manner, it cannot be considered a word. It will be a few months before the child is producing true words, but he is laying the groundwork at this point by establishing control over the components of his speech mechanism (Sachs, 1989, p. 45). It would certainly be a mistake to assume that the child in Substage Three is not communicating. He is using his vocalizations and gestures to communicate many things from "I'm not a very happy person right now because my diapers are wet—again" to "I would like very much to have that cookie in your hand, and if you don't mind, I am going to grab it while distracting you with my devastating smile."

Scene Four—Substage Four (8 to 12 Months)

As the child moves into the last few months of his first year, he seems more curious about his world. Part of what adults might perceive as curiosity is the further development of the object permanence concept. In the first two substages, if an object was out of sight, it was out of mind. In the third substage, the child would reach for an object if it was partially hidden but would not physically search for it if it was completely out of sight. In the fourth substage, the child shows evidence that he remembers objects. If a playful adult hides his favorite pacifier under a pillow, he will lift the pillow to find it. In addition to understanding that objects are permanent, the child demonstrates an understanding that the shape and size of objects are constant. If a familiar object, such as his bottle, is given to him upside down, he knows that the business end has a nipple on it, and he will turn the bottle around. In other words, he knows the shape has not changed even when his perspective of the bottle is different. He will also recognize his bottle when viewed from a distance, even though the bottle appears smaller from 30 feet away than from 6 inches. The object concept is not yet fully developed, however. For example, the child will look for an object that has disappeared, but often only if he sees it disappear. Piaget (1954, p. 51) observed that his daughter, Jacqueline, in the fourth substage would search for hidden objects where they usually disappeared, not necessarily where she saw them disappear. The object concept is fairly complete by the end of this substage, but there are still some gaps, and we will not see a thorough understanding of object permanence until the sixth substage.

In the fourth substage, we encounter a child who is far less egocentric than in earlier substages. This shift from an egocentric view of the world is most noticeable in the child's more sophisticated understanding of causality. In the third substage, the child had a limited understanding of causality but behaved as though he was the cause of all actions. He now externalizes causality. That is, he understands that other people and other objects can cause activities. Using the same example of bell ringing we employed in the preceding substage, we can create a very different scenario. Earlier the child believed he was responsible for causing the bell to ring even though he did not touch the bell. Now when the child watches me pick up the bell and ring it, he will push my hand toward the bell to indicate that he wants me to ring it again. He understands that I cause the action.

In the third substage, the child showed evidence of a very elementary understanding of means-ends. He used behavior that was goal-oriented, but the goals were set only after behavior was in progress. In the fourth substage, the child plans behavior. He devises a means or strategy before he initiates a behavior, and there is a clear connection between the strategy and the goal. Wadsworth (1971, p. 48) suggests that this behavior is one of "the first clear acts of intelligence" we observe in the developing child. Many of the child's behaviors are now intentional, and they reflect thoughtful planning. In an earlier example related to object permanence, the child searched for his pacifier under a pillow. This same example demonstrates his more sophisticated means-ends understanding. The problem is a missing pacifier. The end is to find the pacifier. The means is to move the pillow. Eureka! There is the pacifier!

Imitation undergoes some interesting and significant changes in the fourth substage. The child now imitates behaviors he has not produced himself, although he is likely to imitate only actions or vocalizations similar to those he has produced on his own (McCormick, 1990). It is not necessary in this substage that he be able to see or hear himself while he is imitating. For example, if while holding the child on my lap, I stick out my tongue, he might imitate this behavior even though he cannot see his own protruding tongue. Owens (1996, p. 142) suggests that this kind of imitation requires some short-term motor memory, which has obvious relevance to the speech skills he will acquire in the near future.

It should be apparent by this point in our drama that play provides the child opportunities to use his developing concepts in activities that are pleasurable. More importantly perhaps, it is through play that the child discovers new aspects of these concepts and demonstrates these new understandings to those who observe him. While playing with his toys, the child in the fourth substage will look for toys that are not in sight. He might demonstrate means-ends by pulling the string on a toy that makes animal sounds, but if this action is too difficult, he might encourage someone else to pull the string, demonstrating his understanding of external causality,. He might use a few objects in a manner that suggests an understanding of function. For example, he might roll a ball or bang on a toy drum, although it will be some time before he is able to build a small nuclear device or create havoc by making contact with NASA's computer system.

In the early months of the fourth substage, the child is still babbling. By the end of the substage, he may actually produce his first meaningful words. Whether or not there are true words during this time, it is evident that the child is communicating, vocally and gesturally, in an intentional manner. Even without speech, children in the latter months of this substage link gestures and vocalizations to convey fairly specific messages. Bates, Camaioni, and Volterra (1975) studied a girl in this substage who, on one occasion at least, vocalized "ha" to her mother while looking in the direction of the kitchen. When her mother carried her into the kitchen, the girl pointed at the sink, prompting her mother to give her a drink of water. The child did not use words, but she certainly communicated.

Scene Five—Substage Five (12 to 18 Months)

The child in this substage is tantalizingly close to having a complete understanding of object permanence. In the last scene, the child would search for an object if he saw it disappear, but even if he saw it disappear, he would look for it where it is usually hidden, not always where he actually saw it hidden. In the fourth substage, he cannot accommodate sequential displacements (Wadsworth, 1971, p. 55). If I usually hide his pacifier under a pillow, but I now hide it under his blanket, he will look for the pacifier under the pillow, even if he watches me hide it under the blanket. This seems strange from an adult point of view, but remember the developing child's perspective. He is a physical and sensory creature who only gradually acquires the ability to deal with objects in an abstract sense. For him, what you see is what you get, and through the fourth substage, what you see is what you get only if what you get is where you expect it to be! In the fifth substage, we see a giant step forward. He is now capable of following sequential displacements. If I hide his pacifier under the pillow, he will look under the pillow. If I then hide it under his blanket, he will look under the blanket, and if I put it in my shirt pocket, he will search for his pacifier in my pocket, undoubtedly ripping my shirt in the process. Why then is the concept not complete? Although the child can handle sequential displacements if he can see them, he cannot handle a displacement he cannot see. If, for example, I hide his pacifier under the pillow, and while I have my hand under the pillow, I slip the pacifier between the sofa cushions, the child will look for the pacifier under, over, and around the pillow, but will not search between the sofa cushions. The object permanence concept becomes complete in the sixth and final substage when the child is finally able to move an object from its place in the restricted physical world to the mind where it is represented abstractly and is free of all time and space limitations.

The change in causality in substage five is subtle but important. In the last substage, the child was aware that people and things other than himself can be agents of cause, but he demonstrated this understanding only in relation to people, things, and actions with which he was familiar. In this substage, the child's understanding of causality becomes more sophisticated in that he sees other people and objects as agents for causality in new situations. If, for example, the child is given a new toy unlike anything he has seen before, he might examine it carefully and,

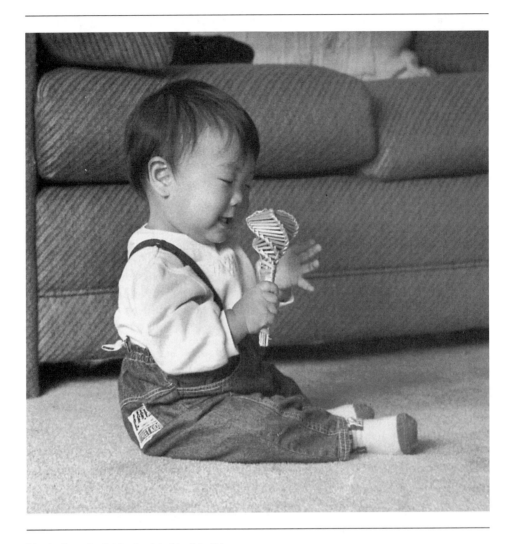

My, look at the intricate detail in this thing.

deciding he does not know what to do with it, push it into an adult's hand. He is seeking the adult's assistance as an agent of causality. In essence, "Show me what this thing does!" In another example, we have a child who, when playing with his mother's lipstick got the sticky red goo all over his fingers. He now approaches a fire hydrant painted the same bright red as the lipstick. He touches the hydrant and examines his fingers, expecting to see them colored red. In this example, the child is able to transfer his understanding of causality from one situation to another, and in the process learns that red does not always icky fingers make. In both examples, we see evidence that the child's understanding of external causality has increased.

Means-ends in the fifth substage can be characterized as more creative or experimental in comparison to the fourth substage. The child is becoming a problem-solver, and in the process of learning to solve problems, he experiments with objects and actions. The child, for example, has a toy workbench. He uses a play hammer to drive a large wooden peg through an opening in the bench. Banging the hammer is the means by which to reach the end, defined as making the peg move. He now picks up a banana. It weighs about the same as the hammer, and it has a convenient "handle," so the child hits the peg with the banana. The banana breaks, and the peg does not move. This means did not accomplish the desired end because, as the child learned through his trial and error, the banana is too soft. As his experimentation proceeds, he will learn that things other than the hammer can be used, like Dad's shoe, or Mom's skillet, to drive the peg through the bench because, like the hammer, they are hard. As you might imagine, this experimentation business can be interesting and dangerous. Parents are well advised to observe their children carefully as they identify their goals and map their strategies for attaining them. A peanut butter sandwich might be approximately the same size as a VHS cassette, but pushed into the loading device of the VCR, the peanut butter sandwich has a markedly different effect than the cassette. Yech!

The same willingness, perhaps eagerness, to experiment observed in means-ends experiences is observed in imitation. The child is an excellent and uninhibited imitator in this substage.. The accuracy of his imitations is limited only by his motor abilities (Owens, 1996, p. 142), but he will try almost anything. According to McCormick (1990), this child imitates to better understand his world and the things in it. He will imitate animal noises, for example, and will attempt to imitate even complex speech productions. When my own children were in this substage, I modeled words like *encyclopedia, electroencephalographic,* and *diadochokinesis,* which they gladly tried to imitate. Their productions of these words were not accurate, but they produced excellent imitations of words and actions that were within their motoric capabilities.

The child's play in this substage clearly reflects his cognitive advances. He thoroughly examines his toys and quickly figures out the operative pieces. If the toy is relatively simple to operate, he figures out how to make it work through trial and error. If there is a string, he pulls it. If there is a lever, he pushes it. If there is a dial, he turns it. If he cannot figure out what to do with the toy, as mentioned in the causality discussion, he hands it to someone else for consultation and demonstration. The child also combines toys in a functional manner. He might, for example, use his toy hammer to make a ball roll across the floor.

It is during this substage that we typically see children producing their first meaningful words. These words are monosyllabic (e.g., "go," "no") or duplicated disyllabic forms (e.g., "mama." "wawa"). There is no question that communication during this substage is intentional. For example, the child might say "bye-bye" to indicate that he wants to leave or wants someone else to leave. Toward the end of this substage, it is not uncommon for the child to say "nite-nite," while shaking his head from side to side, to suggest that he has no intention of going to bed now, under any circumstances, not until "Monday Night Football" is over or until the strained popcorn is all gone, whichever occurs first. Communication continues to be heavily dependent on nonverbal messages in the voice, face, and gestures, but there is very little of importance, as defined by the child's own needs and desires, that he cannot communicate.

As Scene Five closes, we leave the last of the truly sensorimotor substages. The child is now ready for an important transition. Through the first five substages, he has evolved from a creature tied completely to his physical world by his senses and his oral and manual manipulation of objects to a creature who has gradually distanced himself from direct contact with objects. In the fifth substage, we have seen a child who understands that he is only one of many people in the world. He understands that other people and other things are agents of cause. He is a curious creature who tests and expands his understanding of causality and means-ends by exploration and experimentation. He freely and happily interacts with other people by imitating their vocalizations and their actions, including behaviors totally unfamiliar to him, and he communicates with other people. He sends and receives messages nonverbally, and for the first time, verbally. This has been an exciting scene in our drama, the transitional scene that sets the stage for the final scene, Substage Six, during which we will see the completion of the concepts and the elaboration of the behaviors we have been following in the first five scenes.

Scene Six—Substage Six (18 to 24 Months)

The common denominator underlying all the significant changes in the sixth substage is representation. That is, the child's understanding of his world moves from the sensorimotor level to a level in which he is able to represent objects internally and to manipulate these internal representations of reality to solve problems. He is becoming, in a word, a cognitive thinker instead of a touchy-feely experiencer.

The child now has a fully developed concept of object permanence. Not only can he follow sequential displacements, but he can accommodate invisible displacements. If I move the pacifier out of sight under the pillow and then slide the pacifier between the sofa cushions, the child will first look under the pillow, but not finding it, will continue to look in and around the area where it disappeared until he finds it. He now has a mental image of the pacifier that is entirely free of his senses and his physical contacts with it. He knows that the pacifier and all objects are permanent, do not disappear just because they are out of sight, and do

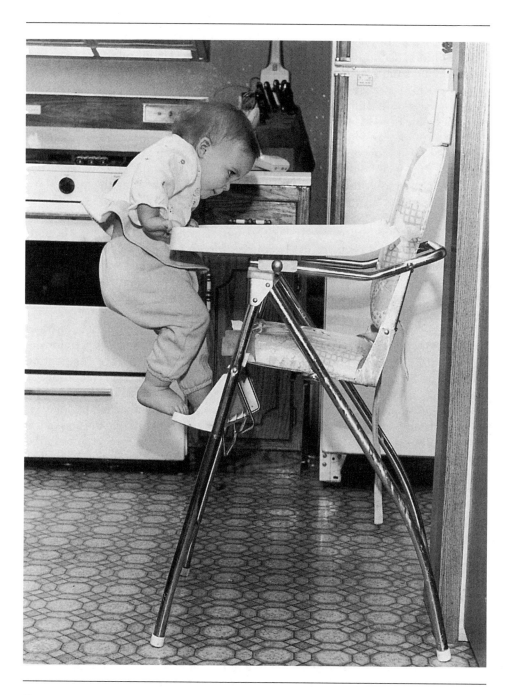

Executing an imperfect and perhaps dangerous plan of action.

not change in size or shape just because they are viewed from different angles or distances. When the object is out of sight, it is now firmly in mind. It is, in reference to the common denominator of this substage, *represented* in his mind.

The child's understanding of causality is also enhanced by this ability to represent objects and cause-effect relationships in his mind. A child in the early substages, for example, might simply react with frustration when trying to remove a play telephone from his toy box, the receiver of which is tangled on another toy at the bottom of the box. He cannot see what has tangled the receiver, and he does not have the ability to conceptualize the cause-effect relationship that is preventing the removal of the telephone. After tugging a few times, he might give up or cry, but he will not try to solve the problem by identifying and eliminating the cause. If we move this same child forward to substage six, we see a much different performance when faced with the same problem. After tugging on the phone a time or two, he reaches into the toy box to discover what is tangling the receiver. He eliminates the tangle and removes the telephone. He was able to solve this problem because, even without seeing what was catching the receiver, he was able to mentally represent a physical obstacle of some kind. He understood the principle of cause and effect that was operating, and he applied this intellectual understanding to the solution of a physical problem.

Means-ends, in its fully developed form, is about intentionality. It is a process of identifying goals and planning strategies for attaining those goals. Obviously, the more fully the child understands causality, the more capable he is of creating sophisticated means-ends strategies. In the sixth substage, the child can represent the goal mentally, and can map out plans for reaching that goal in his mind's eye. In earlier substages, the child might get a cookie out of the unreachable cookie jar by pointing and grunting until someone gets the cookie for him. By the end of the sensorimotor stage, this child might push a chair to the counter, climb onto the counter, and stand on tiptoes to reach the cookie jar on the shelf his mother thought was safely beyond reach. He set a goal. He invented a means for reaching the goal, and he put the plan into action. This kind of creative planning is just part of what is waiting for parents during the stage of child development often called The Terrible Twos.

Imitation undergoes significant changes as we proceed through the six substages. In the early substages, the child imitates only those actions and vocalizations he produces spontaneously. In the fourth substage, he imitates behaviors that are similar to those he produces, and in the fifth substage, he imitates new behaviors. In the sixth substage, the child produces what are called "deferred imitations" (McCormick, 1990). This means that the child can imitate a behavior modeled for him earlier, an action or vocalization that he has represented mentally and stored in his memory. Now when someone asks the child what sound the cow makes, he retrieves the model from his own mental catalog of animal noises and imitates that model by saying, "Moo!" When someone leaves the house, he does not need to have someone prompt a wave by demonstration and exhortation. He remembers the action and produces it spontaneously, a deferred imitation of a model he has stored in his memory.

In addition to seeing the child apply his more complete conceptual understandings in play, we observe some fundamental changes in the nature of the child's play in the sixth substage (Westby, 1980). Early in this substage, the child might pretend to drink out of a cup or glass, or pretend to sleep, but all of his pretending behaviors are autosymbolic. That is, he limits pretending to his own actions. About midway through the final substage, he extends pretending to other objects during symbolic play, but the objects must be realistic. The child will pretend he is feeding a doll with a real or toy spoon, for example, but will not pretend that a popsicle stick is a spoon. By the end of the sixth substage, the child will engage in play activities that represent real-life experiences. He might play house, but the toys used must still be realistic in terms of function, and to some extent, even in terms of size. He will not be ready for representational toys, like a Fisher-Price house or barn, until he is about three years old.

All the changes we have identified in the sixth substage have direct implications for what is happening to the child as a communicator as he completes this phase of his cognitive development and prepares to move forward. Until the child has some understanding that objects are permanent, he cannot represent them in words. Only when the child understands that all people and many objects can be agents of cause, will he be ready to use communication as an agent for causality. If intentionality is the key to means-ends, it is clearly the key that opens the door of communication, both verbal and nonverbal. As the sensorimotor stage unfolds, the child learns that gestures can be used to make needs and desires known, and he eventually learns that words can be even more effective because they allow greater specificity. Language has been described as a tool for many years, and in the context of means-ends, that is an apt description. As the sensorimotor stage comes to a close, the child is using words and combinations of words to get things done. Imitation, especially deferred imitation, is critical to the development of communication. The child learns gestures by imitation, and as mentioned earlier, will use a gesture to label an object "by carrying out an action typically associated with it" (Bates & Snyder, 1987). Imitation also plays a role in the acquisition of speech. By the end of the fourth substage, the typical child is producing his first meaningful words which, although they may be only approximations of adult utterances, are evidence of internalized models. In the fifth substage, the child is imitating adult utterances unlike anything he has produced on his own, and by the end of the sixth substage, he is imitating and spontaneously producing multiple word utterances. The essential contribution of imitation is that it helps the child develop the ability to internally represent behaviors, and eventually to produce these behaviors even when the models are not present. This is the essence of language, a system of communication based, in part, on a huge inventory of internalized models. As the child's play progresses from a solitary, physically limited activity to a more interactive and representational activity, language plays a more

TABLE 3-1 Highlights of Sensorimotor Development

Substage (and Months)	Object Permanence	Causality	Means-Ends	Imitation	Play	Communication
1 (0 to 1)	Out of sight, out of mind.	No concept of causality.	No understanding of means-ends.	None.	None.	No communicative intent.
2 (1 to 4)	Uses senses to make and maintain contact with objects.	No concept of causality.	No understanding of means-ends.	Pre-imitation. Repeats his own behavior that has been imitated by someone else.	Produces behaviors preliminary to play including grasping and looking at objects.	Cries, coos, and laughs.
3 (4 to 8)	Watches object move and anticipates its future position. Reaches for partially hidden object.	Does not understand cause-effect. Behaves as though he is the cause of all actions.	Produces goal-oriented behaviors but only after activity has begun.	Imitates only behaviors he has spontaneously produced at an earlier time.	Still very sensory but begins to interact with other people.	Babbles.
4 (8 to 12)	Looks for an object if he sees it being hidden.	Externalizes causality. Knows other people and objects can cause activities.	Evidence of planning and the production of intentional behaviors.	Imitates behaviors he has not spontaneously produced.	Uses developing concepts in his play activities.	Links gestures and vocalizations to convey fairly specific messages.
5 (12 to 18)	Follows sequential displacements to find hidden object.	Sees other people and objects as agents for causality in new situations.	Uses experimentation to solve problems.	Uninhibited imitation to facilitate his own understanding.	Play reflects cognitive growth. He figures out how to make toys work.	Produces first meaningful words. Communication is intentional but still heavily nonverbal.
6 (18 to 24)	Fully developed concept of object permanence. Can now accommodate invisible displacements.	Causality enhanced by ability to represent objects and cause-effect relationships in his mind.	Can mentally represent a goal and his plan for achieving the goal.	Deferred imitation. Imitates a behavior he has represented mentally and stored in his memory.	Progresses from autosymbolic to symbolic play.	Imitates and spontaneously produces multiple word utterances.

important role. We have to go beyond the sensorimotor stage to observe speech as a primary play activity, but in the latter months of this first stage of cognitive development, we see communication becoming an increasingly important part of play.

As the curtain slowly falls on the sensorimotor drama, the reader should be reminded that this is but the beginning of the cognitive development story. Piaget's theory has three more stages, which might be viewed as sequels to the sensorimotor drama. Unlike sequels to bad movies, which typically only compound the badness of the original, however, the cognitive sequels are improved dramas because each stage is based upon and incorporates the preceding stage. We are pausing after the sensorimotor phase, not to indicate intellectual closure, but to indicate that the stage has now been set for the part of the child development story that is the primary focus of this book—speech and language acquisition. (Table 3-1 reviews the highlights of the child's sensorimotor development.) We will provide closure to our discussion of Piaget's theory of cognitive development, however, by reviewing reservations about some of his views precipitated by research data gathered in recent years.

Recent Research: A Critical Review of Piaget's Sensorimotor Stage

Because the Piagetian view of cognitive development was so widely accepted and so heavily influenced our understanding of many aspects of early child development (with direct and indirect connections to cognitive development), researchers have tried to verify Piaget's observations about what happens during the sensorimotor stage and when. The results of this research suggest that children exhibit some cognitive abilities at much earlier ages than Piaget indicated. The reader should note, however, that reservations about what Piaget proposed should not be construed as criticisms of the man. Today's researchers understand that Piaget did not have access to modern research methodologies that would have allowed him to conduct the kind of carefully designed and rigorously implemented studies the human behavioral research community demands today. Piaget suggested, for example, that the infant shows evidence that he is exploring his world and making preliminary efforts to control aspects of his environment when he is about four to eight months old. Using basic operant conditioning principles, researchers have demonstrated that the child is displaying this level of cognitive awareness immediately after birth. This conclusion is drawn from evidence that the neonate will enthusiastically suck on a nipple in order to produce a wide range of sounds and sights he finds interesting. This experiment demonstrates that the newborn child is aware of these auditory and visual stimuli and that he is able to exercise rudimentary control to make them happen. Similar research strategies, based on operant conditioning principles, have been used to help us understand what the sensorimotor-stage child knows about object permanence and mental representation and when he knows it.

Object Permanence

The reader may recall that during substage three of the sensorimotor period, when the child is four to eight months old, he is beginning to demonstrate an awareness of *object permanence,* the idea that even if an object is out of sight, it still exists. At this point, however, the child does not try to locate an object that is hidden. According to Piaget, trying to locate a hidden object is a behavior that provides evidence that the child knows object permanence. The suggestion from Piaget is clear. Until the child is older than eight months, he believes that an object that is out of sight has ceased to exist, an idea so widely accepted that we often use a maxim based on this assumption, *Out of sight, out of mind.* Is Piaget's assertion about when the child's knowledge of object permanence emerges supported by research? It is not.

Baillargeon (1987) and Baillargeon and Devos (1991) provide evidence that children may have object permanence as early as three-and-a-half months. The method used to make this determination involves what is called the *habituation-dishabituation response.* The subjects were first habituated to two events. The first event involved a picture of a short carrot moving from left to right behind a yellow screen. This event was alternated with a second event, which involved a tall carrot moving from left to right behind a yellow screen. After the subjects were *habituated* to these events, which essentially means that they paid attention to them, two test events were introduced. Two changes were made to the test event scenes: (1) Each scene now had a wall with an inserted window in the middle of the visual field, and (2) The color of the screen was changed from yellow to blue to help draw the subjects' attention to the wall and window. The two test events involved a *possible event* and an *impossible event.* In the *possible event,* the short carrot moved from left to right behind the wall and below the lowest margin of the window and reappeared on the other side. In real life, this is exactly what would happen. That is, an object shorter than the bottom frame of the window could be seen before reaching the wall, would be out of sight as it crossed behind the wall and below the window sill, and would reappear only when it reached the right side of the wall. In the *impossible event,* the tall carrot moved from left to right behind the wall, and even though the tall carrot was higher than the window sill, it also disappeared until it reached the right side of the wall. In real life, any object taller than the lowest boundary of the window would be visible when it moved by the window, so what the subjects saw in this second event was not possible, not realistic. Although it seems incredible, subjects as young as three-and-a-half months habituated to the possible event and dishabituated to the impossible event, suggesting that they understood object permanence. It is reasonable to wonder why there is such an age discrepancy between what this research indicates about when the child understands object permanence and what Piaget asserted. Baillargeon, Graber, DeVos, and Black (1990) concluded that it is possible that the child understands object permanence even if he is not yet capable of implementing the means-ends strategies necessary for locating an object when it is moved out of sight. It is one thing, after all, to know that an object still exists even when it is no longer visible, and it is quite another to push aside, lift up, or reach behind whatever is hiding the object. The child might know object permanence, therefore, even if he is not yet demonstrating that knowledge in his searching or locating behaviors.

According to Piaget, when the child is in substage four of the sensorimotor period, which extends from about eight to twelve months, he begins to search for objects when they are hidden. When an object is hidden several times in different locations, however, he sometimes looks in the wrong place. At one time, there was general agreement that these searching errors reflected the child's inability to remember where an object is hidden if it is hidden in several places. Baillargeon, DeVos, and Graber (1989) offer an alternative explanation based on their finding that the child at eight months does remember the last location of an object that is hidden in several different places. That is, prior to his first birthday, the child might look in the wrong place because he has difficulty incorporating what he knows about an object's being moved from location to location into a viable searching strategy. We must remember that there are two different factors operating here: (1) Knowing that an object is permanent and that it is being moved from place to place, and (2) Developing a strategy for finding the object. Baillargeon et al. (1989) suggest that prior to twelve months, the child has a pretty good handle on *knowing* but is still struggling with *finding*.

Mental Representation: Deferred Imitation and Categorization

According to Piaget's cognitive theory, the child cannot represent experience until he is about eighteen months old. Meltzoff (1988a) has demonstrated, however, that deferred imitation occurs in children as young as nine months. In this study, nine-month-old subjects were introduced to three toys they had not seen before, three toys that could be manipulated in specific ways. They included a bendable L-shaped piece of wood, a box equipped with a button that could be depressed, and a plastic egg containing metal nuts that could be shaken like a rattle. These actions were modeled for the experimental subjects. Control subjects were introduced to the toys but did not receive the modeling exposure. When all the subjects were tested the next day, those who had observed how the toys functioned demonstrated the toys' actions much more frequently that those who did not have the benefit of modeling. The subjects who reproduced the actions modeled for them were demonstrating deferred imitation, a form of mental representation, and they exhibited this behavior almost one year earlier than Piaget suggested it should be produced. Meltzoff's findings went even further, however. He found that the child at nine months can retain several actions in memory at the same time. By the time the child is fourteen months old, according to another Meltzoff (1988b) study, he can hold in memory as many as six modeled actions over the course of a week. In view of these findings, Piaget's predictions relative to deferred imitation are much too conservative.

According to Piaget's theory of cognitive development, we do not see evidence of mental representation, including deferred imitation and categorization, until the end of the sensorimotor period. Recent evidence indicates that mental representation is probably not the end product of sensorimotor development as Piaget's theory suggests. Mandler (1992a, 1992b) believes that it is more plausible to conclude that sensorimotor schemes and symbolic schemes develop simultaneously. This view would certainly be consistent with research findings relative to categorization. Hayne, Rovee-Collier, and Perris (1987), for example, have found that infants as young as three months can categorize the physical characteristics of mobile elements, and they are able to distinguish one mobile from another based on the categories they have developed. In one of the experiments that led to this conclusion, three-month-old subjects were introduced to a mobile constructed of blocks, each of which was marked with the letter "A." The subjects discovered that they could make the mobile move by kicking the blocks. When this activity was interrupted and then resumed, the subjects would enthusiastically kick the blocks only if they were marked with the letter "A." If the mobile was changed so that each block was marked with "2," the subjects' kicking behavior was drastically reduced in frequency and vigor. The investigators concluded that during their first experiences with the mobile, when the subjects kicked the mobile to make it move, they grouped the elements of the mobile together into an "A" category, and they associated their kicking with this category. When the elements of the mobile were changed to "2," they differentiated between the "A" category and the "2" category by kicking the "A" elements and by not kicking the "2" elements. This is a rather primitive application of categorization, but there is no question that these children were exhibiting behaviors based on their abilities to mentally group and differentiate.

The same habituation-dishabituation strategy that was used in the short carrot–tall carrot study has been used in experiments designed to determine whether or not infants can categorize. Using this strategy, subjects might be shown a series of pictures of different kinds of birds. After reasonable exposure time to pictures of members of the "bird category," the subjects are shown pictures of birds along with pictures of things that clearly do not belong to this category. These might include pictures of buildings or trains. The investigators then observe the subjects to determine whether they pay greater or lesser attention to pictures of things outside the "bird category" than to pictures of birds. Using this habituation-dishabituation strategy, researchers have found that children as young as nine to twelve months habituate, or look longer, at pictures of things within the category to which they have been exposed than to pictures of objects foreign to that category. They have found that children in this age range can place things into a wide range of categories, including birds, food, and stuffed animals

(Oakes, Madole, & Cohen, 1991; Roberts, 1988; Sherman, 1985). By the time children are just eighteen months old, they can categorize objects into two classes (Gopnik & Meltzoff, 1987). This means that an eighteen-month-old child, given a mixture of blocks and dolls, has the ability not just to know that there is "block category" and a "doll category," but to physically group all the blocks together and all the dolls together. All of these mental representation abilities are manifested at ages far earlier than Piaget predicted, suggesting to those who question Piaget's theory that the emergence of these abilities cannot be explained solely within the context of sensorimotor development.

What Does All This Suggest about the Sensorimotor Stage?

The findings of current research on the cognitive abilities of young children make it impossible to escape the conclusion that many essential and basic cognitive abilities, at least in preliminary form, are exhibited by children considerably earlier than Piaget predicted. To some, this might seem grounds enough to dismiss Piaget's theory, but we should react cautiously to the apparent contradictions between what Piaget proposed theoretically and what researchers have found in actual behavior. Berk (1994, p. 231) notes, for example, that "when these (cognitive) capacities first appear, they may not be secure enough to make a large difference in the baby's understanding of the world or to serve as the foundation for new knowledge." It is also important to affirm, as Berk and others have affirmed, that the general developmental timeline established by Piaget's sensorimotor stage holds in terms of when many basic cognitive abilities are fully emerged even if Piaget did not accurately predict the earliest manifestations of these abilities.

The most significant differences between what Piaget proposed and what researchers have found center on the emergence of specific cognitive abilities, such as object permanence, and on how early cognitive development takes place. That is, some cognitive abilities do emerge earlier than Piaget asserted. These include the abilities we have highlighted in this discussion, object permanence and mental representation. A more important gap between the theory and current research focuses on **how** this development occurs. Piaget believed that in this first stage of cognitive development, the acquisition of all knowledge is facilitated by the child's sensorimotor experiences. Even those who have serious reservations about Piaget's theory concede that some of the child's knowledge in these early months of life is established by motor and sensory contact with his environment. These same people suggest, however, that some of the child's cognitive abilities, including object permanence and the ability to imitate, may be genetically determined, and that other abilities may be products of innate perceptual processing of auditory and visual information. That is, some of the knowledge the child demonstrates during the first year, and even the first half year, of his life comes through watching and listening, not through direct physical contact with the things in his world.

Some critics believe that recent research findings suggest that cognitive development does not progress in the fairly rigid, step-by-step manner implied by Piaget's stages. According to Piaget's theory, a range of cognitive abilities develop together within each substage of the sensorimotor period, and they undergo comparable changes within each succeeding stage. The research evidence suggests that the specific cognitive abilities of a given child might be at different levels of maturity at the same time, and that when there is a change in one ability, there will not necessarily be a directly correlated change in another. Cognitive development, these critics argue, is variable because it depends on biological maturation interacting with environmental experiences. The most extreme of these critics believe we should completely dismiss the notion of stages in our understanding of cognitive development. They believe that the bases of cognitive abilities are constant at all ages and that, over time, each child gradually figures out how to apply each ability to the completion of thought-related tasks (Gelman & Baillargeon, 1983). Others take a more moderate view. They believe that Piaget's stage concept, with appropriate modifications, remains viable. Flavell (1985), for example, has difficulty accepting the idea that cognition and its development is as widely variable as some have suggested. He believes that the varying cognitive abilities all theorists and researchers recognize in developing children must somehow be tied together in a coherent manner. These connections among cognitive abilities, in combination with maturational changes, suggest to Flavell that there must be some stage foundation to cognitive development.

So, where does this leave us? There is little doubt, even among the most ardent critics of Piaget's theory, that Piaget has appropriately identified the cognitive abilities the child acquires, and there is consensus that Piaget's general timeframe for the maturity of cognitive abilities is, for the most part, on target. It is clear that some of Piaget's estimates about when certain cognitive abilities first appear were not correct. Children show the first signs of certain cognitive abilities much earlier than Piaget predicted. It also seems fair to conclude, based on recent research evidence, that early knowledge is not the product of sensorimotor experience only, that some cognitive abilities may be genetically predetermined, and that others may be influenced at least as much by innate perceptual abilities and experiences as by direct environmental contact. On the issue of stages, there is still legitimate debate. It would not be unreasonable to assume, however, that when the dust from this particular battle settles, we will have concluded that some semblance of a stage model is still useful in understanding cognitive development, even though any future stage model will almost certainly accommodate wide individual variations.

The Sensorimotor Stage and Language: A Summary

In closing this section on Piaget's theory of cognitive development, it will be useful to return to our primary focus, language. Even though, as we noted earlier,

Piaget did not specifically theorize about language development, he and others who have endorsed his theory have related aspects of cognitive development, as Piaget has described it, to language. What follows, in Table 3-2, is a brief summary of key aspects of cognitive development that are related, or appear to be related, to language development. In processing this information, the reader should keep in mind that *relationship* does not necessarily mean *cause-effect*. In fact, most of the research data do not suggest that the connections between cognitive and language factors are more than correlational relationships. Nevertheless, it is intriguing to think about what these relationships might mean relative to both cognitive and language functions.

Vygotsky's Theory of Cognitive Development: A Sociocultural Perspective

The question we posed at the beginning of this chapter has significant relevance in relation to Vygotsky's theory of cognitive development: *Does thought shape language or does language shape thought?* Hold that question in mind as this section unfolds, and try to determine how Lev Vygotsky would answer it.

Like Piaget, Vygotsky believed that the child is an active agent in his quest for knowledge. Beyond this general agreement, however, there is a striking difference in the views of the two men. While Piaget believed that the child operates independently, especially during the early stages of cognitive development, Vygotsky was convinced that the child's cognitive development is heavily influenced by his environment and by his culture from the very beginning of knowledge acquisition. In fact, Vygotsky believed that the developing child interacts with his environment in order to develop cognitive abilities that will allow him to adapt to his culture. In other words, during the course of intellectual development, there is a synergistic relationship between what the child brings to the cognitive table in terms of innate abilities and self-directed exploration and what his environment and culture bring to the table.

Vygotsky's views about cognitive development were not merely the result of academic musing, but were forged in his own life experiences. We will best understand the theory, therefore, if we take a brief look at the man. In an interesting coincidence, the two men who have exercised the most profound influences on our understanding of cognitive development, Jean Piaget and Lev Vygotsky, were born in the same year, 1896. Tragically, Vygotsky's life was cut short at 37 years by tuberculosis. The brief professional life he had was exceptionally productive, but he did not have the same long-term opportunity for reflection that Piaget had. For that reason, his theory is not as fully developed and not as detailed as Piaget's theory.

Vygotsky's own boyhood experiences related to learning shaped his views of cognitive development. As a youngster, he did not attend a formal school. He was taught at home by a tutor who believed that education involves more than simply

TABLE 3-2 Sensorimotor and Language Events: A Summary

Sensorimotor Concept/Behavior	Language Behavior
Object Permanence	1. Object permanence appears to be related to early semantic functions, including nonexistence, disappearance, and recurrence. 2. Brown (1973) suggests that the understanding of object permanence reflected in substage four may be adequate for the acquisition of the child's first productive words.
Causality	1. An understanding of causality is a cognitive prerequisite for communication (Bates & Snyder, 1987; Greenwald & Leonard, 1979; Snyder, 1978). 2. There appears to be a significant relationship between causality and the child's ability to understand verbs and semantic relations (Miller, Chapman, Branston, & Reichle, 1980).
Means-Ends	1. An understanding of means-ends is critical to language development. 2. There is a significant correlation between an understanding of mean-ends and language development during the early portion of substage four (Bates et al., 1975; Bates, Benigni, Bretherton, Camaioni, & Volterra, 1977; Bates et al., 1979). This cognitive ability is particularly important to the development of communicative intentionality. 3. The understanding of means-ends reflected in substage six appears to be significantly related to the emergence of two-word utterances (Zachary, 1978).
Imitation	1. Imitation is significantly correlated with gestural development at nine to 10 months. 2. Deferred imitation is significantly correlated with naming and with recognitory gestures (i.e., gestures that represent the functions or uses of objects) (Bates & Snyder, 1987). 3. When the child produces deferred imitation, we can assume that he has a true understanding of symbolic function because in deferred imitation, the referent for the imitation need not be present.
Play	1. There is a significant correlation between object play and language at 10 to 13 months (Bates et al., 1979; James, 1980). 2. Children who show a propensity for using a variety of schemes for objects in their early play experiences tend to progress more dramatically in language development than children who are more limited in their use of object schemes (Bates et al., 1975; Greenwald & Leonard, 1979; Sugarman, 1978). 3. A child will produce meaningful words as symbols for people, things, and events before he has demonstrated complete competence in symbolic play.

filling an empty intellectual vessel. The tutor challenged the young Russian boy to be fully engaged in the process of learning, to answer questions, pose questions, process answers, to think about how one piece of knowledge is integrated with established knowledge, to consider how one question leads to another. His was a truly interactive learning experience, and he came away from this personal experience believing that knowledge acquisition and intellectual development must necessarily proceed in this interactive manner. Vygotsky's later educational experiences resulted in another critical difference between his views about cognitive development and Piaget's. Piaget, you will recall, did not give language any unique status in the process of cognitive development. He viewed language as simply one of a number of symbolic abilities the child acquires over the course of intellectual development. Vygotsky always viewed language as a key player in cognitive development, a perspective that was undoubtedly enhanced by his academic interest in literature, his major field of study at the University of Moscow. It is not surprising that when he shifted his attention to the study of cognitive development, he retained a focus on language.

One might well ask why there is so much interest in Vygotsky's views about cognitive development today. After all, this man's views about cognition were published more than 50 years ago. According to Wertsch and Tulviste (1992), the present interest in Vygotsky's theory can be traced to his belief that the child is not an independently operating agent, that the child's cognitive development is the product of an interaction between the child's innate abilities and his social experiences. It is noteworthy that Vygotsky's view of intellectual development is generally consonant with the dominant view of language development today, the social interactionist view. The marriage between a sociocultural view of cognition and a social interactionist view of language is a natural and eminently logical phenomenon.

Even though some people might be tempted to park Vygotsky at the nurture end of the nature-versus-nurture continuum, that would be an oversimplification of his views about development. Vygotsky begins, in fact, with a nature base. He believes that human children are born with fundamental cognitive and perceptual abilities, including capacities for memory and for attending, abilities that human beings share with other animals. During the first two years of the human child's life, these abilities develop and mature according to a mostly biological calendar, and as a result of the child's primitive contacts with his environment. The nature of cognitive development changes radically, however, as soon as the child can mentally represent the environmental phenomena he is experiencing. This mental representation includes, as a primary component, language. At this point, armed with naturally developing cognitive and perceptual abilities and with emerging language skills, the child is able to engage in the social dialogues that are so inextricably connected to cultural activities. The groundwork is now laid for the component of Vygotsky's theory of cognitive development most closely associated with his name, *private speech*. When the young child begins to talk to himself, he crosses an important threshold in his cognitive development.

From this point forward, and as a direct result of the power of language, the child's mental abilities will be shaped into the higher-order cognitive processes of an intelligence that clearly separates human beings from animals with lesser cognitive capacities. That is, the child uses language to direct his actions and to learn how to get things done (Wertsch & Tulviste, 1992).

Before we take a closer look at private speech and other critical elements of Vygotsky's theory, there is another basic difference between Piaget and Vygotsky that must be stressed. Piaget, as we have noted at a number of junctures in this chapter, believed that cognitive development proceeds in a predictable stage-by-stage manner. Vygotsky's view was that cognitive development does not proceed through exactly the same progressive sequence for all children. He argued that while each child experiences progressive changes in the way he thinks and behaves as a cognitive creature, the progression is continuous rather than stage-by-stage. More importantly, each child's cognitive development is shaped by the influences of the important adults and peers in his social environment and by the experiences unique to his culture. While Vygotsky and Piaget would agree that there are systematic changes in cognitive development, Vygotsky would argue that these systematic changes vary widely across cultures because the nature of social interactions between children and the important people in their lives vary widely by culture. The tasks around which learning occurs differ from culture to culture. In some cultures, for example, girls are expected to perform domestic tasks at a young age. In other cultures, boys are expected to learn how to hunt and fish. In our culture, children are free of these kinds of responsibilities and are encouraged to play and "have fun." It is not difficult to imagine significant differences in the kinds of interactions that will occur between adults and children in each of these cultural situations. If little girls are expected to perform domestic tasks at an early age, they will be taught these skills by their primary caregivers and other significant adults. These lessons will involve communicative exchanges unique to the tasks being taught. Learning the skills inherent to the tasks will involve unique problem-solving challenges. Little boys who must learn how to hunt, fish, and forage will have radically different interactions with their caregivers than little boys whose caregivers teach them how to play baseball and fly kites. Children who live in cultures that place a premium on written language will face different cognitive challenges and will experience different social and communicative interactions with their significant others than children who live in cultures that depend mostly or solely on spoken language. A list of possible major cultural differences that might affect the way children acquire knowledge relative to cultural expectations and to the social/communicative interactions that facilitate the acquisition of knowledge would be impressive in its length and breadth. Vygotsky's point is that cognitive development does not occur in isolation, but is a function of a person's social and cultural environment. That there are cross-cultural differences in the nature of social/communicative exchanges between young children and adults has been demonstrated by research that lends support to Vygotsky's argument (Bakeman, Adamson, Konner, & Barr, 1990; Saxe, 1988; Childs & Greenfield, 1982; Draper & Cashdan, 1988). We will now turn our attention to some of the critical elements in Vygotsky's theory, beginning with private speech.

Private Speech

Anyone who has watched young children play has heard private speech. A preschool child who is trying to construct a building out of blocks might say to himself, "This piece is too big. It sticks out. I need a smaller one." A child with a fistful of crayons and a coloring book might mutter to herself, "What color should the house be? I think I'll make it purple. No, that's not right. Houses aren't purple. It should be white. Where's the white crayon?" Yet another child, trying to put plastic pieces of varying geometric shapes into a box with holes corresponding to these shapes, might be heard to say to herself, "This one is round, so it won't fit here, but it will fit here. Whoops, it didn't fit because it's too big. I need to find the small round one. There it is!"

What is all this self-talking about? The answer to that question depends on the expert to whom it is addressed. Piaget referred to this self-directed talk as *egocentric speech,* which he believed is nonsocial and relatively purposeless. It is speech produced by the individual child for the individual child who cannot mentally represent the viewpoints of other people. Based on what we have already established about Vygotsky's theory, you would expect a very different response from his perspective, and your expectation will be realized. Vygotsky (1986) believed that when children speak to themselves, they are guiding themselves through their actions. Especially early in their lives, children use self-directed speech, or private speech, to literally help themselves think through problems and tasks, to help themselves choose actions that are most appropriate to doing whatever it is they are trying to do. Private speech is a first step toward more elaborate cognitive skills. It helps the child learn how to pay attention, how to memorize and recall bits of information from memory, how to formulate and execute plans in solving problems, and in a very real sense, how to think, ponder, or muse. As the child gets older, the nature of self-directed talking changes. In the beginning, the child talks out loud. As he gets older, he might whisper or mutter under his breath. Eventually, his private speech will be truly private. It will be silent and internalized. In short, it will become exactly the kind of private speech you use every day to think through your problems, to choose plans of actions for solving your problems, to reflect on the meaning of life and the futility of the Chicago Cubs.

The weight of the research evidence relative to self-directed talking comes down heavily on the side of Vygotsky. For that reason, most people who refer to self-directed talking today refer to it as *private speech* and no longer as *egocentric speech.* The most telling evidence supporting Vygotsky's view about private speech shows that children are more likely to talk to themselves when they are engaged in difficult tasks, when they are struggling with tasks and making mistakes, or when they are unsure about what they should do next (Berk, 1992). The research also confirms that Vygotsky was correct about the changes that occur to private speech as children mature. That is, it becomes less overt and more private until it becomes essentially speech in thought form (Berk & Landau, 1993; Frauenglass & Diaz, 1985). From a cognitive development point of view, Vygotsky's most crucial assertion is that private speech provides a foundation for higher-order cognitive functions. Research findings appear to confirm this assertion as well. Studies conducted by Bivens and Berk (1990) and Behrend, Rosengren, and Perlmutter (1992) demonstrate that children who are uninhibited self-talkers when they are confronted with challenging tasks are more attentive, more fully engaged, and more likely to complete tasks successfully than children who are more reticent self-talkers.

Social Keys to Cognitive Development

Keep in mind that Vygotsky believed that the establishment of higher-order cognitive functions begins in the child's social interactions with the important people in his environment, interactions that reflect the culture of which he is a member. This means that, from Vygotsky's point of view, we cannot talk about cognitive development without taking these social interactions into account. The child learns how to do things, and he learns how to process his thoughts in ways that appropriately reflect the culture in which he lives by interacting with adults who already know how things should be done and how to think in ways that are culturally acceptable. The child might be able to handle some tasks with which he is confronted without any direct intervention or assistance. That is, he will figure some things out, just as Piaget suggested, by independent discovery. There are many other tasks, however, that the child cannot manage on his own. He needs help from people who have greater knowledge, experience, and skill than he possesses. These tasks fall into what is called the *zone of proximal development.* Within this zone are those tasks with which the child needs help, and the help typically comes in the form of language. As a child and adult work together to learn a skill or solve a task problem, they talk to one another. The child retains language from these exchanges that he incorporates into his private speech. At some later time, he will use his private speech, now enhanced by the language he has garnered from these dialogues, to solve problems on his own.

If he had lived longer and continued to revise and elaborate his theory, Vygotsky would have probably tried to identify the features of adult–child dialogues that would most effectively facilitate the development of the child's cognitive abilities. In the absence of direction from Vygotsky himself on this subject, researchers have identified at least two attributes of these dialogues they believe are crucial in transferring the adult's cognitive competence to the child's cognitive development. The first of these attributes is *intersubjectivity*. An interaction is characterized by intersubjectivity if two people working together on a common task with different levels of understanding about how the task can or should be accomplished manage to merge what they know into a shared understanding as the task is completed. In this kind of interaction, each partner accommodates the viewpoint and competence of the other partner. An adult-to-adult dialogue characterized by intersubjectivity might include comments such as these: "What I hear you saying is . . ." or "I think I understand what you are saying . . . , but have you considered . . .?" Each adult partner tries to understand the other partner's perspective, tries to gauge the other partner's knowledge base, tries to take from that knowledge base what he does not understand, and tries to impart knowledge he has that his partner might lack. In this kind of dialogue there is mutual respect and a shared determination to solve a problem for which the partners feel a united ownership. In an interaction shared by an adult and a child, the adult will convey what she knows to the child in a manner that fits what the child already knows and that does not exceed the child's ability to understand. You will recognize that this is exactly what occurs in any good teaching–learning situation even when the teacher and learner are both adults. That is, the teacher conveys her knowledge to the student by drawing upon what the student already knows, by taking into account the student's abilities to understand, and by challenging the student to expand his own knowledge. In an interaction characterized by intersubjectivity, therefore, the child is challenged by the adult's dialogue and demonstrations to extend his understanding so that he develops a more mature, adult-like, strategy for completing the targeted task (Rogoff, 1990).

The second attribute that characterizes facilitating dialogues is *scaffolding* (Bruner, 1983; Wood, 1989). In order to understand this feature of dialogues, we should first consider the literal meaning of the word *scaffold* and consider how scaffolds are used in real life. According to the dictionary tool in my trusty Encarta '95 computerized encyclopedia, *scaffold* is defined as *a temporary platform on which workers perform tasks at heights above the ground.* We have all seen painters and window washers on scaffolds. At one time, scaffolds were no more than planks of wood attached to ropes. Today they are more sturdy mechanisms made of steel and protected by back-up safety systems to guard against mechanical failures, but the general idea of a scaffold has not changed. When the window washer completes the windows on the third floor of a building, the scaffold is raised to the fourth floor, and it continues to be raised until all the windows on all the floors are squeaky clean. How does scaffolding relate to cognitive development and to the dialogues and interactions that facilitate cognitive development? Just as a real-life scaffold is adjusted to the height necessary for the completion of a task such as washing windows, an adult can provide scaffolds for the child when he is trying to reach new heights of cognitive competence. If the child has little idea about how to accomplish a targeted task, the adult will set the scaffold low in the sense that she provides direct instruction. At this level, the adult might try to segment the task into

smaller tasks, building upon what the child does know and can do, and then helping him master the next level, and then the next, until he can compete the whole
task. When we teach children to write, for example, we do not expect the child to
move from no writing skill to adult mastery in one step. We begin by asking the
child to draw vertical lines, horizontal lines, and circles, skills he already has or
that he can easily master. We scaffold the skills upward from the easiest and most
basic of drawing skills to increasingly more elaborate writing skills until the child
is actually producing written letters. As the child's cognitive competence increases,
his need for direct support decreases. The adult who is a skillful scaffolder will
gradually withdraw cognitive supports as the child gradually demonstrates less
need for them, but the same sensitive scaffolder will be prepared to introduce the
supports again if the child's independent efforts are producing more frustration
and failure than success. The general rule in effective scaffolding, therefore, is to
adjust support so that it meets the changing cognitive needs of the child. Does
effective scaffolding make a difference? There is research evidence that indicates
it does. In studies focusing on the possible benefits of this strategy, some mothers used scaffolding more effectively than others in the process of teaching their
children how to solve a particularly difficult puzzle. The children of the more
effective scaffolders used more private speech and were more successful in independently solving a similar puzzle than the children of mothers who were less
skillful in the use of scaffolding (Behrend, Rosengren, & Perlmutter, 1992; Berk &
Spuhl, 1992.)

   During his tragically brief life, Vygotsky gave us much to think about relative
to cognition, cognitive development, and the synergistic relationship between cognition and language. Researchers continue to test the principles and concepts of his
theory, and so far at least, his view that cognitive development occurs within the
larger context of social and cultural experiences, and his view that language directs
cognition as much as cognition directs language are holding up well to empirical
scrutiny.

The Perceptual Groundwork for Communication

Before we proceed to a detailed description of speech and language development
in the next three chapters, we must more fully address the perceptual preparation
for communication, a topic briefly introduced when we discussed the principle of
distancing earlier in this chapter. **Perception,** you may remember, refers to the
processes by which a person selects, organizes, integrates, and interprets the sensory stimuli he receives. Since the child must somehow make sense of the sensory
information he receives related to communication in general and speech specifically before he can create his own communicative output, we should know something about what he receives and what catches his attention during the preparation
period. What follows then is a brief summary of what we believe are the child's
earliest perceptual abilities as they pertain to communication.

The Relationship Between Cognition and Perception

It should be fairly obvious that perception cannot be completely separated from cognition. To understand, think, solve problems, and engage in all other activities associated with cognition, I must be able to sort through the stimuli my senses are receiving, recognize important stimuli, ignore unimportant ones, and then categorize, integrate, and interpret the stimuli I have selected. The further into perception I proceed, the closer to cognition I get until the line between them becomes effectively blurred to the point of virtual elimination.

Stern (1977) makes a useful distinction between **perceptual stimulation** and **cognitive stimulation.** As a result of perceptual or sensory stimulation, a child recognizes that stimuli are present, and reacts to the major characteristics of the stimuli. If they are auditory stimuli, for example, he reacts to the loudness and pitch changes of the sounds he is receiving. If they are visual, he reacts to things like size and shape. This level of perception develops early. As the child develops intellectually, he shows evidence of cognitive stimulation, which means he not only recognizes stimuli by their sensory characteristics, but he understands what they mean and how they compare to other stimuli he has received. He understands, for example, the difference between the ringing of the doorbell and the ringing of the telephone. When the doorbell rings, he runs to the door because he knows someone will be there. When the telephone rings, he picks up the receiver because he knows someone will answer. He combines his ability to make discriminations among similar and dissimilar bits of sensory information with his ability to make mental judgments about what this information means. This complex marriage of perception and cognition continues throughout the child development years and beyond. In fact, as long as a person can receive new information, process it, and think about it, the marriage thrives.

Visual Perception

You might wonder what visual perception has to do with language and especially with speech. Actually, what the child sees can be very important in the language acquisition process. Sachs (1989, p. 38) contends that visual and tactile stimuli "play a great role in establishing the bond between adult and child." This in no way minimizes the importance of auditory stimulation, but it does suggest that what the child sees helps to direct and fix his attention. Presumably, once the speaker has gained the child's attention by whatever visual or tactile stimuli are required, the child will gain more from the auditory stimuli produced by the speaker. Even though we have no proof that this connection of sensory modalities is necessary for speech development, it is probably more than coincidental that infants are interested in the kinds of visual stimuli that are characteristic of early child-adult interactions.

Vision is the first sensory system the child controls (Tiegerman, 1989). Within hours after birth, the infant can follow movement visually (Greenman, 1963), and is able to focus on a target 7½ inches removed, the distance at which vision achieves its optimal focus (Owens, 1996, p. 160). This is potentially significant because when the child is being fed, his mother's eyes are almost exactly 8 inches away, and his mother watches him almost constantly during feeding (Stern, 1977) while he returns the visual favor. It is tempting to conclude, as some observers have, that the child is genetically preprogrammed for this visual coupling which, it is further assumed, leads to bonding between the child and mother.

By the time the child is three months old, he can control eye movements sufficiently to determine the visual information he chooses to receive. He looks at things and people he finds interesting, and he turns away when he is no longer interested. The infant prefers objects of contrasting colors, and he likes things that move (Haith, 1976). He is attracted to objects with designs of varying angles and curves, and visually complex objects that reflect light variably (Fantz, 1964; Freedman, 1964; Haaf & Bell, 1967). What makes this fascinating is that the infant shows strong interest in the human face, an object that meets all these criteria for preference and interest. The face can consist of many colors when you include all the parts: hair, eyes, eyebrows, lashes, lips, and cheeks. The face is capable of almost infinite movement, and has many angles and curves that reflect and shade light. Again, it is tempting to conclude that the child is born with visual interests that perfectly match the facial characteristics of his primary object of attention and affection, his caregiver.

Much attention has been paid by researchers and theorists to the child's interest in the human face in general, his caregiver's face in particular, and to the eye contact or gaze between child and caregiver. There has been much speculation about what all this might suggest about bonding the child-caregiver relationship. Certainly no one questions the newborn's preoccupation with looking at his caregiver's face. So fixed is he on looking at the caregiver's face in the first few weeks of his life that it is difficult to direct his visual attention anywhere else. By the time he is just two weeks old, he may be able to distinguish, on the basis of face and voice, his caregiver from other people (Bower, 1977). When he is three weeks old, he will respond to his caregiver's face and other human faces by smiling (Trevarthen, 1979). By the time he is three months old, the infant and his caregiver exchange gazes in a manner that suggests adult-like conversational turn-taking (Jaffe, Stern, & Perry, 1973). At the very least, this is intriguing stuff. At most, contingent on more research that would allow for more confident conclusions, it might suggest that the child is genetically tuned to certain visual stimuli that are important in capturing his attention and in helping to establish a communicative relationship with his caregiver, a relationship many social interactionist theorists believe is important, if not vital, to normal communication development.

Auditory Perception

Just as the child seems to have a special interest in the visual characteristics of the human face, he seems to be especially attracted to the human voice and speech.

It is important to establish, however, that there are characteristics of sounds in general that appeal to the infant, characteristics found in human speech. This could mean that the child is interested in these characteristics because he is born with speech perceptual abilities and finds these sound characteristics interesting whether they occur in speech or nonspeech sounds. It could mean that the child is born with an auditory system designed to make discriminations among sounds we believe he finds interesting and is not designed to make discriminations among sounds we assume he is ignoring. It could, of course, be only coincidental that the child reacts to sound features that happen to be characteristic of human speech. Much more research needs to be conducted before we know *why* the child reacts as he does to specified features of sound. In the meantime, we can account for at least some of *what* he seems to find appealing in the sounds he hears.

It would seem important to first assess the very young infant's ability to determine the direction from which a sound is coming. An early study by Wertheimer (1961) indicated that a child just after birth moved his eyes in the direction of clicking sounds, but other studies since have not confirmed this finding. A more reasonable suggestion of the localization of sound in young infants is turning the head, a behavior studied by Muir and Field (1979). Using headturning as a criterion for localizing sound, they found that infants ranging in age from two to seven days turned in the direction of a rattling noise about three-fourths of the time. This consistency allows us to conclude that newborns can determine at least the general direction of sound sources.

From the time the child is born, perhaps even while he is still in the uterus, he can make many kinds of auditory discriminations. Some newborn children, for example, can discriminate between a pure tone at 400 Hz and another at 1000 Hz (Bridger, 1961), and there is evidence that they seem to make their best discriminations among frequencies characteristic of human speech (Eisenberg, 1976).

The newborn can make gross discriminations about the loudness levels of sounds. When he listens to white noise (a mixture of a wide range of frequencies) that is varied in loudness, there are noticeable changes in heart rate and in the startle reflex (Bench, 1969). Similar changes in behavior occur when the child hears pure tones varied by loudness (Bartoshuk, 1964).

Although it is important to remind the reader that we are dealing with only the broadest judgments of differences, there is some evidence that infants respond differentially to sounds of varying durations (Clifton, Graham, & Hatton, 1968; Ling, 1972). In reference to the Ling study, Reich (1986, p. 15) cautions that it "does not demonstrate that the infant can detect these differences, only that it reacts more to signals of longer duration." At the least, this research indicates that infants are aware of when sounds begin and end and how long they are sustained, and it is probable that infants are able to make some discriminations concerning durations.

An Early Interest in the Human Voice and Speech

One of the most exciting general findings of the research related to the early perceptual abilities of children is that infants show a greater interest in human speech than other noises (Eisenberg, 1976; Jensen, Williams, & Bzoch, 1975). There is evidence that a child may prefer the acoustic characteristics of a speech passage his mother recited while she was pregnant over the acoustic characteristics of something she did not read (DeCasper & Spence, 1986), and there is evidence that a child as young as three days recognizes his mother's voice and discriminates it from the voices of other mothers (DeCasper & Fifer, 1980). All of this can be interpreted to mean that, just as a child is born with basic biological abilities to produce speech and language, he is born with biological perceptual abilities to receive and interpret speech and language. Whether or not a conclusion as sweeping as this is warranted, we can conclude that a newborn infant is able to distinguish between speech and nonspeech sounds, that he seems to prefer speech, that he recognizes his mother's voice very early, and that he seems to be aware of differences between sounds to which he was exposed while in the uterus and sounds to which he was not exposed. These are significant perceptual abilities.

As impressive as the infant's general speech discrimination are, it is perhaps even more impressive that as early as one month, he can discriminate among speech sounds. One of the methods used to assess this ability in infants is known as non-nutritive sucking or high amplitude sucking and was developed at Brown University (Eimas, Siqueland, Jusczyk, & Vigorito, 1971). In this procedure, the infant sucks on a specially designed pacifier connected to a sound generator. When he sucks on the pacifier with enough vigor, he hears a predetermined sound. Since the only thing that changes in this exercise is the sound produced by the sucking, it is reasonable to assume that, if the infant does not recognize the difference between the first sound and the second, there will be no change in the rate of sucking, but this is not what happens. When Eimas et al. (1971) presented "ba," the one-month-old infant sucked vigorously and quickly, but after a few minutes lost interest and decreased the rate of sucking. When a new sound, "pa," was introduced, he increased the rate of sucking. A number of studies reviewed by Aslin, Pisoni, and Jusczyk (1983) have shown the same reaction with a variety of speech sounds.

Since this ability is demonstrated at such a young age, it appears to be an innate ability rather than environmental. In an attempt to answer this particular nature-nurture question, Trehub (1976) tested the ability of Canadian infants and English-speaking adults to discriminate between two Czechoslovakian sounds. Although the infants discriminated between the Czech sounds as well as between English sounds like "p" and "b," the adults had great difficulty with the Czech sounds. Trehub concluded that children are born with the ability to discriminate among sounds found in all languages. As speakers become more immersed in their own languages, they lose some of this discriminative ability.

Taking the question to the next logical level, Werker and Tees (1984) tried to determine how quickly the infant loses this open-ended ability to discriminate speech sounds. They presented non-English sounds to English-speaking children ranging in age from six months to twelve months. Infants between six and eight months had little difficulty making the necessary discriminations. Those between eight and ten months had more difficulty, and those between ten and twelve months had the most difficulty. It appears then that the ability to discriminate a wide range of sounds representing many languages declines early in the child's life. Werker and Tees suggest that it is probably not coincidental that the child's discrimination abilities become more narrow as he is acquiring his own sound system and language. Environment does play a role in shaping discrimination abilities, therefore, but rather than expanding these abilities, the child's environmental experiences make his discriminations more selective, more consistent with the speech sounds native to his language.

I'm Ready! Let's Talk!

There is much we still do not know about the child's preparation for language, but it should be obvious that the child does not just sit in his crib waiting for that thrilling moment when he begins to speak. From the time the child is born, even before he is born, he is receiving sensory information about his world. From the moment of his birth, he processes all of this data in attempts to understand the nature of objects, people, and sounds. From the earliest moments of his life, he can make distinctions among things he sees and things he hears, and many of these distinctions seem to be relevant to his future social and communicative development. Over the first two years of his life, he progresses from an almost completely reflexive and sensory creature to a person who is able to think and solve problems. He progresses from an intellectual view of the world that is strictly *reality-based* and hands on to a view that allows for *mental representation* of all that is real and even some that is not. When the child is able to capture the world in his brain and in his thought processes, when he is able to transform things, people, places, events, and actions into abstract, representational forms, he is ready for language. Readiness does not come in one magic moment, of course, and language does not spill out of the child in a complete package. Language, like the cognitive and perceptual abilities upon which it is based, emerges in a progressive manner, in steps and stages that are as interlocking and integrated as are the stages of cognitive development. Even in this chapter, which has focused on the preparation for speech and language, we have seen substantial evidence of communicative ability and output. In the next three chapters we will look more closely at speech and language development, a progression that amounts to an explosion in the preschool years, but slows down and becomes more evolutionary in nature as the child moves toward adolescence.

If this were a roller coaster, we would just now be at the top of the highest crest getting ready for a wild and woolly ride. Hold on! It's getting exciting now!

Review Questions

1. What does common sense suggest about the relationship between language and thought?

2. Define and provide examples for the following concepts included in Piaget's theory of cognitive development: schema, assimilation, accommodation, and equilibrium.

3. Identify and briefly describe each of Piaget's four stages of intellectual development from birth through adolescence.

4. What is the principle of distancing? What does this principle contribute to our understanding of cognitive and language development?

5. Define each of the following key concepts and behaviors as the primary players in the sensorimotor stage of cognitive development: object permanence, causality, means-ends, imitation, play, and communication.

6. There are six substages in Piaget's sensorimotor stage of intellectual development. Identify what you believe are the most important developmental changes in each substage, and justify your selections.

7. How are the cognitive theories of Piaget and Vygotsky similar? What are their major differences?

8. What does recent research suggest about Piaget's predictions regarding the emergence of *object permanence?* Why is there such a disparity between what Piaget predicted and what empirical evidence seems to suggest about the emergence of this cognitive ability?

9. What does the evidence suggesting that *mental representation* occurs earlier than Piaget predicted suggest about the explanation of early cognitive abilities solely within the context of sensorimotor experiences?

10. Why do some critics of Piaget's theory believe that the stage concept of cognitive development is no longer viable? Why do others believe that the stage concept, in some form, still has value in understanding how intellectual development occurs?

11. How did Vygotsky's own life experiences shape his views about cognitive development?

12. Why is Vygotsky's theory referred to as a *sociocultural* theory of cognitive development?

13. Differentiate Vygotsky's *private speech* from Piaget's *egocentric speech.* Why is *private speech* the preferred label for self-directed talk today?

14. What is meant by the *zone of proximal development?*

15. Identify and describe the two attributes of adult–child dialogues that presumably facilitate cognitive development.

16. How are cognition and perception related to one another?

17. How is visual perception related to speech and language development?

18. What auditory perceptual abilities does the newborn child have that seem to be related to early communication development?

19. Summarize what is known about the infant's interest in the human voice and speech.

References and Suggested Readings

Anisfeld, M. (1984). *Language development from birth to three.* Hillsdale, NJ: Erlbaum.

Aslin, R., Pisoni, D., & Jusczyk, P. (1983). Auditory development and speech perception in infancy. In M. Haith & J. Campos (Eds.), *Handbook of child psychology: Vol. 2. Infancy and developmental psychobiology.* New York: Wiley.

Baillargeon, R. (1987). Object permanence in 3.5- and 4.5-month-old infants. *Developmental Psychology, 23,* 655–644.

Baillargeon, R., DeVos, J., & Graber, M. (1989). Location memory in 8-month-old infants in a non-search AB task: Further evidence. *Cognitive Development, 4,* 345–367.

Baillargeon, R., Graber, M., DeVos, J., & Black, J. (1990). Why do young infants fail to search for hidden objects? *Cognition, 36,* 255–284.

Baillargeon, R., & DeVos, J. (1991). Object permanence in young infants: Further evidence. *Child Development, 62,* 1227–1246.

Bakeman, R., Adamson, L. B., Konner, M., & Barr, R. G. (1990). !Kung infancy: The social context of object exploration. *Child Development, 61,* 794–809.

Bartoshuk, A. (1964). Human neonatal cardiac responses to sound: A power function. *Psychodynamic Science, 1,* 151–152.

Bates, E., Benigni, L., Bretherton, I., Camaioni, L., & Volterra, V. (1977). From gesture to the first word: On cognitive and social prerequisites. In M. Lewis & L. Rosenblum (Eds.), *Interaction, conversation, and the development of language.* New York: Wiley.

Bates, E., Benigni, L., Bretherton, I., Camaioni, L., & Volterra, V. (1979). *The emergence of symbols: Cognition and communication in infancy.* New York: Academic Press.

Bates, E., Bretherton, I., Snyder, L., Shore, C., & Volterra, V. (1980). Vocal and gestural symbols at 13 months. *Merrill-Palmer Quarterly, 26,* 407–423.

Bates, E., Camaioni, L., & Volterra, V. (1975). The acquisition of performatives prior to speech. *Merrill-Palmer Quarterly, 21,* 205–224.

Bates, E., & Snyder, L., (1987). The cognitive hypothesis in language development. In I. Uzgiris & J. Hunt (Eds.), *Infant performance and experience: New findings with the ordinal scale.* Urbana, IL: University of Illinois Press.

Behrend, D. A., Rosengren, K. S., & Perlmutter, M. (1992). The relation between private speech and parental interactive style. In R. M. Diaz & L. E. Berk (Eds.), *Private speech: From social interaction to self-regulation.* Hillsdale, NJ: Erlbaum.

Bench, J. (1969). Audio-frequency and audio-intensity discrimination in the human neonate. *International Audiology, 8,* 615–625.

Berk, L. E. (1992). Children's private speech: An overview of theory and the status of research. In R. M. Diaz & L. E. Berk (Eds.), *Private speech: From social interaction to self-regulation.* Hillsdale, NJ: Erlbaum.

Berk, L. E. (1994). *Child development* (3rd ed.). Needham Heights, MA: Allyn and Bacon.

Berk, L. E., & Landau, S. (1993). Private speech of learning disabled and normally achieving children in classroom academic and laboratory contexts. *Child Development, 64,* 556–571.

Berk, L. E., & Spuhl, S. (1992). *Maternal teaching, private speech, and task performance.* Paper presented at the First International Conference on Sociocultural Research. Madrid, Spain.

Bivens, J. A., & Berk, L. E. (1990). A longitudinal study of the development of elementary school children's private speech. *Merrill-Palmer Quarterly, 36,* 443–463.

Borden, G., & Harris, K. (1984) *Speech science primer: Physiology, acoustics, and perception of speech* (2nd ed.) Baltimore: Williams and Wilkins.

Bower, T. (1977). *The perceptual world of the child.* Cambridge, MA: Harvard University Press.

Bridger, W. (1961). Sensory habituation and discrimination in the human neonate. *American Journal of Psychiatry, 117,* 991–996.

Brown, R. (1973). *A first language: The early stages.* Cambridge, MA: Harvard University Press.

Bruner, J. S. (1983). *Child's talk: Learning to use language.* Oxford: Oxford University Press.

Bryen, D. (1982). *Inquiries into child language.* Boston: Allyn & Bacon, Inc.

Childs, C. P., & Greenfield, P. M. (1982). Informal modes of learning and teaching: The case of Zinacanteco weaving. In N. Warren (Ed.), *Advances in cross-cultural psychology,* Volume 2. London: Academic Press.

Clifton, R., Graham, R., & Hatton, H. (1968). Newborn heart-rate response and response habituation as a function of stimulus duration. *Journal of Experimental Child Psychology, 6,* 265–278.

Cole, M., John-Steiner, V., Scribner, S., & Souberman (Eds.) (1978). *Mind in society: The development of higher psychological processes.* Cambridge, MA: Harvard University Press.

DeCasper, A., & Fifer, W. (1980). Of human bonding: Newborns prefer their mothers' voices. *Science, 208,* 1174–1176.

DeCasper, A., & Spence, M. (1986). Prenatal maternal speech influences newborns' perception of speech sounds. *Infant Behavior and Development, 9,* 133–150.

D'Odorico, L. (1984). Nonsegmental features in prelinguistic communications: An analysis of some types of infant cry and noncry vocalizations. *Journal of Child Language, 11,* 17–27.

Draper, P., & Cashdan, E. (1988). Technological change and child behavior among the !Kung. *Ethnology, 27,* 339–365.

Dunst, C. (1980). *Clinical and educational manual for use with the Uzgiris and Hunt scales of infant psychological development.* Baltimore: University Park Press.

Eilers, R., & Oller, K. (1983). Speech perception in infancy. In E. Lasky & J. Katz (Eds.), *Central auditory processing disorders: Problems of speech, language, and learning.* Austin, TX: Pro-Ed.

Eimas, P., Siqueland, E., Jusczyk, P., & Vigorito, J. (1971). Speech perception in infants. *Science, 171,* 303–306.

Eisenberg, R. (1976). *Auditory competence in early life: The roots of communicative-behavior.* Baltimore: University Park Press.

Fantz, R. (1964). Visual experience in infants: Decreased attention to familiar patterns relative to novel ones. *Science, 146,* 668–670.

Flavell, J. (1977). *Concept development.* Englewood Cliffs, NJ: Prentice-Hall.

Flavell, J. H. (1985). *Cognitive development* (2nd ed.). Englewood Cliffs, NJ: Prentice-Hall.

Frauenglass, M. H., & Diaz, R. M. (1985). Self-regulatory functions of children's private speech: A critical analysis of recent challenges to Vygotsky's theory. *Developmental Psychology, 21,* 357–364.

Freedman, D. (1964). Smiling in blind infants and the issue of innate vs. acquired. *Journal of Child Psychology and Psychiatry, 5,* 171–184.

Gelman, R., & Baillargeon, R. (1983). A review of some Piagetian concepts. In P. H. Mussen (Ed.), *Handbook of child psychology: Volume 3.* Cognitive development (4th ed.). New York: Wiley.

Gopnik, A., & Meltzoff, A. N. (1987). The development of categorization in the second year and its relation to other cognitive and linguistic developments. *Child Development, 58,* 1523–1531.

Greenman, G. (1963). Visual behavior of newborn infants. In A. Solnit & S. Provence (Eds.), *Modern perspectives in child development.* New York: Hallmark.

Greenwald, C., & Leonard, L. (1979). Communicative and sensorimotor development in Down's Syndrome children. *American Journal of Mental Deficiency, 84,* 296–303.

Haaf, R., & Bell, R. (1967). A facial dimension in visual discrimination by human infants. *Child Development, 38,* 893–899.

Haith, M. (1976, July). *Organization of visual behavior at birth.* Paper presented at the 21st International Congress of Psychology, Paris, France.

Hayne, H., Rovee-Collier, C. K., & Perris, E. E. (1987). Categorization and memory retrieval by three-month olds. *Child Development, 58,* 750–767.

Jaffe, J., Stern, D., & Perry, C. (1973). "Conversational" coupling of gaze behavior in prelinguistic human development. *Journal of Psycholinguistic Research, 2,* 321–330.

James, S. (1980). *Language and sensorimotor cognitive development in the young child.* Paper presented at the annual convention of the New York Speech-Language-Hearing Association.

James, S. (1990). *Normal language acquisition.* Austin, TX: Pro-Ed.

Jensen, P., Williams, W., & Bzoch, K. (1975, November). *Preference of young infants for speech vs. nonspeech stimuli.* Paper presented to the annual American Speech and Hearing Association convention, Washington, DC.

Johnston, E., & Johnston, A. (1984). *The Piagetian language nursery: An intensive group language intervention program for preschoolers.* Rockville, MD: Aspen.

Ling, D. (1972). Acoustic stimulus duration in relation to behavioral responses of newborn infants. *Journal of Speech and Hearing Research, 15,* 567–571.

Mandler, J. M. (1992a). The foundations of conceptual thought in infancy. *Cognitive Development, 7,* 273–285.

Mandler, J. M. (1992b). How to build a baby: II. Conceptual primitives. *Psychological Review, 99,* 587–604.

McCormick, L. (1990). Bases for language and communication development. In L. McCormick & R. Schiefelbusch (Eds.), *Early language intervention: An introduction* (2nd ed.). Columbus, OH: Merrill/Macmillan.

Meltzoff, A. N. (1988a). Imitation of televised models by infants. *Child Development, 59,* 1221–1229.

Meltzoff, A. N. (1988b). Infant imitation after a 1-week delay: Long-term memory for novel acts and multiple stimuli. *Developmental Psychology, 24,* 470–476.

Miller, J., Chapman, R., Branston, M., and Reichle, J. (1980). Language comprehension in sensorimotor stages 5 and 6. *Journal of Speech and Hearing Research, 4,* 1–12.

Moerk, E. (1977). *Pragmatic and semantic aspects of early language development.* Baltimore: University Park Press.

Moore, K., & Meltzoff, A. (1978). Object permanence, imitation, and language development in infancy: Toward a neo-Piagetian perspective on communicative development. In F. Minifie & L. Lloyd (Eds.), *Communicative and cognitive abilities—Early behavioral assessment.* Baltimore: University Park Press.

Muir, D., & Field, J. (1979). Newborn infants orient to sounds. *Child Development, 50,* 431–436.

Muma, J. (1978). *Language handbook.* Englewood Cliffs, NJ: Prentice-Hall.

Oakes, L. M., Madole, K. L., & Cohen, L. B. (1991). Infants' object examining: Habituation and categorization. *Cognitive Development, 6,* 377–392.

Owens, R. (1996). *Language development: An introduction,* (4th ed.). Needham, MA: Allyn and Bacon.

Piaget, J. (1952). *Origins of intelligence in children.* New York: International Universities Press.

Piaget, J. (1954). *The construction of reality in the child.* New York: Basic Books.

Piaget, J. (1963). *The origins of intelligence in children.* New York: Norton.

Reed, V. (1986). Bases of language functioning. In V. Reed (Ed.), *An introduction to children with language disorders.* New York: Macmillan Publishers.

Rees, N. (1975). Imitation and language development: Issues and clinical implications. *Journal of Speech and Hearing Disorders, 40,* 339–350.

Reich, P. (1986). *Language development.* Englewood Cliffs, NJ: Prentice-Hall.

Rice, M. (1983). Contemporary accounts of the cognitive/language relationship: Implications for speech-language clinicians. *Journal of Speech and Hearing Disorders, 48,* 347–359.

Roberts, K. (1988). Retrieval of a basic-level category in prelinguistic infants. *Developmental Psychology, 24,* 21–27.

Rogoff, B. (1990). *Apprenticeship in thinking.* New York: Oxford University Press.

Sachs, J. (1989). Communication development in infancy. In J. Berko-Gleason (Ed.), *The development of language*. Columbus, OH: Merrill/Macmillan.

Saxe, G. G. (1988). Candy selling and math learning. *Educational Researcher, 17*, 14–21.

Sherman, T. (1985). Categorization skills in infants. *Child Development, 56*, 1561–1573.

Snyder, L. (1978). Communicative and cognitive abilities and disabilities in the sensorimotor period. *Merrill-Palmer Quarterly, 24*, 161–180.

Stark, R. (1979). Prespeech segmental feature development. In P. Fletcher & M. Garman (Eds.), *Language Acquisition*. New York: Cambridge University Press.

Stern, D. (1977). *The first relationship*. Cambridge, MA: Harvard University Press.

Sugarman, S. (1978). A description of communicative development in the prelanguage child. In I. Markova (Ed.), *The social context of language*. New York: Wiley.

Tiegerman, E. (1989). The cognitive bases in language development. In D. Berstein & E. Tiegerman (Eds.), *Language and communication disorders in children* (2nd ed.). Columbus, OH: Merrill/Macmillan.

Trehub, S. (1976). The discrimination of foreign speech contrasts by infants and children. *Child Development, 47*, 466–472.

Trevarthen, C. (1979). Communication and cooperation in early infancy: A description of primary intersubjectivity. In M. Bullowa (Ed.), *Before speech*. New York: Cambridge University Press.

Vygotsky, L. (1962). *Thought and language*. Cambridge, MA: MIT Press.

Vygotsky, L. S. (1986). *Thought and language* (A. Kozuhn, Trans.). Cambridge, MA: MIT Press. (Original work published 1934).

Wadsworth, B. (1971). *Piaget's theory of cognitive development*. New York: David McKay Company.

Werker, J., & Tees, R. (1984). Cross-language speech perception: Evidence for perceptual reorganization during the first year of life. *Infant Behavior and Development, 7*, 49–64.

Wertheimer, M. (1961). Psychomotor coordination of auditory and visual space at birth. *Science, 134*, 1692.

Wertsch, J. V., & Tulviste, P. (1992). L. S. Vygotsky and contemporary developmental psychology. *Developmental Psychology, 28*, 548–557.

Westby, C. (1980). Assessment of cognitive and language abilities through play. *Language, Speech, and Hearing Services in Schools, 11*, 154–168.

Wood, D. J. (1989). Social interaction as tutoring. In M. H. Bornstein & J. S. Bruner (Eds.), *Interaction in human development*. Hillsdale, NJ: Erlbaum.

Zachary, W. (1978). Ordinality and interdependence of representation and language development in infants. *Child Development, 49*, 681–687.

In the Beginning: Communication Development from Birth to Two Years

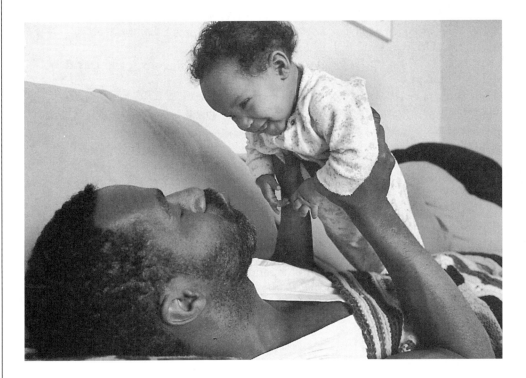

Chapter Objectives

Three chapters trace language development from birth through the school-age years. In this chapter, we consider language development from birth through two years. We emphasize that the child is a communicator from the beginning of his life, and that the changes in his communication system over the first two years are dramatic. He begins by crying, and by the time he is two years old, he has already been talking for a year. As a framework for our discussion of language acquisition in this chapter and the next, we use a stage view of development. Although we focus primarily on speech and language *production*, we also consider the vital role of *comprehension* in communication development. Specifically, this chapter is designed to facilitate understanding of the following topics:

- The *receptive* component of the infant's communication system, including the early discrimination abilities that appear to be linked in a preparatory sense to speech production.
- Infant–adult interactions that create a communication environment conducive to speech and language development.
- Speech production during infancy from first cries to first words.
- The stage concept of language acquisition, including the strengths and potential dangers in this view of human development.
- *Morphology, morphemes*, and *mean length of utterance (MLU)*.
- *Stage One* (12 to 26 months) of language development, with special attention to the classification and functions of first words, early conversational skills, and the emergence of word combinations.

- The relationship between comprehension and production in an emerging communication system.
- The role of the caregiver in Stage One of language development.

To the casual observer, the child's first year of life is fairly uneventful. It seems to be a succession of days marked by sleeping, eating, spitting up, crying, and soiling diapers. The more educated observer understands that much more is going on than this. The child comes into the world genetically programmed to become a whole person, a thinking, acting, reacting, speaking human being, and he does not wait until his first birthday to begin his growth into personhood. He is born with an enormous intellectual capacity that begins to develop immediately. He has fairly sophisticated perceptual abilities that he uses within the first hours and days of his life. Much of his first year is devoted to making contact with his world, first through his senses. He absorbs the sights, sounds, and textures of this new environment into which he has been hurled. He makes immediate connections to those people who will be most important in his early development. In the beginning, he does not understand his relationship to the people and things in his environment, but in a very real sense he *relates* to these people and things by looking at them, listening to them, by grasping them, and putting them into his mouth. The newborn child is not a mass of tissue simply waiting to be molded. During the first year of his life, he is a vital, active, exploring, thinking creature, and from the very beginning he is a **communicator**.

From the Beginning . . . the Infant Communicates

Before the child develops language, he communicates. Before he sends *intentional* messages, he communicates. As we noted in the opening chapter of this book, human beings communicate even when they do not intend to communicate. We cannot help ourselves! When the newborn infant cries, he is sending a message. It is not always a clear message, and he does not send it with any sense of purpose, but those within hearing distance receive something they perceive as a message. A listener will likely interpret this reflexive cry to mean, "I am hungry," "I am sleepy," or "I am in pain." When the child responds to stimuli with the startle reflex by kicking his legs and pumping his arms, the observer interprets the action to mean, "I'm excited," or "I'm frightened." When the child smiles, the listener senses that the child is communicating something like, "I see you. You're really special to me, and I love you." There are no boundaries when these signals, most of which are reflexive responses to specific stimuli, are interpreted by people who are anxious to connect to the child. Some adults even attach messages to noises like sucking, gurgling, and burping—"Oh, he's telling us he's hungry," or "He really enjoyed those strained peas!"

In the preceding chapter, we traced cognitive development over the first two years, and we considered the perceptual abilities the child has from the earliest days of his life. The infant uses his perceptual abilities to receive and process sensory data. As he uses this information to develop an understanding of objects, cause-effect, and means-ends, he moves closer to intentional communication. Before the first year ends, we see evidence of communicative intent. Over the next few years, the child becomes an amazingly sophisticated and effective communicator. This chapter and the next will trace the impressive progression in communicative ability and the emergence of language that characterize the child's development through the preschool years. We begin by taking a closer look at communication development during infancy.

I May Be Naked, But I Have All My Parts and They Work!

It is important to keep in mind as we trace the development of communication in general and language specifically, that the child is born with all the anatomical equipment he needs for receiving and producing speech and language. Even though growth and neuromuscular maturation must occur before these structures are used with intricate skill, the child uses all of his communication equipment from the beginning. He uses his ears to hear. He uses his larynx first to make crying noises and within just a few weeks to make sounds of pleasure as well. The adjustments he makes with his articulators during the first year are mostly random and meaningless, but within just a few months he is making vowel-like adjustments in the speech mechanism, and by the end of the first year, he is making the kinds of movements and contacts that are necessary to produce consonants. The point to be made here is that the human child is born ready to talk, and he wastes no time in preparing for that day when his communication strategy will include **language.**

Perhaps the most impressive part of the infant's communication system is the *receptive* component. He has very good hearing, and he is able to process the auditory stimuli he receives in ways that suggest a strong innate interest in speech. This is important because there seems little question that speech and language development depends on the ability to receive and process sensory data, especially auditory data. Owens (1996, p. 154) suggests that speech and language development depends on six perceptual abilities:

1. The ability to attend specifically to speech.
2. The ability to discriminate speech sounds.
3. The ability to remember a sequence of speech sounds in the correct order.
4. The ability to discriminate between sequences of speech sounds.
5. The ability to compare a sequence of speech sounds to a model that has been stored in memory.
6. The ability to make discriminations among intonational patterns.

These six abilities will provide a framework for our discussion of *speech perception*, an essential component in the process of language development. You may recognize that we have already discussed the first two of these abilities in the final section of the preceding chapter. We established that the infant can not only make gross discriminations among sounds relative to the direction of the sound source, pitch, loudness, and duration, but he seems to have a special and discriminatory interest in speech and the human voice. In addition, the child as young as one month can make discriminations among speech sounds. At first this speech sound discrimination ability is fairly open-ended. That is, the six-month-old infant can discriminate among a wide range of sounds, but by the end of his first year, his discrimination skills are already becoming more focused on the speech sounds of his native language.

Remembering a Sequence of Sounds in the Correct Order

It will be immediately obvious to anyone who listens to young children that the child does not begin to talk by producing speech sounds in isolation. From the beginning. he produces sounds in sequences. The first sequences are very simple, of course, but he does link sounds together. It would seem logical, therefore, that in processing the speech he hears, the child would need to hear not only the specific sounds in the models presented to him, but the correct order of sounds as they are sequenced.

Since this is a matter of memory as much as perception, we need to know when the infant begins to develop a memory. There is evidence that the infant as young as one month can remember an object if it reappears within 2-½ seconds, and by the time he is four months old, he can remember the object after 5 to 7 seconds (Owens, 1996, pp. 77–80). Although this may not be impressive by adult standards, it does represent the beginning of the short-term memory that is essential in processing speech.

Discriminating Between Sequences of Sounds

Imagine what it would be like to listen to speech and not know where words begin and end. What if you could not distinguish differences between sequences of sounds? It you have listened to a language you do not speak, you should be able to relate to this experience. I do not speak Japanese. When I listen to Japanese being spoken, I cannot tell which sequences of sounds are words. I cannot tell where sentences begin and end. I certainly cannot make any meaningful discriminations among the sequences of sounds I am hearing. It is reasonable to assume that the newborn child's experience with speech is very similar to this. He hears continuous strings of sounds with no idea about where the boundaries are and with no ability to make *meaningful* discriminations among strings of sounds in the sense that he associates the strings of sounds with specific people, things, events, or ideas. The ability to make this kind of discrimination must develop. When does it begin?

We have already established in the preceding chapter that the infant as young as one month can discriminate among individual speech sounds (Aslin et al., 1983; Eimas et al., 1971). There is additional evidence that by the time the infant is 6.5 months old, he can discriminate differences in strings of syllables (Goodsitt, Morse, VerHoeve, & Cowan, 1984), although there is much we do not understand about how the infant makes these discriminations. The point to be made and understood in the context of our discussion is that the infant possesses the ability to discriminate among sounds and among sequences of sounds within the first six or seven months of his life. Since words are sequences of sounds, the ability to recognize differences among strings of sounds is crucial to the acquisition of language. Since some words are identical except for one sound, it is also essential that the language-acquiring child be able to recognize differences among individual speech sounds. By nine months, the child can make distinctions among the speech sounds specific to his language in the models presented to him, and he is on the threshold of being able to produce words that reflect his understanding of speech sound differences.

Comparing Sequences of Sounds to Stored Models

By the second half of his first year, the child is beginning to understand words. Consider what this means in terms of memory and sequences of sounds. When someone produces the right sequence of sounds, like "mama," the child recognizes the sequence because it matches a combination of sounds he has stored in his memory, a combination he associates with a person or object in his environment. We need to be reminded that the sound sequence-meaning association may not be the same for the child as for an adult, but that does not minimize the significance of the association. The child at eight or nine months, for example, might understand the word "mama" to mean "any female person who hangs around the house a lot." Within the next eight or nine months, through the cognitive processes of accommodation and assimilation, he will sort out female persons into narrower and more appropriate schemata. He will recognize other sequences of sounds that are used to refer to these schemata, sequences that will be stored in his progressively more powerful memory. Notice how cognitive development, memory, and perceptual abilities interact as the child takes his first steps in language acquisition. These interactions are absolutely essential and increasingly obvious as language development accelerates.

Discriminating Intonational Patterns

Have you ever thought about how much of the meaning in the messages you send and receive depends on variables of speech like rate, rhythm, stress, and intonational patterns? Calculating an exact percentage is impossible because how much meaning is sent verbally and nonverbally depends on each utterance. In some communications, the words are of such great importance that other variables do not really matter. If a speaker is simply providing information, for example, non-verbal variables would not contribute much to the total meaning. In other situations, the word or words are almost superfluous. Imagine a situation in which I see you do something I think is a little suspicious. I look at you and say, "So?" It's difficult to imagine this scenario without imagining the intonational pattern which would be superimposed on the "So?"

Now think about how important these nonverbal variations are in communications with young children or even in communications with the family dog. If I say to my dog, "I'm going to take you outside and beat you with a stick," but say it in a manner that suggests this is going to be happy occasion, my dog will wag his tail and jump up and down in joyful anticipation. In much the same way, the infant responds more positively to speech with "happy" and "friendly" intonational patterns than to speech that sounds stern, angry, or threatening. We noted in the preceding chapter that a newborn child can discriminate among pure tones (Bridger, 1961), and he makes his best discriminations among frequencies characteristic of speech (Eisenberg, 1976). By the time he is 6 months old, the infant recognizes and even imitates intonational patterns (Kessen, Levine, & Wendrich, 1979). The "melody" of speech created by pitch changes and intonational patterns is an important element in creating and receiving messages from the earliest days of the child's communicative life, and it continues to be important as language emerges and communication becomes more sophisticated. In many cases, for children and adults, *what* is said may be less important in determining the ultimate meaning of a message than *how* the words are spoken. Depending on the intonational pattern used and other elements of speech like loudness, rate, and stress, the sentence "Get out of here" might be interpreted as an urgent threat to one's health and safety, or it might be interpreted as a light-hearted, "You're kidding me, aren't you?"

Creating a Communication Environment: Infant-Adult Interactions

It is interesting that not only is the child ready and able to communicate from the beginning of his life, but those who take care of the child seem eager to communicate with him, often even before birth. We have all heard about parents who talk to their children in utero, who read to them, or play music for them. These parents are so anxious to connect to their babies, they cannot wait for their births! They want to establish meaningful interpersonal relationships with these new humans, and they want to talk to them. Parents often attach messages to the movements of the child in the uterus, and after he is born, as we have already mentioned, they are likely to associate meaning with every noise the child makes from cries to burps. It is not surprising, therefore, that parents and other adults do talk to babies. The speech directed at infants, as you know from your own experiences, is not the same as speech directed at adults. In fact, we sometimes call the speech we use with infants, "baby talk." We all recognize this kind of speech when we hear it, but have you ever considered what baby talk really is? Are certain characteristics of baby talk the same in all cultures? Does baby talk serve a purpose for the child or for the adult? Is baby talk an important, perhaps necessary, part of language acquisition?

Baby Talk, Motherese or Parentese

When we say that parents use "baby talk," we do not mean language forms we typically ascribe to the speech of young children, as in the utterance, "doe to 'tore" for "go to store." Baby talk refers to the special way parents talk to their children. Many language people believe that the unique characteristics of baby talk facilitate the acquisition of language. There is evidence, in fact, that the input provided in this kind of language enables deaf children to reach normal developmental milestones when they are presented from birth with sign language comparable in form to baby talk (Petitto, 1984, 1985a, 1985b, 1986, 1987, 1988; Pettito & Marentette, 1990, 1991).

Sachs (1989, p. 36), in summarizing some of the relevant research findings, has identified some of the unique characteristics of speech directed to babies. In talking to babies, for example, speakers place more emphasis on components of speech such as pitch, rate, loudness, stress, rhythm, and intonation than on the words themselves. Kaye (1980) noted that mothers use considerable repetition in their speech, and that each successive utterance is semantically similar to the preceding utterance. Most early topics tend to focus on objects children can see and hear (Bruner, 1975; Phillips, 1973). When children reach the sixth month of life, their mothers tend to employ an informational style of talking, a style that is less centered on objects and more centered on their infants' surroundings and behaviors (Penman, Cross, Milgrom-Friedman, & Meares, 1983). Although there may be exceptions, baby talk in most languages is produced at higher than normal pitch levels, and intonational patterns include greater extremes of high and low pitches than are used in adult-to-adult speech. In addition, the rhythm of speech directed to babies is more regular than adult speech, resulting in what some researchers describe as a "singsong cadence." It is interesting, and probably not coincidental, that mothers who sign to their deaf children incorporate rhythms with their hands that are remarkably similar to the rhythms underlying the speech directed to hearing children (Fernald, 1994).

Based on what we know about the infant's perceptual abilities, the characteristics of talk directed to babies are not surprising. The child is able to make distinctions among pitch levels at an early age, and he prefers pitches in the speech range. There is also evidence that infants can make at least gross discriminations among loudness levels, sounds of varying durations, and different consonants in consonant–vowel–consonant (CVC) syllables (Moon, Bever, & Fifer, 1992). It is important to note that infants not only prefer speech over other kinds of sounds, but according to some research (Fernald, 1985; Sullivan & Horowitz, 1983), they prefer speech with baby talk characteristics to adult speech. One must be careful, however, about the conclusions drawn from these findings. It is possible that infants prefer baby talk because they are innately tuned to the characteristics of baby talk,

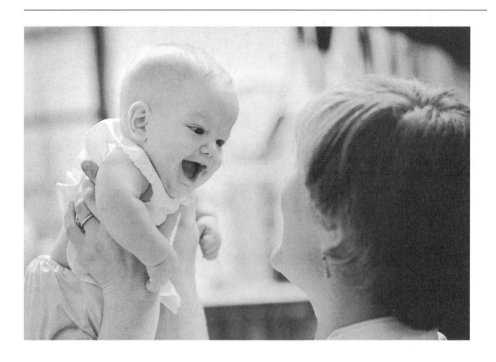

Infant–adult interaction, a precursor of communication.

but it is also possible that the preference is an environmental phenomenon that develops because infants associate baby talk with their caregivers. Why do adults use this kind of speech with babies? It is unlikely that parents make a conscious decision to use higher than normal pitches, widely varying intonation contours, and singsong cadences because they are familiar with the research literature that suggests these characteristics are appropriate for speech directed at babies. It may simply be that through trial and error, adults have learned that they are better able to gain the attention of an infant by using baby talk, and it would be difficult to argue against the idea that each generation "learns" how to use baby talk by observing members of the preceding generation communicating with babies.

Even if we cannot determine if baby talk is the product of genetics or environment, we can appreciate its role in child-adult interactions. In the preceding chapter, we indicated that the infant has an early and powerful interest in the caregiver's face. He has a similar interest in the caregiver's voice and speech. The caregiver quickly learns that she can use her face, voice, and speech to capture the infant's attention. On the basis of our present knowledge, it would not be appropriate to argue that this kind of contact is essential for speech and language development, but there seems little doubt that during these special moments when the caregiver gazes into the baby's attentive eyes and fills his discriminating ears with the lilting, soothing sounds of speech, an important bond is being formed, a bond that certainly has the potential to facilitate communication acquisition.

Working Together: A Mother–Child Partnership

An implication shared by words such as *communication* and *interaction* is that both partners are involved in the process . . . and that is one of the most important points to be made about infant communication. It is noteworthy, for example, that in addition to their interest in baby talk or motherese, researchers have directed their attention to the "joint" nature of the interaction between caregiver and child. The word "joint" suggests a sense of togetherness, and the behaviors that are exhibited in this joint venture may play a role in the language acquisition process (Bruner, 1975). The importance of these behaviors will become clear as we examine several specific "joint" applications.

Joint focus of attention, sometimes called *joint reference,* suggests that the caregiver and child are focusing on the same object or event at the same time. Owens (1996, pp. 188–189), referring to research by Bruner & Sylva (in press), notes that there are four phases in the development of establishing joint focus of attention. During phase one, which extends from about four to six weeks, the caregiver might place an object where the child can see it, move it to make certain the child focuses on it, and say the child's name or something such as "Look!" to ensure that the child is paying attention. Even though these exchanges may initially be meaningless to the child, he will pay attention to the caregiver's utterances by three months, and by six months, he may recognize that the caregiver's pitch pattern is a signal to establish joint attention (Ryan, 1974). The child enters phase two at about seven months. At his point, the child begins to demonstrate an intention to communicate and may create joint referencing by pointing to an object or event of interest. By eight months, the child may reach for an object and look to his caregiver for a response. It is not difficult to imagine that in this scenario, the caregiver enthusiastically responds by handing the object to the child and providing him the kind of accolades we might expect from cheerleaders at a basketball game. Well, it might not be quite that dramatic, but there is no doubt that the caregiver will be pleased and proud, and will convey that message to the child with considerable verve. During phase three, which ranges from about eight to twelve months of age, the child produces gestures, such as pointing, showing, and reaching, accompanied by vocalizations. When the caregiver observes the child using a gesture, she might seize the opportunity to ask the child about his intention, and she might incorporate the same gesture in her response. When the child reaches his first birthday, he is entering the final phase of joint focus of attention. He can now name objects and events. He is beginning to exercise more control over the topics of his communicative exchanges with other people. As the child begins to take more initiative in these exchanges, his caregiver reduces the number of questions she asks him, and she provides more labels for the objects and events on which the child is focusing his attention.

Constructing a conversation is another joint venture. Experts who focus on such matters believe that the physical and talking routines involved in infant–caregiver interactions make important contributions to the child's acquisition of conversational skills. The turn-taking inherent in the daily routines associated with mealtime and taking a bath, for example, and the turn-taking that is structured into playing games help form a framework in which the child can find where his behavior *fits* into a given communicative exchange. This framework is referred to as a *script* or *scaffold.* As the child repeatedly experiences these activities and the routines or scripts associated with them, his knowledge about the events themselves increases, and he develops a greater understanding about the kinds of communicative dialogues that are appropriate in varying circumstances. This is all part of learning what can and should be said and done in a range of situations that call for certain actions and certain kinds of talking. We all know that what might be appropriate in one circumstance is not appropriate in another, and we probably all know from personal experience that it takes some time to sort out what is proper and when it is proper. The sorting begins at a young age, and some folks never seem to get it quite right.

Snow (1977) described the evolution of conversation between two mothers and their babies as they moved toward their second birthdays. When the children were about three months old, the communicative exchanges were very simple and were directed primarily by the children. When the children smiled or burped, for example, the mothers reacted with comments, sometimes in the form of questions. The mothers' utterances were short and simple, but there was no expectation on their parts that the babies understood the content. Even at this stage, however, the exchanges were conversation-like in the sense that each mother treated the behaviors of her child as though they were intentional messages. It was interesting that these mothers offered considerable courtesy in these "conversations." Whereas adults often make it difficult for one another to have their turns in conversation, these mothers tried to prompt responses from their babies, and they paused expectantly, waiting for responses. There was a clear attempt to encourage and allow the turn-taking that characterizes real conversation, even though these children were not processing words as linguistic units.

As their children matured, the mothers in Snow's study developed greater expectations and made greater demands. Midway through the first year, the mothers were more selective in their responses to the noises their babies were making. They no longer treated bodily noises like burps as equal to vocalized sounds like cooing and babbling. The mothers tried to build conversations based on vocalized sounds and essentially ignored other noises. In order to maintain conversational turn-taking, the mothers often imitated their babies' utterances. When the children responded by repeating their original vocalizations, these utterances were treated like appropriate turns in the conversations.

By the time the children in Snow's study reached the end of their first year, the communicative stakes had been raised considerably. There was an even stronger emphasis on speech-like behaviors in terms of what was judged to be conversationally acceptable, and the mothers often interpreted their babies' utterances as real words, even when they probably were not. Since children begin to produce true words at about twelve months and begin to combine words into multiple-word utterances by about eighteen months, conversation becomes much more adult-like as the second year unfolds.

We have yet to answer the most important question posed in the opening of this section. Is speech directed to the infant an important or necessary component of speech and language acquisition? No one has offered evidence that normal children who receive little speech from their caregivers *cannot* develop normal speech and language. On the other hand, there is evidence that communicative stimulation from caregivers is helpful. One study directly applicable to this question was conducted by Clarke-Stewart (1973), who found that a child's language competence is correlated with the amount of speech and language stimulation the child receives from the caregiver. It is interesting that Clarke-Stewart found that the caregiver's speech to others, speech to which the child is also exposed, does not have an influence on the child's language competence. This suggests that it is not the total quantity of speech to which a child is exposed that has an impact on communicative development but the amount of speech which is intended specifically for the child. After reviewing the Clarke-Stewart study and related research, Sachs (1989, p. 40) reached this conclusion about the importance of baby talk in the acquisition process: "It would seem that baby talk, the way adults communicate with infants, is not simply a culturally transmitted, functionless style but rather a well-founded mode of speech that helps develop communication abilities in the child."

Speech Production in Infancy: From Cries to Words

To this point, we have emphasized the importance of *reception* in the infant's earliest communication experiences, and we have addressed the issue of *infant-caregiver interaction*. If you think about speech production in the context of an input-output model, we have concentrated so far on the *input* portion of the model. Caregivers provide the speech and language stimuli that the infant feeds into his linguistic processor. The input portion is more complicated than simple absorption, however, because the infant does not simply *receive* information. He *interacts* with the sender and, as we have just noted, there is evidence that linguistic information specifically directed to the child is more meaningful and more important than linguistic information directed to other people in the child's presence. The output portion of communication does not begin with speech but with nonlinguistic behaviors. As the child matures intellectually, perceptually, and neuromuscularly, he is able to use the linguistic information he receives from his caregivers and others to make his communications more specific, more intentional, and more language-like. The beginning of the child's communicative output is very simple, sometimes very loud, and it sometimes interferes with a peaceful night's sleep. He cries!

Reflexive Cries and Other Biological Noises

The first sounds the infant makes, including his first cries, are **reflexive,** which means **unlearned.** In addition to crying, he will also burp, sneeze, and cough. These noises are sometimes called **vegetative** sounds to indicate that they are natural sounds made by a passive but living organism. The infant's first cries have often been described as "undifferentiated," which immediately after birth is undoubtedly true, but by the end of the first month, the infant's caregiver can usually differentiate among several basic cries (Wolff, 1969). When the child is hungry, he produces a repeating pattern of loud cry, silence, inhalation, and a resting period often accompanied by sucking noises. When he is in pain, he produces a cry best described as long, loud, and piercing. This cry may be followed by a silence during which he seems to be holding his breath. He may then produce a few whimpers before shrieking again. When the infant is in pain, he might also clench his fists and contort his face with tightened muscles and a frown. He is not a pretty sight and the sounds of his anguish are often unmistakable. The infant's anger cry is similar in many respects to the pain cry, but when he cries in anger, he moves a greater volume of air, and most listeners have no difficulty recognizing the underlying message of vexation and irritation.

Sounds of Comfort and Pleasure

By the time the infant is two months old, caregivers notice that crying behaviors are decreasing in frequency, but the cries become more varied and differentiated. According to D'Odorico (1984), the infant at four months is producing distinctive cries to signal discomfort, call, and request. The cries of discomfort would include the cries of pain and probably some of the cries of anger described earlier. At this stage, the child will cry to call someone as in, "Hey, somebody get in here quick!" He will also cry to make a request as in, "I'm hungry, and I'll thank you to give me a bottle."

The most positive change occurring at this time is the emergence of sounds communicating pleasure and comfort. By two months, the infant is **cooing.** Cooing is usually understood as the production of vowel-like sounds, but there may also be brief consonant-like sounds resembling *k* or *g*. Although these sounds are sometimes produced by the infant when he is alone, they are often elicited when the caregiver talks to the infant or smiles during gaze-coupling. In a typical exchange, the caregiver smiles and says something like, "Aren't you a sweetheart." The infant responds with "O-o-o-o-u-u-u-u," and the caregiver imitates the coo. This cooing-imitation-cooing exchange can sometimes continue for 15 minutes or longer, and most adults find it as delightful a communicative experience as the infant. The child at four months is not only cooing but laughing (Stark, 1979), and the laughter is at times sustained long enough that there is no question about the nature of the behavior. It may be difficult to determine what the child perceives as the punch line, but he finds something worthy of laughter.

Introductory or Transitional Babbling

According to Stark (1979) and Sachs (1989), "true" babbling does not begin until the child is six months or older. Beginning at about five months, however, the infant is producing vocalizations that seem to bridge cooing and true babbling. These are single-syllable productions consisting of vowel-like and consonant-like sounds, and we can think of them as transitional behaviors that extend beyond cooing and prepare the way for babbling. Stark (1979) refers to these sequences as "marginal babbling."

True Babbling

We traditionally use the term **babbling** to describe repeated consonant-vowel syllables, like "mamama" or "nanana," productions which tend to appear at about six or seven months. The more specific term for this kind of production is *reduplicated babbling.* According to Stark, Bernstein, and Demorest (1993), reduplicated babbling occurs most often when the infant is investigating his environment or holding an object. The consonants most frequently incorporated into these utterances are produced at the front of the mouth, for example, *m, p, b, t, d,* and *n.* Some of the intonational contours the infant produced during cooing have disappeared (Stark, 1979), but the production of consonants suggests an increasing maturity in the child's control of the speech mechanism. Whereas cooing is often elicited by social interaction between the infant and the caregiver, the infant will often babble most when he is by himself (Nakazima, 1975; Stark, 1981). Many researchers and writers have observed that during babbling, the infant produces a wide variety of sounds, many of which are not included in the sound system of his native language. Ferguson (1978) suggests that the sounds the child produces are largely the product of the limitations of his speech mechanism. As the structures of speech mature physiologically and as the infant becomes more absorbed in the sounds of his own language, his babbling more closely resembles his native language (Rees, 1972).

In addition to babbling, the infant between eight and twelve months produces an interesting behavior called **echolalia.** Echolalia is the immediate, parrot-like imitation of sounds, syllables, or words produced by someone else. The term "parrot-like" suggests that the infant does not understand what he is saying even though his imitations may be fairly accurate. If for no other reason, this behavior is important because it represents a change in the nature of imitation in speech and language development. In the cooing stage, communication is maintained when the caregiver imitates the infant. In echolalia, the infant imitates the caregiver. In the months and years to come, the child's imitations of the speech models he hears become increasingly important in terms of acquiring the sound system, vocabulary, and structure of his language.

It is important to emphasize that during true babbling, the infant's productions become more heavily dependent on self-hearing. For this reason, infants who are deaf sound very much like hearing children until they reach this point. Deaf infants cry, laugh, coo, and produce some marginal babbling, but when hearing infants begin to produce true babbling, deaf infants begin to restrict their output and they use fewer consonant sounds than hearing infants at about eight months of age (Oller, Eilers, Bull & Carney, 1985; Stoel-Gammon & Otomo, 1986).

Variegated Babbling and Jargon

Beginning at about nine months and continuing through eighteen months, the nature of babbling changes in the sense that it becomes more varied within a single utterance. Instead of simply repeating the same syllable as he did in the earlier stage, the child now produces successive syllables that differ from one another, as in "madagaba." This more advanced babbling is known as *variegated* babbling. Stark (1986) found that some variegated babbling productions are consonant–vowel–consonant (CVC) combinations, in which the consonant is replicated, and vowel–consonant–vowel (VCV) combinations, in which the vowel is replicated. That is, the child might say, "gug" (CVC) or "ugu" (VCV). As the name suggests, variegated babbling is characterized by a wider range of sounds, especially consonants, than reduplicated babbling. It should be noted that not all researchers are convinced that the variegated babbling period necessarily follows the reduplicated babbling period (Mitchell and Kent, 1990), but there is a certain logical appeal to the progression.

The seven- or eight-month-old infant attends to the intonational contours of adult speech. It makes sense then that, as he continues to experiment with sounds and sound combinations, he begins to incorporate intonational contours into his vocalizations, producing what is called *jargon* babbling. Jargon babbling productions are distinguished by melodic patterns. In fact, this form of babbling has many of the characteristics of real speech. If you attend just to the melody of jargon babbling utterances, they sound adult-like. The child produces the rhythm, stresses, rate variations, and intonational contours of his language, even though he produces few, if any, meaningful words. Jargon babbling is to speech as humming or "la-la-la"ing is to singing when we do not know or cannot remember the lyrics. When the child produces these vocalizations, adult listeners hear what they believe are questions, commands, expressions of joy, statements of concern, and virtually every kind of communication imaginable. The son of a friend in graduate school was particularly proficient in jargon babbling. His father was a great storyteller. The son would "tell stories" in jargon babbling, some "funny" as evidenced by his laughter and some "serious" as reflected by the tone of his voice and the look on his face, using the same speech melodies as his father used. These vocalizations were delightfully entertaining, and if the truth be told, many of the son's stories were better than the father's!

Although jargon babbling is interesting and clearly indicates that the child is paying attention to and imitating the melodic characteristics of adult speech, it is not language. Early in this same nine to eighteen month period, however, there is evidence that the child is moving from prelinguistic communication to language. The child will not produce his first conventional words until he is about twelve months, but by the time he is nine or ten months old, he may be producing what are called **vocables, phonetically consistent forms, performatives,** or **protowords.** All of these terms refer to productions, unique to a given child, which are consistent patterns of sounds used in reference to particular things or situations. The son of von Raffier Engler (1973), for example, produced the sound "e-e-e" to signal that he wanted an object, and he produced "u-u-u" to signal disapproval. These are not words, of course, but they represent an important transition from vocal play and babbling, vocalizations that are random and devoid of specific meaning, to productions that are purposive, consistent, and meaningful. Carter's (1975) analysis of vocables in one child suggests there may be a fairly direct connection between some vocables and corresponding true words. She found, for example, that vocables beginning with *m,* accompanied by a gesture to indicate "I want," gradually evolved into the words *more, my,* and *mine.* Recent evidence suggests that vocables are present in children's productions, no matter which language they are acquiring (Blake & deBoysson-Bardies, 1992).

The Development of Communication Functions: Using Communication to Get Things Done

Although it is true that human beings talk even when they have nothing to say and even when no one, perhaps even the speaker, is listening, humans usually communicate for a purpose. We use speech intentionally to accomplish specific goals. We use speech to inform, to persuade, to direct, to flatter, to manipulate, to request, to express, to argue, to impress, to complain, and the list goes on. The study of the functions, purposes, or intents of communication is called **pragmatics.** The term makes sense. "Pragmatic" means "practical," and pragmatics is the study of the practical aspects of communication. Does the infant show an awareness of pragmatics or communicative function before he begins to produce language? Of course he does. In this section, we will briefly examine the stages of communicative function development in children.

As we noted in Chapter Two, the pragmatics revolution stimulated interest in the functions served by communicative efforts. The work of Austin (1962) and Searle (1969), which focused on adult speech, suggested that there are three components to all speech acts: (1) perlocutions, which are concerned with how listeners interpret speech acts, (2) illocutions, which involve the intentions expressed by the speaker, and (3) locutions, which include the meanings of utterances. Bates,

Camaioni, & Volterra (1975) borrowed these terms from Searle and applied them to the developing communication functions of children.

We will consider three stages of communication function development based on Searle's terms. To fully appreciate what happens in this development, the reader must understand that the child is developing the ability to produce goal-directed, intentional communication behaviors. The child is able to do this only to the extent that he takes into consideration the persons with whom he is communicating, and only to the extent that he is able to formulate messages for people other than himself.

How does the child learn to use communication intentionally? Although there is probably not a clear and definitive answer to that question, you should not find it difficult to speculate about how communicative intent evolves. In the preceding chapter, we traced cognitive development through infancy. It should come as no surprise that there is a relationship between cognitive development and the developmental stages of early communication functions.

The *perlocutionary stage* of development extends from birth to approximately eight months of age. At the beginning of this stage, the infant is producing only reflexive cries. By the end of this stage, he is producing the goal-directed behaviors described in substage three of Piaget's sensorimotor period. By the end of the perlocutionary stage, the infant is using gestures to indicate that he recognizes the functions of common objects. He might lift a glass to his mouth, for example, or he might put a spoon into his mouth. The production of these gestures demonstrates that the infant is organizing his world into conceptual categories. These early gestures have been called *recognitory* because they reflect the infant's ability to "recognize," albeit in a primitive way, the functionality of objects (Bates, Bretherton, Shore, & McNew, 1983).

The *illocutionary stage* extends from eight to twelve months of age. During this stage, the infant uses gestures or vocalizations to signal intentionality. By using a variety of gestures including pointing, showing, and requesting, the infant can convey differentiated intentions. At the same time, the infant might use vocables, those phonetically consistent forms of vocalization we referred to earlier in this chapter, to express a range of specific and recognizable communicative functions.

Halliday (1975) concluded that his son, Nigel, between the ages of nine and sixteen months, produced a number of nonlinguistic utterances or vocables to convey meanings with four identifiable communicative intents. Nigel communicated to satisfy needs and wants, to control the behavior of others, to interact with others, and to express an emotion or interest.

Bates (1979) uses the term **protodeclarative** to describe the communicative gestures that are used to point out objects or events to which the child and adult attend together. The child might point to a cow, for example, not to request the cow or to ask about the cow, but simply to say, "Hey, Mom, look at that big thing standing over there with a multi-fingered bubble on its belly!" Bates uses the term **protoimperative** in reference to gestures used by the infant to control or manipulate the behaviors of others. The child might point to an object to indicate that he wants the object. He might use a similar gesture to indicate that he wants a light

TABLE 4-1 Early Communicative Functions

Function (Definition)	Example
Instrumental[a] (to have needs and wants satisfied)	"Uh-uh-uh" while pointing at refrigerator to get food or drink
Regulatory (to control the behaviors of other people)	"Kuh-kuh" while moving the caregiver's hands together to suggest the continuation of patty-cake
Interactional (to establish or maintain interpersonal contact)	"Muh-muh" while holding the caregiver's face to maintain attention on an object of shared interest
Personal (to express an emotion, interest, or attitude)	"Ga-ga" in angry tones while playing with a toy the child cannot manipulate properly

[a]The italicized terms are used by Halliday (1975).

turned off or on. He might shake his head vigorously and produce a different kind of vocalization to indicate that he does not want to eat any more strained peas. These are all protoimperatives.

The *locutionary stage* is the final stage. The child, who is now beyond his first birthday, is producing his first meaningful words. Words and gestures are now combined to express the same basic meanings or intentions that were previously conveyed by gestures or vocalizations.

Like Halliday (1975), Bruner (1981) found infant communications that reflect an interest in establishing contact with others. Bruner refers to this communicative function or intent as **social interaction.** These communications include behaviors used to greet another person, to attract and maintain the attention of another person, and to establish the shared attention of the child and another person. As we have already noted, adults and especially parents react to virtually all of a child's behaviors as though they are purposive and have communicative intent. Harding (1983a, 1983b) suggests that infant–adult interactions may help the infant learn about the practical nature of communication. She suggests that when caregivers reinforce and expand on behaviors such as eye contact, gesturing, crying, babbling, and other vocalizations (interpreting them as communication), infants are better able to recognize such behaviors as intentional communications, and produce them more often. In summary then, the infant most likely acquires the ability to use nonverbal behaviors and vocalized behaviors with specific communicative intents as a result of overall biological maturation, cognitive development, and his social interactions with caregivers.

The first year of life has not been passive. The child has matured considerably. His intellectual abilities have progressed rapidly. He has interacted with his world and his caregivers with enthusiasm and unbridled curiosity. He has communicated unintentionally and intentionally, but all of this has been merely prologue for what is about to occur. He is now ready for the magic and wonder of true language. As his first year comes to an end, he is about to become a linguistic communicator beginning with his first real words.

Beyond Infancy: The Emergence of Language

The issue of stages was briefly discussed in the context of cognitive development. It is important to keep in mind that we trace the development of many behaviors through stages because stages provide a convenient framework for understanding the changes that occur during the development of a behavior or, in the case of language, an aggregate of behaviors. Consider for a moment how stages of speech and language development might be compared to grade levels in the study of mathematics. The mathematic skills you acquire and practice in first grade are clearly different from the skills you acquire and learn in trigonometry and precalculus as a senior in high school, but you reach advanced mathematic skills by acquiring and building upon knowledge and skills that are progressively more sophisticated and complex as you move through the grade levels of elementary, junior high, and senior high school math courses. You begin by learning what numbers are and what they represent. You learn to add and subtract, and then you learn to multiply and divide, and you understand that multiplication is an advanced version of addition, and division is an advanced version of subtraction. You continue to add layer upon layer of mathematic knowledge, but each layer rests upon all the layers below. Learning mathematics then is really a continuous process that involves learning new concepts, reviewing old concepts, and applying old concepts in new ways. The stages of mathematic acquisition are represented by grade levels and course names, but grade levels and course names are merely conveniences to help us organize the process of learning and to categorize the basic skills that are acquired at certain junctures in the overall development of mathematic competence.

TABLE 4-2 Synopsis of Infant Communication

Age	Type of Communication
Birth	Reflexive cries and other biological noises
2 months	Cooing—sounds of comfort and pleasure
5 months	Marginal/transitional babbling
6 months	True babbling
8 to 12 months	Echolalia
9 to 18 months	Variegated and jargon babbling and vocables/protowords

In very much the same way, human beings learn speech and language in a continuous, uninterrupted manner. As the child acquires new words and new language forms, he is constantly reviewing prior language knowledge, and he is using language he has already acquired in new ways. We will consider speech and language development in stages because it is a useful and convenient way to organize our discussion and because stages help us to understand how, and to some extent, when changes occur in language acquisition. It needs to be emphasized that the *order* in which changes occur is far more important than the *ages* we will attach to these changes. All children will go through these stages in the same order, and as was true of Piaget's cognitive stages, children do not skip stages of language development. *When* children go through these stages, however, might differ considerably. The age ranges associated with the stages are broad enough that most children will fit, but you should be careful not to read too much into the fact that a given child is either "ahead" or "behind" the normal age range for a given language behavior.

The specific stage model we use in our discussion of speech and language acquisition was developed by Roger Brown (1973). Brown's stages are widely used by researchers and authors to describe *syntactic* or structural development in children, and Brown's conclusions relative to these stages have been supported by the research of deVilliers and deVilliers (1978). Brown traced the development of syntax through five major stages. We will describe these stages, but in addition to syntax, we will include information about *semantic* or meaning development and about *pragmatic* development. Brown tracked syntactic development by measuring the *mean length of utterance* (MLU), a concept more fully explained in the next section. Although age is not as reliable a measure of syntactic development as MLU, Miller and Chapman (1981) found that age and MLU are positively related. Because most people think about development in terms of ages, approximate age ranges will be provided as we move through Brown's five stages (Bernstein, 1989,

TABLE 4-3 Overview of Brown's (1973) Stages of Syntactic Development

Stage	Age Range in Months	Mean Length of Utterance (MLU)
I. Semantic Roles and Grammatical Relations	12 to 26	1.0 to 2.00
II. Grammatical Morphemes and the Modulation of Meanings	27 to 30	2.0 to 2.50
III. Modalities of the Simple Sentence	31 to 34	2.5 to 3.00
IV. Embedding of One Sentence Within Another	35 to 40	3.0 to 3.75
V. Coordination of Simple Sentences and Propositional Relations	41 to 46	3.75 to 4.50

pp. 108–118; Owens, 1996, pp. 302–304). The rest of this chapter describes the first stage of language development. The remaining four stages are discussed in the following chapter.

Tracking Language Development: Morphemes and Mean Length of Utterance

Before we can understand mean length of utterance, we must understand the units that are being counted, which brings us to morphology. **Morphology** is concerned with words and their parts as units of meaning. A **morpheme** is the smallest meaningful unit of language. It might be tempting to think of a word as being the smallest meaningful unit of language. It is true that a word might be a single morpheme, but some words contain several morphemes. It might seem that a single sound like *s* cannot be a meaning unit, but in some cases, a single sound is a morpheme. It might even seem logical that a morpheme is the same as a syllable, but that is not always true either. Sometimes a syllable is a morpheme, but sometimes it takes two or more syllables in the right combination to make one morpheme. Confused? The confusion is helpful if it helps create the correct mindset about morphemes. Morphemes are **units of meaning.** Morphemes can be sounds, or syllables, or whole words. A sound or sequence of sounds might be morphemes in some contexts but not in others, and they might be different kinds of morphemes depending upon the context. Now let's sort out the confusion by identifying the possibilities.

There are two kinds of morphemes: free and bound. A **free morpheme** can stand alone and be meaningful. The following are free morphemes: *dog, cat, house* and *go*. A **bound morpheme** is a unit of meaning that must be attached to a free morpheme to be meaningful. The word *tie* is a free morpheme meaning *to bind*. Notice what happens if I add *un-* to *tie* to produce *untie*. That word now means *to remove the binding*. By itself, *un-* has no meaning, but when it is attached to certain free morphemes, it means *no* or *not*. Consider words like **un**faithful, **un**reliable, **un**interesting. Does this mean that anytime *un-* appears in a word it is a morpheme? Consider the word *uncle*. In this word, *un-* does not provide meaning, but is one part of a two-syllable free morpheme. In the same way, *in-* in the word *indirect*, means not, but in the word *interest*, *in-* is simply part of a three-syllable free morpheme.

Usually a single sound is not a morpheme, but a sound can be a morpheme. What happens to meaning when I add *s* to the free morpheme, *cat* to produce *cats*? The free morpheme *cat* refers to *one cat*, but *cats* refers to *more than one cat*. The *s* in *cats* is a bound morpheme that means *plurality*. The *s* in *cat's box* means *possessive*.

Bound morphemes can be either **derivational** or **inflectional.** Derivational morphemes are added to the front of free morphemes and are commonly referred to as prefixes or are added to the back of free morphemes and are called suffixes. Derivational morphemes change the class or category of a word. If, for example, I add the derivational morpheme *-ly* to *slow* to create *slowly*, I have changed an adjective to an adverb. I can change the adjective *sad* to a noun by adding *-ness* to create *sadness*. Inflectional morphemes, which occur only as suffixes, change the meaning of words by marking grammatical adjustments for things like plurality, possession, and verb tense. When you add *s* to *bat* to make *bats,* or when you add *d* to *dive* to make *dived,* you have used inflectional morphemes. The child learns to use inflectional morphemes to refine the meanings of words or to make their meanings more exact. When he first begins to produce words, for example, the child might use "cat" to refer to one cat or to several. As he becomes more sophisticated in word usage, he learns that he can add "s" to make "cat" plural. This simple adjustment makes his communication more precise and more meaningful. Since the child does not begin to use morphemes as grammatical markers until the second of Brown's stages, further discussion about the acquisition of these morphemes is reserved until we reach the second stage. At this point, it is important that you understand what morphemes are, however, because morphemes are counted in determining mean length of utterance, one of the measures used to assess progress in language development.

The term **mean** refers to a statistical average. Let's assume we have a sample of a child's language containing 100 utterances. Some utterances consist of single free morphemes. Others consist of four or five morphemes, free and bound. A few utterances contain as many as ten or eleven morphemes. To determine the **mean length of utterance,** we count the morphemes in each utterance, add the total, and divide by the number of utterances, in this case 100. Because this is an arithmetic calculation, the MLU is seldom expressed as a whole number. If a child produces a total of 310 morphemes over 100 utterances, his MLU is 3.1.

Stage One: From Words to Combinations of Words

A child is in the first stage from 12 to 26 months, and he has an MLU range of 1.0 to 2.0 morphemes. In practical terms then, the stage opens when the child is producing his first meaningful words, and it closes as he is beginning to put words together. Although an increase of only one morpheme per utterance does not seem to be much progress, this is an exciting and significant stage because the child is moving from prelinguistic to linguistic communication, and that represents one giant step in the "Mother May I?" of speech and language development.

Because this is a giant step, with significant changes in language including the transition from single-word to two-word combinations at about 18 months, this stage needs to be divided. We have organized our discussion of Stage One, following Roger Brown's (1973) lead, into Early Stage One and Late Stage One.

Early Stage One (MLU: 1–1.5; Age: 12–22 mos.)

Most of us have been around young children enough to be familiar with what speech sounds like in the beginning. The child's first utterances are single-word productions like "wawa" for "water," "mama" for "mother," and "bye-bye" for "good-bye" or "Let's get out of here!" In these examples, the child's words resemble the adult versions, but this is not always the case. A child I observed some years ago referred to cookies and other snacks as "chee-chee." James (1990, p. 40) in her discussion of first words, writes about a child who referred to cats as "gee." These productions are common during this first stage of true speech and language development, and caregivers quickly learn what these unique words mean even if other people do not have a clue.

The child's first words are used in reference to the things that matter most in his own world. He does not reflect on current events, and he does not offer criticisms of art and music. He names people, objects, and actions that are of immediate interest. Most of the child's first words consist of one syllable ("up"), two syllables ("doggie"), or one syllable repeated ("wawa"). First words are usually consonant-vowel ("no"), vowel-consonant ("eat"), or consonant-vowel-consonant-vowel ("mama") forms. Consonant-vowel-consonant forms ("hot") may be produced but are rare (Owens, 1996, p. 245). Lewis (1951) studied the first few words of 26 children and found that 75 percent of these words were either single-syllable productions or two-syllable productions in which one syllable was simply repeated as in "mama" or "dada." Lewis also found that 75 percent of these first words included consonants produced at the front of the mouth like *m, b,* and *w.* There is a wider range of vowels than consonants in the early words of children, although some vowels like the *e* in *"eat"* and the *a* in "mama", "dada", and "wawa" are heard more often than others (Ingram, 1976).

I May Not Mean What You Mean, But I Know What I Mean . . . I Think!

It becomes immediately obvious to anyone who listens to children producing their first words that the meanings attached to these words are often inconsistent with adult meanings. My younger sister, for example, used the word "go-go" in reference to a wide range of motions, but she also used it to refer to cars, trucks, and other objects that moved. A child might use the word "nite-nite" to mean "darkness" as well as "go to sleep" probably because he associates going to sleep with darkness. He might use the word "hot" as a noun, in reference to a flame or the stove, before he uses it as an adjective referring to the temperature of an object.

In our discussion of the child's cognitive development, we identified two processes important to the development of schemata: assimilation and accommodation. We can see the child applying these processes in his first words. When the child assimilates horses, cows, pigs, and elephants into his "doggie" schema, the assimilation is reflected in the way he uses the word "doggie." That is, he uses "doggie" in reference to dogs, horses, pigs, elephants, and probably all other animals with four legs. The application of assimilation to the child's words is called **overextension.** Overextension is very common in the speech of young children. The word "wawa" is often used to refer not only to water, but to any liquid.

"Mama" may be used to name all women, not just mother. Anything edible might be called a "cookie."

Sometimes the child will use a word in a sense that is too narrow from an adult perspective. This is called **underextension.** The child might use the word "doggie" only in reference to Fido, the family pet. Other dogs are something else, but they are definitely not "doggie." The word "cookie" might be reserved for chocolate chip cookies only. If there is a raisin or a nut in the dough, it might be edible, it might even be delicious, but it is not a "cookie." As the child sorts out his cognitive categories by assimilating what should be assimilated and by accommodating when new schemata are needed, his words will be more accurately defined and applied in comparison to adult usage.

There is not universal agreement among language experts about how children attach meanings to words, but there seem to be three basic views: the semantic feature hypothesis, the functional core hypothesis, and the prototype hypothesis.

According to the **semantic feature hypothesis** (Clark, 1975), each word is comprised of bits of meaning information called semantic features. Many words will have some semantic features in common, but each word has its own unique collection of semantic features. The semantic features for a word like *dog* might include *animal, mammal, furry, four legs, wet nose, tail,* and *barks.* You can easily think of other words that would contain one or more of these semantic features. Some are obvious, but think about *four legs* as a semantic feature for *table* or *barks* as a semantic feature for *seal* or for *circus ringmaster.* Consider the possibilities. Words are much more interconnected on the basis of bits of meaning information than they appear on the surface. What must not be missed in this mental exercise, however, is that each word is unique by virtue of its own collection or set of features. Only *dog* includes *all* of the semantic features of *dog* and it is that set of features which separates *dogness* from *catness, pigness,* and all other words which share some but not all of the semantic features of *dog.*

Clark (1973) suggested that the development of meaning for a particular word is a gradual process. The child begins with one or two semantic features, and this accounts for the way the child uses his first words. If, for example, the only semantic feature he has for *dog* is *four legs,* he will call everything he sees with four legs a *dog.* If the only semantic feature he has for *dog* is *that animal who lives at our house and slobbers all over my face,* he will use the word "dog" in reference to that dog and to no other dog. As the child adds more semantic features, his meanings more closely approximate adult meanings, and he uses words in a more adult-like manner. According to Clark, the semantic features of the child's first words are based on perceptual categories like size, shape, texture, taste, and movement. When the child includes a size feature for dogs, he envisions an animal not as large as a horse or as small as a toad. The size feature is a kind of medium, and this works most of the time because most dogs are roughly the same size, but try to imagine the problems created when the child sees a dog like a Chihuahua that is small enough to put into a coffee mug or a giant Great Dane that is large enough to ride. Suddenly the size feature is not as reliable as it once seemed! Clark contends that even if the

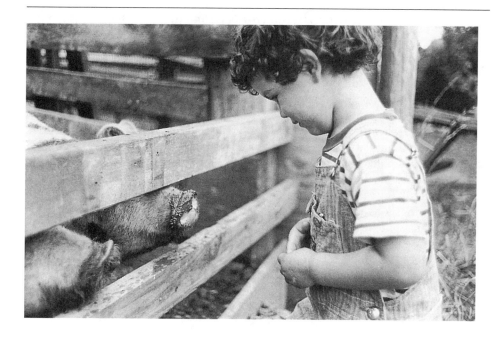

Discovering new things, words, and meanings.

child notices size differences that matter to adults, he is not immediately interested in the semantic significance of the differences.

The reader may recognize that we used the same Chihuahua-Great Dane example in the preceding chapter in the discussion about developing schemata. Developing schemata and acquiring meanings for words by discovering and adjusting semantic features are simply two views of the same process. Cognitive development and the acquisition of language meaning are not so much parallel phenomena as they are integrated phenomena.

Nelson (1974) rejected the notion that the meanings of first words are based on unchanging perceptual features as suggested by Clark. She proposed the **functional core hypothesis,** the argument that the meanings of early words are based on the functions or actions of the things these words represent. Whereas Clark suggested that a child categorizes things according to percepts like size and shape, Nelson proposed that the child places things into categories based upon their actions if they are animate objects, or based on the actions taken upon them if they are inanimate objects. The most appealing aspect of Nelson's hypothesis is that it fits Piaget's explanation of early cognitive development in the sensorimotor phase.

That is, the child's first concepts are based on his sensory contacts with objects and on his manipulation of these objects.

As often happens when there are two substantially different explanations of the same process, someone suggests an option that combines the best features of the opposing views. This is essentially what we find in the **prototype hypothesis** developed by Bowerman (1978). Bowerman contended that both the semantic feature hypothesis and the functional core hypothesis are too narrow in their explanations, that the child relies on both perceptual features and functions in developing the meanings of words. Bowerman proposed that the child develops a **prototype** to represent a given concept. A prototype can best be understood as a model or standard. The idea is that the child will find a model which best represents a concept. The model for "dog," for example, is much more likely to be a Cocker Spaniel or a German Shepherd than a Chihuahua because these dogs are more doglike in size than the Chihuahua. The child's model for "cat" is likely to be the domestic variety, not a lion or tiger. The prototype for "chair" will be the usual four-legged chair we find in our homes, not the bean bag chair that frequently fills the corner of the family room. The model for "fruit" will be an apple, pear, orange, or peach, not a watermelon, grape, or banana. The closer an object comes to matching the child's prototype for a given concept, the more likely he will use the name for that concept. According to this view of meaning acquisition, the child's prototype for a concept will be strongly influenced by the first object or activity he names within the concept. Any new object or activity will be included or not included within the concept depending upon how close it comes to fitting the prototype. The child's initial understanding of a concept will be fairly narrow. As his understanding of the concept develops, the meaning expands, and more and more exemplars are included. At some point, therefore, his understanding of "dogness" is sufficiently broad and refined to include all dogs, in all sizes and shapes, but he is also able to exclude wolves and coyotes because while they are similar and share many traits of dogness, they are not domestic pets. Meaning develops, therefore, as the child expands, fine-tunes, and adjusts his prototype for a given concept. For some concepts and the words associated with them, this process continues throughout childhood, adolescence, and into adulthood.

Classifying the Child's First Words

When adults listen to young children producing their first words, they may be tempted to classify these words according to traditional grammatical categories. If the child says, "doggie," we think *noun*. If he says, "on," we think *preposition*. If he says, "go," we think *verb*. If we listen more carefully, however, we will discover that first words do not always fit adult categories. When the child points to the light switch and says, "on," he may be using the word like a verb to mean "turn on the light." He might use the word "go" like a noun to name a car, bus, or train. It becomes obvious fairly quickly that since children do not use their first words in the same way that adults do, we should probably not classify or categorize these words according to adult grammatical and semantic standards.

Bloom (1973) suggested, based on analysis of her daughter's first words, that early words are of two basic types: substantive and relational. **Substantive words** refer to classes or categories of objects or events that have perceptual or functional features in common. Words like "mama," "dada," "wawa," and "doggie" are substantive. Substantive words can be divided into two more categories based on action. Those words referring to things which cause action are called *agents,* and words which identify things receiving action are called *objects.*

Relational words reflect the child's understanding of object permanence and causality. Relational words refer to actions or states of being that can affect a variety of categories. For example, the child might use the utterance, "allgone," to mean that his "plate is clean" or his "glass is empty" or that "daddy has gone to work." Relational words are most typically used to refer to the appearance or disappearance of objects, the existence or nonexistence of objects, the traits or characteristics of objects, the location of objects, and to note the possession of one object by another (Bloom & Lahey, 1978). Productions like "more," "no," "stop," and "bye-bye" are common relational words in the early vocabularies of children.

Bloom (1973) discovered that when her daughter's speech was confined to single-word productions, she used a limited number of relational words frequently and sustained these words in her vocabulary. She used a much larger number of substantive words, but many of these were not used often and tended to drop out of her vocabulary for weeks or even months. By the time she was about eighteen months old, however, substantive words were no longer dropping out, and since new words were being constantly added, there was an overall growth in her functional vocabulary.

Although Bloom's view of early vocabulary can be considered largely *semantic* in orientation because of her emphasis on the meanings of words, Nelson (1973) interpreted early vocabulary from a *grammatical* point of view. She did not use the traditional adult categories like noun, verb, adjective, adverb, etc., but she did place early words into categories based on grammatical function. Nelson studied the first 50 words of eighteen children, and concluded that these words could be placed into five major categories, one of which was divided into two subcategories: (1) Nominals (Specific and General), (2) Action Words, (3) Modifiers, (4) Personal-Social Words, and (5) Functional Words. **Nominals** are words used to refer to objects. A **specific nominal** is a word that refers to only one thing, as when a child uses "doggie" in reference to the family pet only. A **general nominal** is used in reference to all objects in a category, as when the child identifies all dogs as "doggie" or all females as "girl." It should be noted that if the child uses "doggie" to refer not only to dogs but to cats, horses, pigs, elephants, and other four-legged animals, the word is still a general nominal. It is just more general than the adult version. Nelson found that these children had more nominals than any other category. In fact, 65 percent of their words were nominals, mostly general nominals. Most of the general nominals referred to objects that moved or could be manipulated in some way, like "car" or "ball," or to objects of personal interest to the child like "doggie" or "light." These children were far less likely to identify static objects like buildings or pieces of furniture.

The second most popular category with 13 percent was **action words.** As the name suggests, these are words used to describe or demand action like "go" or "look" or words used to accompany action as when the child says "up" as he is being picked up or "bye-bye" as he waves.

Simple arithmetic indicates that 78 percent, almost eight of every ten words in the early vocabularies of children, are either nominals or action words. What may be surprising is that nominals dominate so much, but this tendency has been noted by a number of researchers, even when environmental differences are taken into account (Schwartz & Leonard, 1984). Perhaps nominals dominate because it is easier for the child to conceptualize things than it is for him to conceptualize how things might be related to one another. In using an action word, he must conceptualize not just an object but how the object might act or be acted upon.

Nelson found that the other categories accounted for far fewer words. **Modifiers,** words such as "hot," "little," and "mine," which were used to identify the characteristics or qualities of things or events, accounted for only 9 percent of the total. **Personal-social words,** including "no" and "please," which express emotions or identify relationships, made up just 8 percent of early vocabularies, and **functional words** like "for" or "that" accounted for only 4 percent of the words in the vocabularies of Nelson's subjects. Benedict (1979), studying the same grammatical categories, essentially confirmed Nelson's percentages. As the child gets older, the percentage of nouns in his vocabulary continues to increase until he is using about 100 words. At this juncture, the number of verbs relative to the number of nouns begins to increase (Bates, Marchman, Thal, Fenson, Dale, Reznick, Reilly, & Hartung, 1994; Marchman & Bates, 1991).

Although it is important to stress that the early words of children are predominantly nouns or object words (Gentner, 1982; Schwartz & Leonard, 1984), it is also appropriate to note that not all early vocabularies are the same. Horgan (1981) identifies some children as "noun lovers" and others as "noun leavers." That is, although some children use so many nouns we might assume they love nouns, others use fewer nouns, but even "noun leavers" use more nouns than other categories of words. The point to be made here is that although nouns dominate the early vocabularies of all children, there are small but noteworthy differences among children. As Nelson (1973) noted, although some children seem to use language primarily to describe and categorize things, others seem to give language a major role in their social and personal interactions. These differences can probably be viewed more as preferential or stylistic differences than major variations in language substance, and they may simply reflect early personality differences. That is, children who use language primarily to describe and categorize may be somewhat less social than children who emphasize language usage in their interactions with other people.

The Functions of Single Words: Pragmatics

Earlier in this chapter, in our discussion of infant communication, we introduced pragmatics, the study of the practical aspects of communication. Pragmatics includes the functions, purposes, or intents of communication. According to Halliday (1975), Bates (1979), and others, children show evidence of communicative intent before they begin to use words, but when the child moves from prelinguistic to linguistic communication, pragmatics undergoes a significant evolution. Words allow for more specific intentions than gestures alone, and as we all know from our adult experiences with language, words provide opportunities for many layers of meaning, including layers of pragmatic meaning. As adults, when someone says something to us, we are often more curious about the intentions of the communicator than about the message itself. We are more inclined to ask questions like, "What did she mean by that?" or "Why did she say that?" than "What did she say?" Figuring out what someone says is usually fairly easy. Determining motive, purpose, or intention is often much more difficult, and in the final analysis, more important because communication ultimately is about getting things done.

The evolution of pragmatics triggered by the onset of language becomes apparent even in the single-word stage of language development. Whereas Halliday (1975) identified four intents in the nonlinguistic utterances of his son, Nigel, the number of intentions expanded to seven with the introduction of his first words. In addition to the earlier functions, which included *satisfying needs and wants, controlling the behavior* of others, *interacting* with others, and *expressing* emotion or interest, Nigel used his early words in his efforts to *explore and categorize* the things in this environment, to *imagine* or pretend, and to *inform* by sharing his experiences with others. You will recognize that these are functions of communication that continue throughout one's life, but these are pretty basic functions or intents. As the child matures and his language becomes more sophisticated, his pragmatic functions expand as well.

Halliday's interpretation of early communicative intents takes into account the reactions of listeners. His categories of functions are based on how well the child's communicative attempts work toward accomplishing specified purposes. Dore (1974, 1975), who analyzed the communicative functions of children during the single-word stage of language development, tried to look at these functions from the point of view of the child. That is, what are the child's intentions and reasons for communicating, regardless of whether they work or do not work from the listener's point of view? According to Dore, children in the single-word stage (twelve to eighteen months) produce what he called **primitive speech acts** (PSAs) to communicate their intentions. A primitive speech act might be a word, a change in the prosodic pattern, or a gesture. Dore found that children could use these communication skills to *label* objects or events, to *answer* questions, to *request an action or answer*, to *address* a person or thing, to *greet* someone, to *protest* or *object*, to *imitate* or *repeat*, and to simply *practice* language.

Bloom and Lahey (1978, pp. 202–203) provide labels that may help to clarify what happens to communicative intentions as the child moves from the prelinguistic stage of communication development to the linguistic stage. They suggest that when the child is using just a few words in combination with gestures, he is using *primary forms.* When his intentions are more consistently communicated through words, he is using *conventional forms.* In some cases, like pointing to something the child wants, the gesture may be just as effective as making a request in words, but when the child begins to use conventional or language-based forms to express his communicative functions, he adds many more options to his repertoire of intentions, and he can express his intentions with much greater clarity and specificity.

Presuppositions and Conversational Turn-Taking

As the child's communicative intentions become more elaborate, the role of the child in speaker-listener relationships becomes more interesting and complex. During the single-word stage, we see evidence of what are called presuppositions. A **presupposition** is an assumption the speaker makes concerning what the listener knows about the subject of the conversation. In a typical communicative exchange, the child will provide information the listener needs and will not comment on what he believes the listener already knows (Greenfield & Smith, 1976). If the child is preparing to push a toy car, for example, he may make the presupposition that the listener knows that the object in his hand is a car. He might comment on what the speaker does not know, which is that he is about to make the car move, so he says, "Go!" while pushing the car across the floor toward Rex, the previously sleeping, now frantic and scurrying family dog. We should keep in mind, of course, that the adult's ability to interpret what the child says is made a little easier because children at this early stage of language development typically talk about the here and now (Greenfield, 1978). Most adults, given even modest communicative assistance from children, are bright enough to figure out communications that focus on what is happening in the present tense in the present place. It must be emphasized that the child in the single-word stage is just beginning to develop presuppositional skills. As we shall see, the child at three and four years is still having difficulty with presuppositions that consider the listener's perspective. Although this aspect of communication begins to emerge early, it continues to develop throughout the preschool and school-age years.

We see evidence of communicative turn-taking before the child begins to use words, but as he moves from prelinguistic to linguistic communication, develops specific communicative intentions, and begins to use presuppositions, he begins to develop a turn-taking style more closely resembling adult conversation. By the time the child is eighteen months old, he is demonstrating some of the basic rules of turn-taking in his conversations with other people (Bloom, Rocissano, & Hood, 1976). If, for example, the child's conversational partner names an object in the child's possession, the child might make a comment about the object, but he will not repeat the label already identified by his partner. He presupposes this knowledge and uses his turn to describe the object or to explain to his partner what is going to happen next. His partner might then comment on the action the child has taken, and the child, presupposing knowledge of all that has been said before, uses his turn to contribute additional information or respond directly to his partner's comments. Turn-taking, assuming knowledge, and taking into account the partner's perspective are some of the bases of adult-like conversation.

Mid-Stage Review: What Is Happening So Far?

To this point, the child's productions have been mostly single words. Before we move to the combination phase of Stage One, it will be useful to review some of what we have discovered so far about the child's earliest language efforts. His first meaningful word appears at about twelve months. By the time he is eighteen months old, he will have about 50 words in his expressive vocabulary, and he will understand many more than that. His first words are mostly nouns, but he does use some action words, and he uses a few modifiers like "big," "bad," or "hot." These first words refer to things, events, people, and actions that are of personal interest to the child. They may not be adult forms of comparable words, and they are often used with wider or narrower meanings than adult versions of the same words. The child might call a dog a "gaga," for example. He might produce an adult-like version such as "doggie," but he might use "doggie" to refer to all four-legged animals, not just dogs, or he might use the word to refer to just one dog, the family pet. His first words are used for fairly specific purposes: to name objects or people, to request something, to control the behavior of someone else, or to express emotion. Even though he is typically using only one word at a time, he shows some understanding of conversation. In a limited way, he takes into account what his listener knows about a subject and tends not to repeat redundant information. He engages in a turn-taking style of communication that allows for comment and the contributions of new information on the parts of both conversational partners. By using basic body language and by varying intonation, the child can indicate that he is asking questions, and he can produce a negative communication by shaking his head or using the word "no," which is likely to show up in his vocabulary very early. Although it is true that adults must be pretty active interpreters to determine the semantic and pragmatic messages in the child's speech, this is pretty impressive stuff for a communicator whose utterances are mostly single words. Try to imagine what will happen to the child's communicative abilities when he begins to put words together.

The First Combinations: True Syntax or Transitional Productions?

Keep in mind that the child acquiring language has been given no instructions about what he is supposed to do next, and it is often difficult for the observer to figure out what the child is doing as he moves from one stage of language development to the next. In the child's first word combinations, we find a perfect example of this kind of problem. What is going on? What do these combinations tell us about the child's knowledge of syntax, semantics, pragmatics? Because these first combinations do not follow adult rules of grammar, because they often seem to be words simply strung together, and because they often appear in the midst of unintelligible productions not unlike babbling or vocal play, it is difficult to know what the child is doing and what he knows.

According to some observers, children do go through a transitional stage between single-word productions and multiple-word productions. Bloom (1973) reported, for example, that her daughter included the meaningless production, "wida," before and after a wide range of meaningful words. Some children repeat a word but vary prosodic elements like stress and intonation. Others produce what appear to be merely strings of single-word utterances. Bloom (1973) provides the example of the child who, while looking at a picture of another child in a play car, said "Go, car, ride." Because each word was produced with equal emphasis and ended with a falling pitch, Bloom concluded that these were three single-word utterances, not one multiple-word utterance. She argued that while these productions indicate that the child knows something about relationships among things, people, and actions, they do not suggest an understanding of the syntactic knowledge that results in the production of true sentences.

Not everyone agrees with Bloom's conclusions, however. Branigan (1979) reports that closer examination of what appear to be successive single-word utterances suggests that, although the pauses between words make them sound like distinct and separate productions, there are other prosodic variations that are more sentence-like. In some cases, not all the words end with a falling pitch, and the last word in the series is often produced with longer duration than the preceding words. These variations suggest that the child is putting the words together in some fashion, even if we cannot recognize the rules or the meaningfulness of the combinations.

Two-Word Productions: The Dawning of Syntax
Late Stage One (MLU: 1.5–2.0; Age: 22–26 mos.)

Whether or not there is a transitional stage between single-word and multiple-word productions, we know that the child typically begins to put two words together between the ages of 18 and 24 months. These combinations represent the beginning of language structure or **syntax**. The child discovers and applies rules for putting words together in a manner that creates meaning greater than the added meanings of the words alone. That's what makes a **sentence**. The meaning of any sentence is the result, not just of the cumulative meanings of the individual words, but of the interactive meanings of words based on their semantic and grammatical relationships with one another, and on how they are ordered in the sentence. The child's two-word utterances do not allow for much complexity in terms of sentence meaning, of course, but they do represent the beginning of syntax and the dramatic extension of meaning made possible by putting words together. Armed with a limited vocabulary and combining only two words at a time, the child is able to make declarative statements ("Daddy go"), and he is able to express negation ("No night-night"). Whereas early in Stage One, the child expressed questions by using a rising intonation on single-word productions ("Doggie?" or "Bye-bye?") or with single-word productions such as "What" or "Where," the child in late Stage One creates primitive interrogative forms by combining those words with other words in productions such as "What doing?" or "Where go?" These are very simple structures to be sure, but they are the embryos of real syntax.

The significance of two-word utterances can be examined and described on three levels: syntactic, semantic, and pragmatic. We consider each level separately, but keep in mind that this separation is for convenience only. When human beings communicate, whether they are adults or children, they do not fragment their messages into structure, meaning, and purpose. The meanings of words are enriched and clarified by the structuring of words into sentences, and our communicative intentions are facilitated, if we use language well, by choosing the right words with the right meanings and putting them in correct and appropriate relationships with one another in effectively crafted sentences.

The Syntactic Level: Arranging Words Appropriately

There are at least two ways to describe syntax in two-word utterances. Crystal, Fletcher, and Garman (1976) suggested that the child chooses two words from four basic sentence constructions: subject, verb, object, and adverbial. These options allow the child to produce clause-like utterances with subjects and predicates as well as phrase-like constructions that include modifications of a subject or predicate. For example, the child might say "Car go," a clause-like production in which "car" is the subject and "go" is the predicate. He might then say, "Go fast," a phrase-like construction in which "fast" is an adverbial modification of the verb "go." He might also produce a phrase like "Daddy car," in which "Daddy" is used to modify the noun "car."

Another approach to describing syntax at the two-word level was proposed by Braine (1963). Braine suggested that the child uses a primitive form of grammar called **Pivot-Open Grammar.** According to this view, the child has just two categories of words: open and pivot. **Open words** can be used alone, in combination with other open words, in combination with pivot words, and in either the first or second position of two-word utterances. **Pivot words** cannot be used alone, cannot be combined with other pivot words, but can be used in either the first or second position of utterances. This means then that the child can produce the following kinds of two-word sentences: Open + Open, Pivot + Open, or Open + Pivot, but he does not produce Pivot + Pivot sentences. One cannot assume that a given word will always be an open word or always a pivot word. Two children might use a given word in different ways so that the word is open for one but pivot for the other.

When Braine's grammar was first published, it seemed a promising way to describe and understand the child's early two-word utterances, but by 1970 some of the limitations of this approach were becoming apparent. One of the first language experts to express concern about the Pivot-Open Grammar was Bloom (1970), who criticized the approach because it did not take into account the meanings of the child's two-word productions. She contended that because the Pivot-Open Grammar considers only structure, it does not give the child adequate credit for his language knowledge. Using one child's productions as examples, Bloom contended that in one context, "Mommy sock" was produced when the child picked up one of her mother's socks. On another occasion when the child's mother was putting a sock on the child's foot, the child produced the same two-word utterance, "Mommy sock." Categorizing these productions as combinations of open and pivot words misses much of what is being communicated, according to Bloom. In the first case, "Mommy sock" is used to mean "This sock belongs to Mommy." In the second case, "Mommy sock" certainly seems to mean "Mommy is putting a sock on my foot." The first utterance focuses on possession. The second utterance is primarily concerned with action performed by an agent (mother) on an object (sock). One of Bloom's primary contentions, therefore, is that one cannot determine how a child is using language, what a child knows about language, or what a child means by the language he is using unless one takes **communicative context** into account. Using context to help determine the meanings of a child's utterances is referred to as **rich interpretation** by Brown (1973). This process has helped guide much of the research on the language of children since the early 1970s.

Semantic Level: Determining the Meanings of Early Sentences

Bloom's objections to a strictly syntactic description of the child's early word combinations, and her emphasis on taking communicative context into account, led to a semantic interpretation of early sentences. Bloom and Lahey (1978) asserted that early two-word utterances reflect an understanding on the child's part about meaning relations and rules for word order. To take this twofold understanding into account, they suggested that the rules the child uses at this juncture in development be referred to as **semantic-syntactic** rules. One might argue that when the child is producing two-word utterances, there is not much opportunity for creating language structure, just as it would be difficult to structure a wall with only two bricks. On the other hand, we have already discovered that the child is able to effectively communicate complete, and sometimes fairly sophisticated, thoughts with single-word utterances. What kind of messages might the child be able to convey if he puts words together with meaning relationships which, when they interact, communicate far more than the additive values of their meanings?

Language experts have proposed several semantic classification systems they believe will more adequately describe children's two-word combinations. Bloom (1970) was the first expert to identify semantic relations in the early language productions of three American children. A few years later, Roger Brown (1973) examined semantic relations in the early productions of children acquiring a range of languages from English to Samoan. Brown suggested that these early productions reflect what children know about the things and actions in their lives, and that the meanings they express are consistent with the level of their intellectual development. The following eight amalgamated meanings were typical of those produced by the late Stage One children who were the subjects in Brown's study:

Semantic-Syntactic Relation	Example
demonstrative (this/that) + entity	*That ball*
entity + attribute	*Kitty nice*
possessor + possession	*My dolly*
entity + location	*Dolly chair*
action + location	*Put table* (Object is being placed on a table)
agent + object	*Baby shoe*
agent + action	*Doggie sit*
action + object	*Drink juice*

Additional two-term relations have been identified by other researchers (Bloom, 1973; Schlesinger, 1971). For example, the child might use a **recurrence +** _____ production if he wants something to occur or appear again, as in "More juice!" He might use a **nonexistence/disappearance** production such as "Allgone juice" to proudly announce that he has finished his drink, that it has disappeared, that it no longer exists. He might use a **rejection** production such as "No 'tatoes!" when he exercises what he thinks is his right to refuse an order to finish his helping of mashed potatoes. He might use a **denial** production such as "Not kitty" in response to his mother's incorrect reference to the family dog as a "kitty." Among the forms children use to express negative semantic relations, nonexistence/disappearance is used by children more frequently than rejection or denial. The use of denial involves some fairly complicated cognitive and perceptual manipulations. That is, the child must compare the object or being described by the caregiver to his own perception and understanding of that object or being in order to make a judgment about the validity of the caregiver's observation or question. If the caregiver points to the family dog, for example, and asks, "Is that a kitty?" the child must compare his understanding about what he sees with his understanding about what a kitty is. If there is a mismatch between what he is being asked and what he knows, he produces the denial, "Not kitty!" (Hummer, Wimmer, & Antes, 1993). Researchers have noted that because this kind of production depends on fairly sophisticated perceptual and cognitive processing, it emerges at about 20–25 months, somewhat later than other productions that are otherwise comparable in terms of meaning and function (Bloom, 1970, 1973; Choi, 1988; Vaidyanathan, 1991).

Research has provided some information about the developmental order of a few semantic relations. According to Wells (1985), for example, when children express **entity + location,** they generally refer to the location of a static or stationary entity or object before they refer to the movement or action of placing an object *in* or *on* something. That is, the child will typically say something like, "Doggie chair," to indicate that a dog is sitting on a chair, before he manages a comment about an activity in progress involving the movement of an object from one place to another. Caregivers must patiently wait for the child to make a statement such as, "In box," to indicate that he is in the process of dumping a spoonful of mashed potatoes into his mother's sewing basket. This kind of utterance, in addition to creating a sense of excitement for mother, expresses an entity + location semantic relation in which there is the movement of something (mashed potatoes) from one place (the child's plate) to another (Mom's sewing basket). Wells' (1985) findings suggest that the child will produce location relations by 21 months, and that the typical child will be using two-word combinations to express attribute (attribute + entity) by the time he is two years old.

Using this kind of analysis, one might reasonably conclude that the child is able to talk about things, where they are, what actions they perform, what actions are performed on them, and who creates these actions. He is also able to identify characteristics or attributes of things, and he can express ownership or possession. We should not lose sight of the fact that the child in early Stage One can use single-word utterances to express relations such as **existence, nonexistence, disappearance,** and **recurrence,** but the successful communication of these relations during early Stage One depends heavily on the interpretative powers of adult listeners. When the child begins to use two-word combinations, interpretation remains difficult, but it is somewhat less murky because the child is now employing syntactic rules for ordering words in combination with the stress patterns of his language to help convey his intended meanings. Interpretation is also facilitated by context. That is, if the adult takes into account what was said prior to the utterance being interpreted, and if she considers the nonlinguistic circumstances surrounding the production, she is more likely to correctly interpret the meaning of the child's message.

As the child develops into late Stage One (22–26 months), he continues to make steady, if not always dramatic, progress in terms of semantic-syntactic relations. There is evidence that the child will begin to produce three- and even four-word combinations at approximately 24 months. Only about half of his productions at this point are two-word utterances (Owens, 1996, pp. 265–266). Productions such as "Baby push truck" (agent + action + object), and "Daddy put box" (agent + action + location, to indicate that Daddy is putting something in the box), are not uncommon utterances for the late Stage One child.

The Pragmatic Level: An Emphasis on the Functions of Early Sentences

Throughout this chapter we have cited the work of Dore (1974, 1975) and Halliday (1975) to trace the development of communicative intents during Stage One of language development. Before the child begins using words, he is able to express four communicative intentions, according to Halliday. When the child uses words, he expands his repertoire of intentions to about seven. When the child begins to put words together, between the ages of 18 and 24 months, we see additional changes in communicative intentions. The child now engages in what can properly be considered dialogue. That is, he understands that in two-way communication, the participants fill and exchange certain roles. One speaks and the other listens, then the listener speaks and the speaker listens. When one speaks, the other sometimes responds to the message expressed by the speaker, sometimes by simply acknowledging the message, sometimes by adding information, sometimes by agreeing or disagreeing. Sometimes the speaker is a questioner and the listener is a responder. There are many roles to be filled in communication, and even with a limited expressive vocabulary and only single-word and two-word utterances, the child is able to fill these roles.

The functions or intentions we identified earlier from Halliday's work are now combined and modified into at least three new functions: pragmatic, mathetic, and informative. The **pragmatic** function of language is undoubtedly the most basic. That is, the child uses language to get things done. He uses language to make requests and demands, to satisfy his needs, to interact with and control the behavior of other people. The **mathetic** function of language is manifested in communications concerned with learning. The child uses language to learn about himself and about his world. He comments, questions, predicts, and remembers. He uses language to express his developing understanding of how people, things, and events are connected. His language, however limited, is a reflection of his intellectual development. The **informative** function emerges when the child uses language to give new information to others. Adults often think of the informative function as the most basic function of language and probably the first to emerge, but it is actually one of the last. Why? One cannot use language to inform until he knows something others do not or until one thinks he knows something he assumes others do not know. In the beginning, everyone knows more than the child! Before Stage One ends, however, the child is more than happy to use language to tell others what he knows, even if what he "knows" is incorrect, incomplete, or irrelevant. He uses language to inform the dog, brothers and sisters, Mom and Dad, Teddy Bear, and anyone else who cares to profit from his wisdom. This is one of the most delightful functions of early multiple-word utterances. When this child speaks, listen, learn, enjoy, and be prepared to be amazed.

The child at this stage abides by some of the basic rules of conversation. He will address his conversational partner by name to gain his or her attention before speaking. He will listen before he responds, and he understands the turn-taking aspect of conversation. His primary limitation as a conversationalist is a short attention span. He will usually stay on the same topic for only a few turns before he is ready to move on to something else (Bloom, Rocissano, & Hood, 1976). We will see a dramatic change in this aspect of conversation after the child passes his third birthday. It's quite possible that you have already encountered a three-year-old who wanted to talk about a topic long after your knowledge and/or interest was exhausted.

Comprehension and Production: A Critical and Evolving Relationship

Before we conclude our description (of language development in Stage One, we need to include a brief review of what the child comprehends at this time. Expressive language cannot be separated from receptive language, of course. As the child matures, what he understands dramatically impacts what he is able to express and how he expresses it.

For as long as people have systematically studied language and language development, there have been questions about the relationship between comprehension and production. There is appealing logic in the assumption that comprehension must precede production, and that view has been held by many linguists through the years. In fact, one notable linguist of the present era, Ingram (1974, p. 313), makes the clear assertion that "comprehension ahead of production is a linguistic universal of acquisition." Others are not sure that the relationship is this simple. Bloom (1974), for example, argues that although we do not know the precise character of the relationship between comprehension and production, we know it is a relationship, of shared dependence. Whatever the true nature of this relationship, it seems clear that it changes as language develops, and it is not the same for all components of language. As we noted in the opening section of this chapter, the infant comprehends differences among speech sounds, sequences of speech sounds, and intonational patterns long before he produces sounds and superimposes intonational patterns on sequences of sounds. These discriminations are made within the first half of the first year (Goodsitt et al., 1984; Kessen, Levine, & Wendrich, 1979), while comparable productions do not occur until after the first birthday.

When the child begins to produce his first meaningful words, we see a changing relationship between comprehension and production. The child produces words *before* he has a complete understanding of them. We have already noted, for example, that the child might use the word "doggie" to refer to only the family pet, or he might use "doggie" to refer to any four-legged animal. There is some comprehension associated with this production, of course, but it is not a complete comprehension according to adult standards. Only after the child experiences sufficient intellectual development to understand "doggie" as a category that includes all dogs but only dogs, and only after he acquires additional words in his vocabulary to reflect this understanding will his comprehension of "doggie" be complete. In the meantime, the child's ability to understand is greatly influenced by all the nonlinguistic cues that surround the words spoken to him. Because adults

often fail to take this nonlinguistic information into account, they may overestimate what the child really comprehends in the words spoken to him, and they may
overestimate, based on the child's language production, the child's real language
competence.

According to Benedict (1979), comprehension does precede production to a
significant extent for the first 50 words. The eight children in her study compre-
hended about 50 words before they were able to produce 10 words. They com-
prehended 50 words at 13 months, but did not produce 50 words until they were
19 months old. Their receptive vocabularies increased by about 22 words per
month, but their expressive vocabularies grew by only 9 or 10 words each month.
Based on these findings, it is reasonable to conclude that in early language development, the gap between comprehension and production is substantial.

In the beginning, comprehension is not language-based. That is, the child
does not understand a word like "doggie" in reference to a dictionary definition.
The child's first understandings are based on nonverbal insights about things,
actions, and the relationships among things and actions (Huttenlocher, 1974).
Paul (1990) referred to this type of understanding as knowledge based on routines, or scripts of events, in which repetitions of the event itself in combination
with adults' repetitive linguistic and nonlinguistic behaviors associated with the
event facilitate word comprehension. The child understands important and basic
categories of things like food, people, and pets. He understands basic actions like
eating or sitting, and he understands obvious relationships like putting food into
the mouth. The child conceptualizes these things, actions, and relationships apart
from language, but as he hears certain sequences of sounds produced in connection with these mental representations, he associates the sequences of sounds, or
words, with the things, actions, and relationships. When the connections become
established, the words serve to help the child recall the things, actions, and relationships to which the words refer. It is important to notice the sequence in comprehension Huttenlocher is suggesting. The child first understands aspects or
characteristics of things and actions in his environment. He then creates mental
pictures or concepts of these things and actions, and he gradually associates these
mental pictures with spoken words. The words help him to retrieve the mental
pictures.

As one might guess, the child comprehends names for things and people
before he comprehends words that describe actions and relationships. As one
might also guess, the child understands words for things and people in the here
and now before he understands words for things and people that are absent in
time and/or space. The findings of a study of children between the ages of 10 and
21 months by Miller, Chapman, Branston, and Reichle (1980) suggest a fairly consistent sequence of comprehensions. All of the twelve-month-old subjects understood names for people in sight, and about half understood words for things in
their presence. Words describing actions were understood by most of the subjects
older than 15 months. A little more than half of the children between 19 and 21

months understood words referring to people and things not present. Semantic relationships in two- and three-word utterances were understood only by those children over eighteen months. Among the semantic relationships studied, the most often understood was possessor + possession as in "My doggie" or "Mommy shoe."

Just as adults may overestimate the child's understanding of single words, they may overestimate what the child is able to comprehend in the sentences he hears. Chapman (1978) suggests that when the child responds to utterances, he may use comprehension strategies that give the impression of greater understanding than the child actually possesses. For example, when an adult says, "Throw the ball," the child might pick up the ball and throw it. The adult assumes the child understands the words "ball" and "throw" and the relationship between them. If the adult then says, "Hide the ball," or "Kiss the ball," or "Hit the ball," the child is likely to throw the ball again. If the child has selected the ball from among several objects, it might be safe to assume he understands the word "ball," but he may not understand the rest of the words in any of these sentences. What he does know is that balls are for throwing, so whenever he hears "ball" in an utterance, he throws it. His comprehension strategy, therefore, is to perform the action on an object most commonly associated with that object. Assuming he understands the words "milk," "cookie," and "ball," he *drinks* milk, *eats* the cookie, and *throws* the ball, no matter what other words happen to surround the words he knows in sentences spoken to him.

Huttenlocher (1974) asserts that when the child *comprehends* language, he uses a word to retrieve the mental image of an object, person, or action. When he *produces* language, he recognizes an object, person, or action, and must retrieve the matching word. Comprehension involves an easier or more direct association between object and word than production, according to Huttenlocher, because the child's understanding of objects, people, and events is more complete than his understanding of the words used to represent them. Adults often have a similar experience with a foreign language. It is easier to comprehend a new language than to speak it because when we listen to the vocabulary of the new language that is not well known, we move to the vocabulary of our native language, which is well understood. When we try to speak the language, we must move from the known to the incompletely known, a much more difficult task. During language development, this difference seems to be reflected in the occurrence of overextensions. The child tends to overextend the meanings of words in production but not in comprehension. In the example we have used several times, the child overextends the word "doggie" to include not only dogs, but cats, horses, cows, and many other four-legged animals. The same child who produces "doggie" to refer to a cow would likely point to the correct animal if, while looking at a cat, dog, and cow, an adult produced each animal's name. In other words, it is easier for the child to retrieve his mental image of an object than to retrieve the word that represents the object.

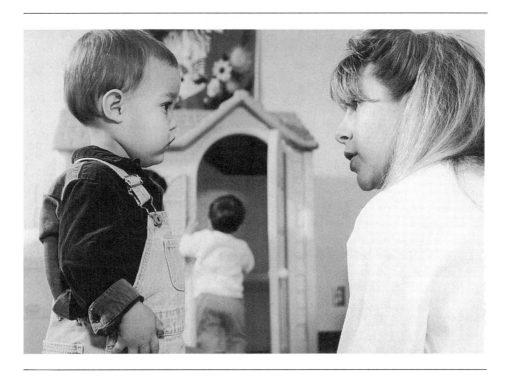

Caregiver–child interactions make important contributions to language development.

The Role of the Caregiver in the Acquisition of Early Language

The reader must keep in mind that language does not develop in a vacuum. The child brings to the acquisition process a strong biological drive to develop language, and the emergence of language is closely associated with cognitive development, but the child will not acquire language unless he is exposed to language models. There is evidence too that simply hearing language is not enough. The child's communicative interactions with his caregivers facilitate vocabulary acquisition (Ahktar, Dunham, & Dunham, 1991) and overall language development. When a caregiver responds to her child's early utterances, she often **expands** them. If the child says, "Daddy work," the caregiver might respond, "Yes, Daddy went to work." The caregiver does not change the order of the words in the child's utterance, and she maintains what she believes is the child's communicative intent, but she expands the utterance into a complete form. According to Hirsch-Pasek, Treiman, and Schneiderman (1984), caregivers expand about 20 percent of their two-year-old children's utterances into more syntactically correct and complete sentences, and children often respond to these expansions by imitating them (Folger & Chapman, 1978).

Although we do not know precisely what expansions contribute to language development, Scherer and Olswang (1984) believe they assist the acquisition of language by helping the child better understand the grammatical functions of words and the rules by which words are combined, by keeping the communicative effort focused on subjects the child has selected, and by reinforcing the turn-taking aspect of conversation. Farrar (1990) suggests that the child may derive different benefits from different types of expansion in learning grammatical morphemes. For example, restating the child's utterances with added or revised grammatical morphemes may assist the child in acquiring plurals and possessives, whereas expanding the topic or general intent of the child's utterance may be more helpful in the acquisition of other grammatical morphemes, including tense markers. Apparently caregivers are sensitive to the length and complexity of their own models even before they expand the child's utterances.. According to Murray, Johnson, and Peters (1990), caregivers actually produce shorter utterances when they talk to toddlers than when they talk to infants. Furthermore, there seems to be a relationship between these shorter adult utterances during the second half of the child's first year and his receptive language abilities at eighteen months. It appears that when adults sense that the child is old enough to benefit from speech and language models, they pay greater attention to the length and complexity of the models they provide in order to give the child clear and attainable language targets. Then when the child begins to produce his own utterances, adults provide additional assistance through various forms of expansion.

Sometimes a caregiver will do more than expand the child's utterance. In an example similar to the one in the preceding paragraph, the child might say, "Daddy go," and the caregiver responds by saying, "Yes, Daddy went to work." In this case, the caregiver is not only providing a more syntactically accurate model, but she is providing additional semantic information. This kind of response is called **extension.** On other occasions, the caregiver will simply imitate what the child has said. Very often when the adult imitates the child's utterance, the child will imitate the imitation to create a simple form of turn-taking. Whether the caregiver expands, extends, or imitates, the child is taking the communicative initiative, but he is being provided models that include enriched syntactic and semantic information. Of no less importance, the child is being encouraged in his language attempts and rewarded for his successful communication connections.

Stage One: A Brief Look Back and a Glimpse Forward

This stage began with the production of first words and ended with the production of combinations of words. The child produces his first word at about 12 months and begins to combine words at about 18 months. His expressive vocabulary grows

TABLE 4-4 Stage One Highlights

Typical Age Range: 12 to 26 Months
MLU: 1.0 TO 2.0 Morphemes

First Words
- Do not always sound like adult words.
- Used in reference to things of greatest importance to the child: people, objects, actions of immediate interest.
- Most are single-syllable words or single syllables repeated.
- May infrequently exhibit overextended or underextended meanings.

Pragmatics
- Uses nonverbal and verbal communication to satisfy needs and wants, control the behavior of others, interact with others, express emotion or interest, explore and categorize, imagine, and inform.
- Demonstrates primitive presuppositional and turn-taking skills.

Multi-Word Productions
- The combining of two words typically begins at 18 to 24 months.
- Three-word and some four-word combinations appear when about half of the child's utterances are two-word productions.
- These productions can be interpreted at three levels: syntactic, semantic, and pragmatic.

Sentence Types
- In early Stage One, the child uses a rising intonation on single words to pose *Yes/No questions,* and he may use approximated forms of *What* or *Where* to ask questions.
- In late Stage One, the child combines two and three words, but still using a rising intonation to pose *Yes/No* questions as in "That + ___?" *Wh* interrogative words are still limited to *what* and *where.*
- In early Stage One, words such as *no, gone,* and *allgone* appear. One of these words may be used in combination with another word (negative + ___).
- In late Stage One, the words *no* and *not* are used interchangeably at the beginning of word combinations. e.g., "No bye-bye!"
- In early Stage One, declarative statements are limited to two constructions: *agent + action* and *action + object.*
- In late Stage One, the child forms declarative statements by combining *subject + verb + object.*
- In late Stage One, the prepositions *in* and *on* are embedded in a sentence.
- In late Stage One, the child uses *and* to form conjoined sentences.

Comprehension
- Comprehension probably precedes production for the first 50 words.
- Understanding names for things and people precedes understanding of words describing actions and relationships.
- Understanding of early words appears to be facilitated by knowledge of event routines or scripts.

Role of Caregiver
- Provides models for language development and opportunities for communicative interactions.
- Assists by expanding and extending the child's utterances.

from one word at the beginning of the stage to 200 to 300 words by the end of the stage. His first words are mostly nouns used to name people or objects. By the end of the stage, he is producing two-word, and even some three- and four-word utterances to make statements, ask questions, express negatives, and make demands. He is using language to get things done, to manipulate the behaviors of other people, and exchange information in a rudimentary form of conversation, complete with turntaking and presuppositional skills, although these skills are just beginning to emerge and are quite primitive by adult standards.

During the remaining stages, the child will learn to produce a greater variety of sentences and to make them more elaborate. He will learn how to put simple sentences together to produce compound sentences and how to put sentences into one another to make complex sentences. He will also become a more sophisticated conversationalist, and of course, his vocabulary will grow, and his understanding of the meanings of words and word combinations will increase. As exciting and full as Stage One has been, the child's language development has truly just begun!

Review Questions

1. Before he has language, how does the child communicate? What are the limitations of these prelinguistic communications?

2. Identify and discuss the infant's perceptual abilities. How do these early perceptual abilities apparently prepare the child for speech production?

3. Describe the prelinguistic interactions of infants and adults. What arguments might be developed to support the importance of infant-adult interactions in communication development?

4. Trace communication production during the infancy months from cries to words. How does each progression appear to build upon behaviors produced earlier to make oral communication more sophisticated and adult-like?

5. What is the value of a *stage* view of language development? What are the potential dangers of adhering too rigidly to this view in studying the development of any set of behaviors in human beings?

6. Define and provide examples for each of the following: morpheme, free morpheme, bound morpheme, derivational bound morpheme, and inflectional bound morpheme.

7. What is mean length of utterance and what is its value in tracing early language development?

8. Briefly describe the following views concerning how children attach meanings to words: semantic feature hypothesis, functional core hypothesis, and prototype hypothesis.

9. Assuming it is not appropriate to classify the child's first words into traditional grammatical categories, how can they be classified?

10. What functions are filled by the child's first words?

11. What does the Stage One child seem to understand about conversational techniques?

12. What are the developmental changes in communication functions associated with the perlocutionary, illocutionary, and locutionary stages?

13. What are the primary semantic-syntactic rules the child expresses in Stage One?

14. How does the child construct the following sentence types as he progresses through Stage One: declaratives, interrogatives, negatives, and conjoined?

15. What is the importance of "joint referencing" in the development of child language?

16. What language knowledge might be reflected in the child's first word combinations?

17. Discuss the evolving relationship between comprehension and production during early language development.

18. Describe Dore's categorization scheme for children's early utterances.

19. What is the role of the child's caregiver during Stage One of language development?

References and Suggested Readings

Ahktar, N., Dunham, F., & Dunham, P. (1991). Directive interactions and early vocabulary development: The role of joint attentional focus. *Journal of Child Language, 18,* 41–49.

Aslin, R., Pisoni, D., & Jusczyk, P. (1983). Auditory development and speech perception in infancy. In M. Haith & J. Campos (Eds.), *Handbook of child psychology: Vol. 2. Infancy and developmental psychobiology.* New York: Wiley.

Austin, J. (1962). *How to do things with words.* London: Oxford University Press.

Barrett, M., Harris, M., & Chasin, J. (1991). Early lexical development and maternal speech: A comparison of children's initial and subsequent uses of words. *Journal of Child Language, 18,* 21–40.

Bates, E. (1979). *The emergence of symbols: Cognition and communication in infancy.* New York: Academic.

Bates, E., Bretherton, L., Shore, C., & McNew, S. (1983). Names, gestures and objects: The role of context in the emergence of symbols. In K. Nelson (Ed.), *Children's language* (Vol. 4). Hillsdale, NJ: Erlbaum.

Bates, E., Camaioni, L., & Volterra, V. (1975). The acquisition of performatives prior to speech. *Merrill-Palmer Quarterly, 21,* 205–216.

Bates, E., Marchman, V., Thal, D., Fenson, L., Dale, P., Reznick, J., Reilly, J., & Hartung, J. (1994). Developmental and stylistic variation in the composition of early vocabulary. *Journal of Child Language, 21,* 85–123.

Benedict, H. (1979). Early lexical development: comprehension and production. *Journal of Child Language, 6,* 183–200.

Bernstein, D. (1989). Language development: The preschool years. In D. Bernstein & E. Tiegerman (Eds.), *Language and communication disorders in children* (2nd ed.). Columbus, OH: Merrill/Macmillan.

Blake, J., & deBoysson-Bardies, B. (1992). Patterns of babbling: A cross-linguistic study. *Journal of Child Language, 19,* 51–74.

Bloom, L. (1970). *Language development: Form and function of emerging grammars.* Cambridge, MA: MIT Press.

Bloom, L. (1973). *One word at a time: The use of single-word utterances before syntax.* The Hague: Mouton.

Bloom, L. (1974). Talking, understanding, and thinking. In R. Schiefelbusch & L. Lloyd (Eds.), *Language perspectives: Acquisition, retardation and intervention.* Baltimore: University Park Press.

Bloom, L., & Lahey, M. (1978). *Language development and language disorders.* New York: Wiley.

Bloom, L., Rocissano, L., & Hood, L. (1976). Adult-child discourse: Developmental interaction between information processing and linguistic interaction. *Cognitive Psychology, 8,* 521–552.

Bowerman, M. (1978). The acquisition of word meaning: An investigation into some current conflicts. In N. Waterson & C. Snow (Eds.), *The development of communication.* New York: Wiley.

Braine, M. (1963). The ontogeny of English phrase structure: The first phrase. *Language, 39,* 1–13.

Branigan, G. (1979). Some reasons why successive single word utterances are not. *Journal of Child Language, 6,* 411–421.

Brazelton, T., & Cramer, B. (1990). *The earliest relationship: Parents, infants, and the drama of early attachment.* Reading, MA: Addison-Wesley Publishing Company.

Bretherton, I. (1988). How to do things with one word: The ontogenesis of intentional message-making in infancy. In M. Smith & J. Locke (Eds.), *The emergent lexicon: The child's development of a linguistic vocabulary.* San Diego, CA: Academic Press.

Bridger, W. (1961). Sensory habituation and discrimination in the human neonate. *American Journal of Psychiatry, 117,* 991–996.

Brown, R. (1973). *A first language: The early stages.* Cambridge, MA: Harvard University Press.

Bruner, J. (1981). The social context of language acquisition. *Language and Communication, 1,* 155–178.

Bruner, J., & Sylva, K. *Acquiring the uses of language.* Manuscript in preparation.

Bushnell, I., Sai, F., & Mullin, J. (1989). Neonatal recognition of the mother's face. *British Journal of Developmental Psychology, 7,* 3–15.

Carpenter, K. (1991). Later rather than sooner: Extralinguistic categories in the acquisition of Thai classifiers. *Journal of Child Language, 18,* 93–113.

Carter, A. (1975). The transformation of sensorimotor morphemes into words: A case study of the development of "more" and "mine." *Journal of Child Language, 2,* 233–250.

Caselli, M. (1990). Communicative gestures and first words. In V. Bolterra & C. Erting (Eds.), *From gesture to sign in hearing and deaf children* (pp. 56–67). New York: Springer-Verlag.

Chapman, R. (1978). Comprehension strategies in children. In J. Kavanaugh & W. Strange (Eds.), *Speech and language in the laboratory, school, and clinic.* Cambridge, MA: MIT Press.

Choi, S. (1988). The semantic development of negation: A cross-linguistic longitudinal study. *Journal of Child Language, 15,* 517–531.

Clark, E. (1973). What's in a word? On the child's acquisition of semantics in his first language. In T. Moore (Ed.), *Cognitive development and the acquisition of language.* New York: Academic.

Clark, E. (1975). Knowledge, context and strategy in the acquisition of meaning. In D. Dato (Ed.), *Developmental psycholinguistics: Theory and application.* Washington, DC: Georgetown University Press.

Clarke-Stewart, K. (1973). Interactions between mothers and their young children: Characteristics and consequences. *Monographs of the Society for Research in Child Development, 38* (Serial No. 153).

Crystal, D., Fletcher, P., & Garman, M. (1976). *The grammatical analysis of language disability: A procedure for assessment and remediation.* London: Edward Arnold.

Davis, B., & MacNeilage, P. (1990). Acquisition of correct vowel production: A quantitative case study. *Journal of Speech and Hearing Research, 33,* 16–27.

deVilliers, J., & deVilliers, P. (1978). *Language acquisition.* Cambridge, MA: Harvard University Press.

D'Odorico, L. (1984). Nonsegmental features in prelinguistic communications: An analysis of some types of infant cry and noncry vocalizations. *Journal of Child Language, 11,* 17–27.

Dore, J. (1975). Holophrases, speech acts and language universals. *Journal of Child Language, 2,* 21–40.

Dore, J. (1974). A pragmatic description of early language development. *Journal of Psycholinguistic Research, 3,* 343–350.

Ebeling, K. S., & Gelman, S. A. (1994). Children's use of context in interpreting "big" and "little." *Child Development, 65,* 1178–1192.

Eimas, P., Siqueland, E., Jusczyk, P., & Vigorito, J. (1971). Speech perception in infants, *Science, 171,* 303–306.

Eisenberg, R. (1976). *Auditory competence in early life: The roots of communicative behavior.* Baltimore: University Park Press.

Farrar, M. (1990). Discourse and the acquisition of grammatical morphemes. *Journal of Child Language, 17,* 607–624.

Fernald, A. (1985). Four-month-old infants prefer to listen to motherese. *Infant Behavior and Development, 8,* 181–195.

Fernald, A. (1994). Human maternal vocalizations to infants as biologically relevant signals: An evolutionary perspective. In P. Bloom (Ed.), *Language acquisition: Core readings.* Cambridge, MA: MIT Press.

Fernald, A., & Morikawa, H. (1993). Common themes and cultural differences in Japanese and American mothers' speech to infants. *Child Development, 64,* 637–656.

Ferguson, C. (1978). Learning to pronounce: The earliest stages of phonological development in the child. In F. Minifie & L. Lloyd (Eds.), *Communicative and cognitive abilities—Early behavioral assessment.* Baltimore: University Park Press.

Folger, J., & Chapman, R. (1978). A pragmatic analysis of spontaneous imitations. *Journal of Child Language, 5,* 25–38.

Gentner, D. (1982). Why nouns are learned before verbs: Linguistic relativity versus natural partitioning. In S. Kuczaj (Ed.), *Language development: Vol 2. Language, Thought, and Culture.* Hillsdale, NJ: Erlbaum.

Ginsberg, G., & Kilbourne, B. (1988). Emergence of vocal alternation in mother-infant interchanges. *Journal of Child Language, 15,* 221–235.

Goldfield, B., & Reznick, J. (1990). Early lexical acquisitions: Rate, content, and the vocabulary spurt. *Journal of Child Language, 17,* 171–183.

Goodsitt, J., Morse, P., VerHoeve, J., & Cowan, N. (1984). Infant speech recognition in multisyllabic contexts. *Child Development, 55,* 903–910.

Gopnik, A., & Choi, S. (1990). Language and cognition. *First Language, 10,* 199–216.

Gopnik, A., & Meltzoff, A. (1984). Semantic and cognitive development in 15- to 21-month-old children. *Journal of Child Development, 11,* 495–513.

Gopnik, A., & Meltzoff, A. (1986). Relations between semantic and cognitive development in the one-word stage: The specificity hypothesis. *Child Development, 57,* 1040–1053.

Gopnik, A., & Meltzoff, A. (1987). The development of categorization in the second year and its relation to other cognitive and linguistic developments, *Child Development, 58,* 1523–1531.

Greenfield, P. (1978). Informativeness, presupposition, and semantic choice in single-word utterances. In N. Waterson & C. Snow (Eds.), *The development of communication.* New York: Wiley.

Greenfield, P., & Smith, J. (1976). *The structure of communication in early language development.* New York: Academic Press.

Grieser, D. L., & Kuhl, P. (1988). Maternal speech to infants in a tonal language: Support for universal prosodic features in motherese. *Developmental Psychology, 24,* 14–20.

Halliday, M. (1975). *Learning how to mean: Explorations in the development of language.* New York: Edward Arnold.

Harding, C. (1983a). Acting with intention: A framework for examining the development of intention. In L. Feagans, C. Garvey, & R. Golinkoff (Eds.), *The origins and growth of communication.* Norwood, NJ: Ablex.

Harding, C. (1983b). Setting the stage for language acquisition: Communication development in the first year. In R. Golinkoff (Ed.), *The transition from prelinguistic to linguistic communication.* Hillsdale, NJ: Erlbaum.

Hickey, T. (1993). Identifying formulas in first language acquisition. *Journal of Child Language, 20,* 27–41.

Hilke, D. (1988). Infant vocalizations and changes in experience. *Journal of Child Language, 15,* 1–15.

Hirsh-Pasek, K., Treiman, R., & Schneiderman, M. (1984). Brown and Hanlon revisited: Mother's sensitivity to ungrammatical forms. *Journal of Child Language, 11,* 81–88.

Horgan, D. (1981). Rate of language acquisition and noun emphasis. *Journal of Psycholinguistic Research, 10,* 629–640.

Hummer, P., Wimmer, H., & Antes, G. (1993). On the origins of denial. *Journal of Child Language, 20,* 607–618.

Huttenlocher, J. (1974) The origins of language comprehension. In R. Soslo (Ed.), *Theories in cognitive psychology: The Loyola symposium.* New York: Wiley.

Ingram, D. (1974). The relationship between comprehension and production. In R. Schiefelbusch & L. Lloyd (Eds.), *Language perspectives—Acquisition, retardation, and intervention.* Baltimore: University Park Press.

Ingram, D. (1976). *Phonological disability in children.* London: Edward Arnold.

James, S. (1990). *Normal language acquisition.* Austin, TX: Pro-Ed.

Kaye, K. (1977). Towards the origin of dialogue. In H. Schaffer (Ed.), *Studies in mother-child interaction.* London: Academic Press.

Kaye, K. (1979). Thickening thin data: The maternal role in developing communication and language. In M. Bullowa (Ed.), *Before speech.* New York: Cambridge University Press.

Kaye, K. (1980). Why we don't talk "baby talk" to babies. *Journal of Child Language, 7,* 489–507.

Kessen, W., Levine, J., & Wendrich, K. (1979). The imitation of pitch in infants. *Infant Behavior and Development, 2,* 93–100.

Lewis, M. (1951). *Infant speech: A study of the beginnings of language.* New York: Humanities Press.

Lynch, M., Oller, K., & Steffens, M. (1989). Development of speech-like vocalizations in a child with congenital absence of cochleas: The case of total deafness. *Applied Psycholinguistics, 10,* 315–333.

Marchman, V. A., & Bates, E. (1991). *Vocabulary size and composition as predictors of morphological development.* Technical Report No. 9103, Center for Research in Language, University of California, San Diego.

Marchman, V. A., & Bates, E. (1994). Continuity in lexical and morphological development: A test of the critical mass hypothesis. *Journal of Child Language, 21,* 339–366.

Marcos, H. (1987). Communicative function of pitch range and pitch direction in infants. *Journal of Child Language, 14,* 255–268.

Mervis, C. A., & Mervis, C. B. (1988). Role of adult input in young children's category evolution: An observational study. *Journal of Child Language, 15,* 257–272.

Miller, J., Chapman, R., Branston, M., & Reichle, J. (1980). Language comprehension in sensorimotor stages V and VI. *Journal of Speech and Hearing Research, 23,* 284–311.

Miller, J., and Chapman, R. (1981). The relation between age and mean length of utterance in morphemes. *Journal of Speech and Hearing Research, 24,* 154–161.

Mitchell, P., & Kent, R. (1990). Phonetic variation in multisyllabic babbling. *Journal of Child Language, 17,* 247–265.

Moon, C., Bever, T. G., & Fifer, W. P. (1992) Canonical and non-canonical syllable discrimination by two-day-old infants. *Journal of Child Language, 19,* 1–17.

Murray, A., Johnson, J., & Peters, J. (1990). Fine tuning of utterance length to pre-verbal infants: Effects on later language development. *Journal of Child Language, 17,* 511–525.

Nakazima, S. A. (1975). Phonemicization and symbolization in language development. In E. H. Lenneberg & E. Lenneberg (Eds.), *Foundations of language: Vol. 1. A multidisciplinary approach.* New York: Academic Press.

Nelson, K. (1973). Structure and strategy in learning to talk. *Monographs of the Society for Research in Child Development, 38.*

Nelson, K. (1974). Concept, word and sentence: interrelations in acquisition and development. *Psychological Review, 31,* 267–285.

Oller, D. (1980). The emergence of the sounds of speech in infancy. In G. Yeni-Komshian, J. Kavanagh, & C. Ferguson (Eds.), *Child phonology, Vol. 1. Production.* New York: Academic Press.

Oller, D., Eilers, R., Bull, D., & Carney, A. (1985). Prespeech vocalizations of a deaf infant: A comparison with normal metaphonological development. *Journal of Speech and Hearing Research, 28,* 47–62.

Oller, D., & Eilers, R. (1988). The role of audition in infant babbling. *Child Development, 59,* 441–449.

Owens, R. (1991). *Language disorders: A functional approach to assessment and intervention.* Columbus, OH: Merrill/Macmillan.

Owens, R. (1996). *Language development: An introduction* (4th ed.). Needham Heights, MA: Allyn & Bacon.

Paul, R. (1990). Comprehension strategies: Interactions between world knowledge and the development of sentence comprehension. *Topics in Language Disorders, 10* (3), 63–75.

Penman., R., Cross, T., Milgrom-Friedman, J., & Meares, R. (1983). Mothers' speech to prelingual infants: A pragmatic analysis. *Journal of Child Language, 10,* 17–34.

Petitto, L. A. (1984). *From gesture to symbol: The relationship between form and the meaning in the acquisition of personal pronouns in American Sign Language.* Unpublished doctoral dissertation, Harvard University, Cambridge, MA.

Petitto, L. A. (1985a, October). *On the use of prelinguistic gestures in hearing and deaf children.* Paper presented at the 10th Annual Boston University Conference on Language Development, Boston.

Petitto, L. A. (1985b). *"Language" in the prelinguistic child* (Tech Rep. No. 4). Montreal: McGill University, Department of Psychology.

Petitto, L. A. (1986). *From gesture to symbol: The relationship between form and the meaning in the acquisition of personal pronouns in American Sign Language.* Bloomington: Indiana University Linguistics Club Press.

Petitto, L. A. (1987). On the autonomy of language and gesture: Evidence from the acquisition of personal pronouns in American Sign Language. *Cognition, 27*(1), 1–52.

Petitto, L. A. (1988). "Language" in the prelinguistic child. In F. Kessel (Ed.), *Development of language and language researchers: Essays in honor of Roger Brown* (pp. 187–221). Hillsdale, NJ: Erlbaum.

Petitto, L. A., & Marentette, P. F. (1990, October). *The timing of linguistic milestones in sign language acquisition: Are first signs acquired earlier than first words?* Paper presented at the 15th Annual Boston University Conference on Language Development, Boston, MA.

Pettito, L. A., & Marentette, P. F. (1991, April). The timing of linguistic milestones in sign and spoken language acquisition. In L. Petitto (Chair), *Are the linguistic milestones in signed and spoken language acquisition similar or different?* Symposium conducted at the Biennial Meeting of the Society for Research in Child Development, Seattle, WA.

Phillips, J. (1973). Syntax and vocabulary of mothers' speech to young children: Age and sex comparisons. *Child Development, 44,* 182–185.

Prutting, C. (1979). Process: The action of moving forward progressively from one point to another on the way to completion. *Journal of Speech and Hearing Disorders, 44,* 3–30.

Reed, V. (Ed.). (1986). *An introduction to children with language disorders.* New York: Macmillan.

Rees, N. (1972). The role of babbling in the child's acquisition of language. *British Journal of Disorders in Communication, 4,* 17–23.

Robb, M., & Saxman, J. (1990). Syllable durations of preword and early word vocalizations. *Journal of Speech and Hearing Research, 33,* 585–593.

Rondal, J., & Cession, A. (1990). Input evidence regarding the semantic bootstrapping hypothesis. *Journal of Child Language, 17,* 711–717.

Ryan, J. (1974). Early language development: Towards a communicational analysis. In P. Richards (Ed.), *The integration of a child into a social world.* London: Cambridge University Press.

Sachs, J. (1989). Communication development in infancy. In J. Berko-Gleason (Ed.), *The development of language.* Columbus, OH: Merrill/Macmillan.

Scherer, N., & Olswang, L. (1984). Role of mothers' expansions in stimulating children's language production. *Journal of Speech and Hearing Research, 27,* 387–396.

Schlesinger, I. (1971). Production of utterances and language acquisition. In D. Slobin (Ed.), *The ontogenesis of grammar.* New York: Academic Press.

Schlesinger, I. (1977). The role of cognitive development and linguistic input in language acquisition. *Journal of Child Language, 4,* 153–169.

Schwartz, R., & Leonard, L. (1994). Words, objects, and actions in early lexical acquisition. *Journal of Speech and Hearing Research, 27,* 119–127.

Searle, J. (1965). What is a speech act? In M. Black (Ed.), *Philosophy in America.* New York: Allen & Unwin, Cornell University Press.

Searle, J. (1969). *Speech acts.* Cambridge: Cambridge University Press.

Siegel, G., Cooper, M., Morgan, J., & Renneise-Sarshad, R. (1990). Imitation of intonation by infants. *Journal of Speech and Hearing Research, 33,* 9–15.

Smith, B., Brown-Sweeney, S., & Stoel-Gammon, C. (1989). A quantitative analysis of reduplicated and variegated babbling. *First Language, 9,* 175–189.

Snow, C. (1977). The development of conversation between mothers and babies. *Journal of Child Language, 4,* 1–22.

Stark, R. (1978). Features of infant sounds: The emergence of cooing. *Journal of Child Language, 5,* 1–12.

Stark, R. (1979). Prespeech segmental feature development. In P. Fletcher & M. Garman (Eds.), *Language acquisition.* New York: Cambridge University Press.

Stark, R. (1980). Stages of speech development in the first year of life. In G. Yeni-Komshian, J. Kavanagh, & C. Ferguson (Eds.), *Child phonology: Vol. 1. Production.* New York: Academic Press.

Stark, R. (1981). Infant vocalizations: A comprehensive view. *Infant Mental Health Journal, 2,* 118–128.

Stark, R. (1986). Prespeech segmental feature development. In P. Fletcher & M. Garman (Eds.), *Language acquisition: Studies in first language acquisition.* New York: Cambridge University Press.

Stark, R. (1989). Temporal patterning of cry and non-cry sounds in the first eight months of life. *First Language, 9,* 107–136.

Stark, R., Bernstein, L., Demorest, M. (1993). Vocal communication in the first 18 months of life, *Journal of Speech and Hearing Research, 36* (3), 548–558.

Stoel-Gammon, C. (1988). Prelinguistic vocalizations of hearing-impaired and normally hearing subjects: A comparison of consonantal inventories. *Journal of Speech and Hearing Disorders, 53,* 302–315.

Stoel-Gammon, C., & Otomo, K. (1986). Babbling development of hearing-impaired and normally hearing subjects. *Journal of Speech and Hearing Disorders, 51,* 33–41.

Sullivan, J. W., & Horowitz, F. D. (1983). The effects of intonation on infant attention: The role of the rising intonation contour. *Journal of Child Language, 10,* 521–534.

Tomasello, M., Conti-Ramsden, G., & Ewert, B. (1990). Young children's conversations with their mothers and fathers: Differences in breakdown and repair. *Journal of Child Language, 17,* 115–130.

Vaidyanathan, R. (1988). Development of forms and functions of interrogatives in children: A language study of Tamil. *Journal of Child Language, 15,* 533–549.

Vaidyanathan, R. (1991). Development of forms and functions of negation in the early stages of language acquisition: A study of Tamil. *Journal of Child Language, 18,* 51–60.

von Raffler-Engel, W. (1973). The development from sound to phoneme in child language. In C. Ferguson & D. Slobin (Eds.), *Studies of child language development.* New York: Holt, Rinehart & Winston.

Wells, G. (1985). *Language development in the preschool years.* New York: Cambridge University Press.

Wolff, P. (1969). The natural history of crying and other vocalizations in early infancy. In B. Foss (Ed.), *Determinants of infant behavior IV.* London: Methuen.

FIVE

The Saga Continues: Language Development Through the Preschool Years

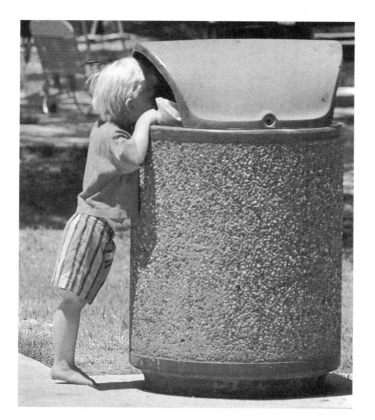

Chapter Objectives

Welcome to the wild and wonderful preschool years, a time of inexhaustible energy, limitless curiosity, and explosive communication development. In this chapter, we examine the phenomenal changes in the child's communication abilities as he runs, jumps, and shrieks through four more stages of language development. At the close of the preceding chapter, the child was just beginning to combine words. By the close of this chapter, he will be an enthusiastic and reasonably competent conversationalist. He will also begin to show evidence of a communication skill we have not seen to this point. He will begin to tell stories, a skill commonly referred to as *narration*. His narrative skills mature during the school years, but they begin to emerge during the preschool years. Specifically, this chapter is designed to facilitate understanding of the following topics:

- **Stage Two (27 to 30 Months)**
- Emergence of grammatical morphemes, pronouns, and auxiliary verbs.
- Using phrases and clauses to create more adultlike sentences.
- Early versions of negation, the interrogative form, and imperatives.
- Cognitive development reflected in vocabulary and semantic advances.
- Struggles with conversational skills such as turn-taking and repair.
- **Stage Three (31 to 34 Months)**
- More consistent use of grammatical morphemes, pronouns, and auxiliary verbs.

- Elaboration of noun phrases in both subjective and objective positions of sentences.
- More adultlike versions of negation and the interrogative form.
- Slow progress on the conversational front.
- **Stage Four (35 to 40 Months)**
- Elaboration of sentences by embedding.
- Improvements in turn-taking, topic maintenance, and presuppositional skills, and learning the art of indirect requests.
- **Stage Five (41 to 46 Months)**
- Mastery of a majority of grammatical morphemes.
- Noun and verb phrases do not increase significantly in length but are more complete and correct, according to adult standards.
- Multiple embeddings and clausal conjoining.
- Struggling with rules of conversational etiquette.
- **The Beginnings of Narrative Discourse**
- **Understanding Language**
- Language comprehension and production supported by cognitive development.
- Understanding active and passive sentences.
- Learning English word order: Does comprehension precede production?
- Understanding words that identify spatial, temporal, quantity, and dimensional relationships.

The "twos" may be terrible for the mother trying to keep track of her increasingly active child, but the twos and threes and the remainder of the preschool years are wonderful and exciting from a language development point of view. As the child exits Stage One, he is already talking, but over the next few years he will experience unbelievable gains in language ability. In this chapter, we trace those changes through four more stages of language development. You will notice that virtually all of these changes are elaborations of abilities that emerged in Stage One.

Stage Two: Elaborating Structure and Refining Meaning

The child is typically in this stage from 27 months to about 30 months, and his MLU is 2.0 to 2.5 morphemes. Brown (1973) has suggested that the greatest change occurring during Stage Two is what he calls the **"modulations of meaning"** in simple sentences, which is accomplished by the use of grammatical morphemes. To modulate means to modify or regulate and both of these synonyms are helpful in understanding what occurs when grammatical morphemes are added to base words. By adding *-ed* to a verb like *show*, I modify the tense from present to past. I use grammatical morphemes to regulate or govern forms of words so that I create the precise meaning I want to express. The timing of *to show* may be just as important to my message as the meaning of the verb itself. In some circumstances, it might be important to distinguish between having one husband or two husbands. In other cases, prepositions like *on* or *in* become critically important to meaning. Did I put my daughter *on* the car or *in* the car? See what I mean?

Most of the terms used to describe grammatical morphemes will be familiar, but some supplementary explanations and terminology may be useful. The term **inflection** is sometimes used to refer to a change in a word created by the addition of a grammatical morpheme. We can inflect nouns, for example, to make them plural or possessive. We can inflect verbs to make them past tense or to make them present progressive. The term **present progressive** is used to describe an action of limited duration that is taking place right now. Think about how you use words like *running, writing, eating.* These are present progressive forms of common verbs. We make some verbs past tense by adding *-ed.* This is known as **regular** past tense. *Looked* is a regular past tense form. Other verbs like *run, sit* and *go* are made past tense, not by inflection but by word changes. These words require **irregular** past tense changes resulting in *ran, sat,* and *went.* The verb *to be* presents some special problems of its own. This verb can be a **main** verb or **copula** as in *He is my dog,* or *I was a bad boy.* The verb *to be* can also be used as a helping or **auxiliary** verb as in sentences such as *He is running,* or *I was eating.* Note that when the verb *to be* is used as an auxiliary, the grammatical morpheme *-ing* is always attached to the main verb that follows the auxiliary. The child must sort out which verb forms can be **contracted** or reduced and which forms cannot be contracted. In the examples above, it is proper to contract *He is* in either the copula or auxiliary form to *He's,* but it is not acceptable to contract *I was.* There is much to learn in the acquisition of grammatical morphemes, and unfortunately the rules sometimes do not make much sense. That children sometimes produce forms that do not match adult forms is not surprising. That they master most of the basic grammatical morphemes by the time they are four years old is a miracle!

Although some grammatical morphemes begin to emerge in the latter part of Stage One, their primary development begins in Stage Two. Several studies have focused on fourteen grammatical morphemes. Brown (1973) and James and Khan (1982) examined the development of these morphemes in longitudinal studies, and de Villiers and de Villiers (1973) looked at them in a cross-sectional study. Although there are some differences among the three studies, especially with regard to the acquisition of irregular past tense, regular past tense, and the contractible copula, the results suggest the following order of acquisition for the fourteen targeted morphemes:

Grammatical Morpheme	Example
Present progressive	She runn*ing*.
In (preposition)	Milk *in* cup.
On (preposition)	Doggie *on* bed.
Regular plural	Girl*s* playing.
Irregular past tense	Mommy *went* work.
Possessive	Billy*'s* ball.
Uncontractible copula	Billy *was* bad.
Articles *(the, a)*	Daddy eating *the* cookie.
Regular past tense	Mommy look*ed*.
Regular third person singular	She *eats*.
Irregular third person singular	Daddy *has* cookie.
Uncontractible auxiliary	I *was* eating.
Contractible copula	Billy*'s* bad.
Contractible auxiliary	He*'s* running.

In all three studies, the criterion for mastery was 90 percent correct usage in *obligatory contexts*. That is, when an utterance *requires* the use of a given grammatical morpheme, and the child uses the appropriate morpheme, he has met the grammatical requirement or obligation for that context. An obligatory context can be linguistic or nonlinguistic. If, for example, the child is watching his mother jump rope, and the mother says, "What is Mommy doing?", a correct response from the child would include the present progressive form of "jump." If the child says, "Mommy jumping" or "Mommy jumping rope," or even if the child says "hopping" or "bouncing" or "running," he has produced the correct grammatical morpheme for that context. The mother's language set up a linguistic obligatory context. The obligatory context might be nonlinguistic, however. Assuming the child has just eaten a cookie and is prepared to comment on this masterful feat of mastication and deglutition, he *should* use the past tense and say something like, "Ate cookie?" If he uses "ate," he has met the obligation for irregular past tense in an opportunity set up, not by the utterance of someone else, but by his own nonverbal, but decidedly oral, actions.

Although researchers have identified age ranges for the mastery of each of these morphemes, it may be more helpful to emphasize what we know about acquisition in general than to focus attention on specific ages. It is important to note, for example, that all of these morphemes begin to emerge during the latter months of Stage One and throughout Stage Two. We see mastery of the earliest grammatical morpheme, present progressive, in some children as young as 19 months. Emergence of the latest of these selected grammatical morphemes, including irregular third person forms of verbs and the correct sorting of contractible and uncontractible copula and auxiliary verb forms, does not occur until about 28 to 30 months. It is also important to stress that although all of these morphemes appear in Stage Two, they are not mastered by some children until Stage Five and beyond. It might be appropriate to remind the reader that some grammatical morphemes are never correctly used by some adults. How often, for example, do adults use the words *data* and *media* as though they are singular noun forms when they are actually plural forms of the words *datum* and *medium?*

One of the interesting, though not surprising, things that happens as children begin to master some of these grammatical morphemes is that they **overextend** or **overgeneralize** their use. When the child begins to make nouns plural by adding *s* to "cat" to make "cats" or the sound *z* to "dog" to make "dogs," he logically concludes that this rule for plural should work on all nouns. His plural form of "man" is "mans" and his plural form of "child" is "childs." At some point in his language development, he is likely to overextend past tense to produce forms like "goed," "runned," "throwed," and "eated." Imagine his confusion when he has to learn that the plural of "deer" is "deer" and the plural of "moose" is "moose" or when he learns that the past tense of "burst" is "burst." Because these productions are unusual and because they catch our attention, we may conclude that they are commonplace in the speech of children at this age. Chapman, Streim, Crais, Salmon, Strand, and Negri (1992, p. 7), in reviewing Cazden's (1968) original data, found that only about five percent of the utterances in the speech samples of her subjects contained overextensions. While it is true, therefore, that a child might occasionally produce an utterance such as, *"Him eated it,"* productions that include overextensions are rare. Keep in mind that while the child is making his own productions, he is listening to the productions of others, and we assume he makes comparisons. In the process of comparing his productions with the productions of those models in his environment who have greater language competence than he does, he will eventually determine how to apply conventional rules. He will figure out, for example, that in some cases the past tense of verbs is indicated by the addition of a grammatical morpheme, as in "tip—tipp*ed."* He will understand that in other cases, past tense is indicated by changing the whole word, as in "run—ran," and that there are some cases in which the word does not change at all, as in "hurt—hurt." Why does the child use overextensions at all? Although it is tempting to view the occurrence of overextensions as evidence that the child is searching for rule-governed patterns, this conclusion is still being debated (Chapman, et. al., 1992). No matter what all this means at this particular stage of development, I think it is fair to reach at least one conclusion. Regular rules make language functional. The exceptions make language interesting and prevent us from becoming overconfident.

Pronouns: Words Used to Represent Nouns

We adults use pronouns so easily we probably do not consider how difficult these words are for children acquiring language. The traditional definition of pronoun in

English grammar textbooks reads something like this: "A **pronoun** is a word used in place of a noun." Actually, there is much more involved than this, and it is the "much more" that should help you understand why children begin to use pronouns in Stage One or Two but may not master the use of some pronouns until Stage Five and beyond. In fact, it is not uncommon for adults to struggle with some pronoun forms, and some of us never get them right!

Consider all the language information conveyed by pronouns. Pronouns convey information about gender or the lack of gender. The child must use pronouns like *she* and *her* to refer to females and *he* and *him* to refer to males, and he must use *it* when the gender is not known or not important. Pronouns convey information about the number of referents, so the child must know the difference between *I* and *we* and between *he* or *she* and *they*, and then there is that ever popular distinction between *you* singular and *you* plural we all love. The child must learn that pronouns differ depending on whether they are used as subjects in sentences or as objects. The pronouns *I, she, he,* and *they,* for example, are **subjective** pronouns, and their **objective** counterparts are *me, her, him,* and *them.* The child must be able to put the right pronoun in the right part of the sentence. This is not an easy task, and it takes the child some time before he gets it right. According to Wells (1985), most subjective and objective pronouns are not mastered until about 36 months, which places the child in Stage Four. In addition to knowing where subjective and objective pronouns belong in the structures of sentences, the child must learn that the number represented by the pronoun determines the verb form to be used. He must say "He is," and "She is," but he must say "They *are,*" and "*I am.*" He must learn the possessive forms of pronouns like *hers, his, mine, their,* and *your,* and he must learn when and when not to use reflexive pronouns like *yourself, himself,* and *herself.* The task becomes even more daunting when one considers that the child must understand that when a pronoun is included in a sentence, the meaning of that sentence will be obscured, or lost entirely, if the listener does not know the informational content of the preceding statement or statements. For example, in order for a listener to properly decode the meaning of the pronoun *it,* as in the sentence "John bought it," he must have heard the previous sentence "John loved that sweater." This type of reference, in which a pronoun is used to refer to something in a preceding utterance, is called an **anaphoric** reference. In the example used here, try to imagine what the listener might conclude without the anaphoric reference. Based on his understanding of common slang expressions, the listener, hearing only that, "John bought it," might conclude that John died, and that would not be a good thing, especially for poor John. This is complicated business! Is it any wonder children get confused and say things like "Me wanna go outside," "Her is eating mine cookie," and "Him wants my ball for hisself"?

Fortunately, there is some order to the potential pronoun chaos. As with all dimensions of language, the child acquires pronouns in a progressive and fairly predictable manner, and we will follow this progress as we move through the remaining stages. In general, you will notice that the child acquires subjective pronouns like *she* and *he* before he acquires objective pronouns like *her* and *him.* He will then acquire pronouns indicating possession like *his, hers, their,* and *our,* and finally he will use reflexive pronouns like *myself, yourself* and *themselves.*

Within the context of Stage Two, we can say this much. Before the child even enters Stage Two, he has probably been using a few pronouns including *I, it,* and *this* and *that.* During Stage Two he will add *my, mine, me,* and *you.* Be aware that the child might not use these pronouns correctly in all situations. He might say "My ball" one time and "Mine ball" at another time. He might use *me* correctly as an objective pronoun when he says, "Kiss me, Mommy," but he might also use *me* as a subjective pronoun when he says, "Me kiss Mommy." It takes time to get all this, that, and the other sorted out.

Auxiliary Verbs

As mentioned earlier, an auxiliary verb is a helping verb. There are **primary** auxiliary verbs like *have* and *do,* and there are secondary auxiliary verbs like *can, shall, may,* and *will* which are also called **modals.** During Stage Two, the child begins to use the verbs *have* and *do* as main verbs and as auxiliary verbs. He also produces what are considered "semi-auxiliary" verb forms like *hafta, gonna,* and *wanna* as in "I hafta go potty," and "I wanna go bye-bye." As we will continue to emphasize with many language forms, children begin to use auxiliary verbs within a wide range of ages (Wells, 1985). So variable are the ages of acquisition that Wells (1985) identified the ages at which only 50 percent of the children studied were producing selected forms. The earliest forms to be used by half of these subjects were *do* and *have,* at about 27 months. *Can, be,* and *will* were being produced at about 30 months, and the last two forms to be used by these children were *shall* at 39 months, and *could* at 42 months, ages which extend beyond Stage Two.

Developing the Parts of Sentences: Phrases and Clauses

Many of us have probably pondered that strange and unanswerable question: "Is our universe just one cell in the fingernail of some greater creature?" It is interesting to consider the parts that make up wholes, and the more we learn about anything, the more we appreciate the smaller parts and the greater wholes. In the production of language, we are confronted with the parts and wholes issue. We have considered morphology, which is the study of the meaning units of language. We have established that a **morpheme** is the smallest unit of language which has meaning. Words are made up of one or more morphemes, but morphemes are made up of smaller parts called **phonemes** or speech sounds, and as we shall see in a later chapter, phonemes are made up of even smaller bits called **distinctive features.**

At this point, we want to move from the small parts of language to the larger parts. At the end of Stage One, the child was combining words in ways that suggested sentences. In Stage Two, he will produce combinations of words that are more recognizable as sentences. To do this, the child must develop an understanding of the basic parts or components of sentences. We call these components phrases and clauses.

A **phrase** is a combination of words that are related to one another, and the combination serves a grammatical purpose, but a phrase does not contain a subject and a predicate. There are two kinds of phrases: noun phrases and verb phrases. As the name suggests, a **noun phrase** contains a noun and words that describe or modify the noun. There are four kinds of modifiers in noun phrases: determiners, adjectivals, initiators, and postmodifiers. A **determiner** is the first unit in a noun phrase and is an article *(a, the)*, possessive pronoun *(my, his, her)*, demonstrative pronoun *(this, that, these, those)*, or a qualifier *(some, most, any)*. An **adjectival** modifies a noun and can be an adjective *(pretty, tall)*, an ordinal *(second, last)*, or a quantifier *(one, couple, few)*. An **initiator** comes before a determiner and places a limit on the noun *(only, all, both, just)*. A **postmodifier,** as its name suggests, is a modifier that comes after the noun. A postmodifier might be a prepositional phrase as in "The fish *in the little tank* is Fred," or it might be a clause as in "The man *who called last night* is my uncle." Although the child is producing noun phrases in Stage Two, he tends to use only determiners and adjectivals as modifiers in these phrases. Not until the end of Stage Four will he consistently use initiators and postmodifiers (Bernstein, 1989, p. 112).

To the surprise of no one, a **verb phrase** contains a verb, and it might contain some other supporting or qualifying words. In the sentence, *The boy is running,* the verb phrase is *is running.* The main verb is *run,* which is in the present progressive form and is supported by *is.* A verb phrase might also contain a **modal,** which is a word indicating the "attitude" of the verb. Common modals are *can, will, must, shall,* and *may.* Notice the difference in the attitudes of the verb phrases in these sentences when we just change the modal: (1) *John **will** go to the party,* and (2) *John **may** go to the party.* The only verb phrase elaboration to be mastered in Stage Two is the present progressive form, but the child does produce primitive infinitive verb forms like "wanna" and gonna" (Miller, 1981), and by the end of Stage Two, the child is typically creating the negative versions of these forms when he produces those sentences we all love to hear: "I can't" or "I won't." The child does not consistently use modals until Stage Four, and he makes further elaborations in his verb phrases in Stage Five (Bernstein, 1989, p. 112). Once again, we see that what begins at an early age is often not finished for many months or several years.

A **clause** is a collection of related words with both a subject and a predicate. Some clauses, called **independent clauses,** can stand alone as simple sentences. When two independent clauses are joined by conjunctions like *and* or *but,* they become one **compound sentence.** A **subordinate clause** has a subject and predicate, but it cannot stand alone as a sentence. When a teacher marks a collection of words on an essay as "incomplete," she is often referring to a subordinate clause. In the sentence, *John wondered if his life would have meaning when his Harley stopped running,* the subordinate clause is *when his Harley stopped running.* The subordinate clause must be attached to an independent clause to create a complete sentence.

The successful merging of an independent clause and a subordinate clause results in a **complex sentence.** Obviously, the Stage Two child is a long way from producing complex sentences. What he does understand by the end of Stage Two is that a sentence must contain a noun phrase and a verb phrase. This knowledge allows the 30-month-old child to produce and understand simple declarative sentences such as "Mommy going work," "Johnny throw ball," and "Doggie eat gerbil!"

Putting the Pieces of Sentences Together

As the child learns to produce and elaborate phrases and clauses, he produces sentences that are more and more complete, syntactically and semantically. Although the most dramatic changes in sentences will not occur until Stage Three and beyond, the child in Stage Two is producing sentences that contain three, four, and more words. Keep in mind that the upper end of the MLU range in this stage is 2.5. The child is still producing single-word utterances, but he is producing fewer of these short utterances and more multiple-word utterances. His sentences become longer because he is expanding his noun phrases and verb phrases. His noun phrases include personal pronouns like "my" and "mine," demonstrative pronouns like "this" and "that," and the articles "a" and "the." His verb phrases include the present progressive form marked by "-ing" as well as semi-auxiliary verb forms like "gonna" and "wanna."

Producing Sentences to Say "NO!!"

By late Stage One, the child begins to express negation, even in sentences as short as two or three words. In an early study of the development of negation, Klima and Bellugi-Klima (1971) identified three periods. In the first period, their subjects expressed negation by putting "no" at the beginning of a statement as in "No kick that!" In the second period, the negative element was placed in front of the verb as in "I no like that!" In the final period, the auxiliary was added and the child transformed the sentence into its proper negative form as in "Daddy is not going to work." The three periods of negation noted by Klima and Bellugi-Klima (1971) emerge in a timeframe that roughly corresponds to the stages described by Brown (1973). That is, the first of these forms of syntactic negation is typically produced by the child in late Stage One and early Stage Two when the MLU range is from approximately 1.5 to about 2.25. The second period of negation is produced by the child in late Stage Two and early Stage Three when the MLU range is from 2.25 to 2.75. It is in Stage Three that the child is likely to position the negative element between the subject and predicate, an accomplishment Brown (1973) considered to be one of the major highlights of Stage Three. The development of additional auxiliaries along with the negative form begins to appear in Klima and Bellugi-Klima's (1971) final period, which includes Brown's late Stage Three and early Stage Four where the MLU ranges from 2.75 to 3.5. Would it be correct to assume that the child has mastered syntactic negation by the time he reaches Stage Four? Not hardly!

The child is probably going to be beyond his preschool years before he starts using questions that contain negative forms such as in the sentence "Why don't you like spinach?" (Owens, 1996, p. 328).

According to Bloom (1970), the child in Stage Two understands the concept of negation well enough to express three variations of the negative theme. He can express the *nonexistence* of something as when he says, "Cookie allgone." He can *reject* as when he says, "No nite-nite," to indicate that he does not want to go to bed, and he can express *denial* as when he says, "No doggie," to indicate that the object being identified by his conversational partner as a "dog" is not a dog. This child does not differentiate between "no" and "not," and sometimes one must consider the situational context in order to determine what the "no" or "not" really means. For example, the child's mother might say to the child, "Let Mommy put you in your chair," and the child responds, "No Daddy." This could mean that the child is rejecting assistance from his father, but depending upon the child's body language and the prosodic variations of his speech, it could mean "I want Daddy to put me into my chair."

By late Stage Two, the child is using "no," "not," "can't," and "don't" in an undifferentiated manner, but he is beginning to put the negative form between the subject and predicate. You should note that even though the child is using "can't" and "don't" in Stage Two, he does not use their positive forms, "can" and "do," until later (Brown, Cazden, & Bellugi, 1969). It is not appropriate, therefore, to conclude that the Stage Two child understands that "don't" is a contracted form of "do not." He simply uses "don't" and "can't" as forms of negation, and he might use "can't" when it should be "don't" and vice versa.

Asking Questions: The First Interrogative Forms

Before we consider what the Stage Two child is able to do in creating question forms of sentences, we should consider the functions of questions. There are essentially two kinds of questions speakers can ask. They can ask questions that elicit *yes* or *no* answers, and they can ask questions beginning with *who, whose, whom, what, where, which, when, why,* or *how.* Questions that begin with *wh-*words or *how* require answers that provide information. If you ask "What time is it?" I will consult my trusty $19.95 Timex and provide you invaluable information about the time of day. Knowing the difference between *yes/no* questions and *wh-* questions should help you understand why the following exchange can be funny: A man asks, *Can you tell me where Grand Central Station is?* The second man answers, *Yes.* The first man intended a *wh-* question because he needed information, but the second man perceived a *yes/no* question. Well, I guess you had to be there.

A *yes/no* question is usually created by moving an auxiliary verb in front of the subject and closing the sentence with a rising intonation. The sentence, *He was going to the store,* is transformed into a *yes/no* question by moving the *was* in front of the *he* to create, *Was he going to the store?* If the statement to be transformed does not have an auxiliary verb, the speaker must add the appropriate form of *do,* so that

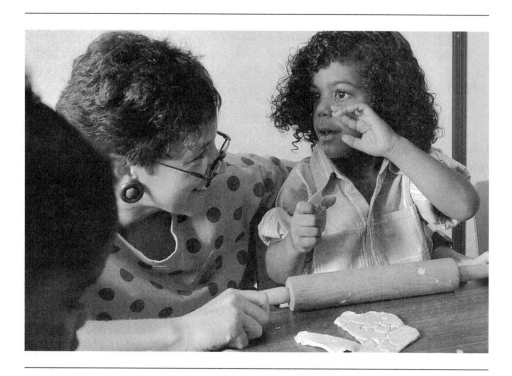

New experiences, new discoveries, and neverending questions.

You have my steak, becomes *Do you have my steak?* or *John plans to come home* becomes *Does John plan to come home?* A *wh-* question is formed by inverting the subject and auxiliary and adding the appropriate *wh-* word or *how* to the beginning of the sentence. *He is sitting* can be transformed into *Where is he sitting?, How is he sitting?,* or *Why is he sitting?*

The Stage Two child is obviously not ready for the sometimes convoluted questions adults as such as, *Where is he sitting, with whom, and why?* He is asking questions, however, and some of these questions call for more than *yes* or *no.* Klima and Bellugi-Klima (1971) have identified three periods in the development of interrogative forms. The first of these periods occurs in the latter part of Stage One and early Stage Two of language development, when we would expect to see MLU values of 1.75 to 2.25. In period one, between the ages of 25 to 28 months, the child is still asking *yes/no* questions by adding rising intonations to simple declarative sentences, the same method he used at the single-word stage of development. By adding a rising intonation to the end of "Go bye-bye," he transforms a statement or demand into a question meaning "Are we going bye-bye?" or "Can we go bye-bye?" In this first phase, he is also asking a few simple *wh-* questions, such as "What this?" or

"Where Mommy?" "What" and "where" questions are most common, probably because they focus on two of the most prominent semantic categories the child uses at this age, naming and locating. In turn, these may be popular semantic categories because they relate to the child's immediate environment and because they are frequently used by the child's caregiver to stimulate speech.

The second period of interrogative development occurs during the latter months associated with late Stage Two and early Stage Three. When the child is approximately 26 to 32 months, and MLU values range from 2.25 to 2.75, he continues to use a rising intonation as the primary means by which he expresses *yes/no* questions. In addition to increased use of "what" and "where" questions, he now adds the infamous "why" question, which will become one of his favorite language forms over the next year or so. The child's questions at this point are more elaborate and typically have subjects and predicates, although he still omits auxiliaries. He poses questions such as "Where Daddy go?", "What Mommy doing?", and "Why he eat that?" Throughout the first two phases, the child experiences some confusion with *wh-* questions. Until he is about two years old, he interprets most *wh-* questions as "where" questions. After two years, he still responds to some "why" questions as though they are "what" questions. The child, for example, throws his food on the floor. The adult asks, "Why did you do that?" The child responds, "I throwed cookie." In this second phase, the child is still forming *yes/no* questions by using rising intonations at the end of statements, but we will see appropriate inverted questions before he reaches his third birthday.

Imperative Sentences: Requests and Demands

Since the child has been making requests and demands even before he started to use language, you may wonder when the imperative form of sentences emerges. The child is about 31 months old before he begins to form true imperative sentences (McCormick, 1990, p. 89). The imperative form has an implied subject and uses an uninflected verb. If I say, *Turn off the light,* it is understood that the subject of the sentence is the person to whom the command is given. The child in Stage One and Stage Two certainly uses the imperative function in his communication system. His body language and his prosodic variations are sufficient to make his request, demand, or command obvious to the listener. When the child in the single-word stage says, "Mommy!" with his arms stretched out and with urgency in his voice, the imperative message is clear. When the Stage Two child says "Go bye-bye" while tugging on his mother's skirt and motioning toward the door, the imperative message is also clear.

Semantic Development in Stage Two

When the child begins to put words together, his vocabulary grows rapidly. Carey (1978) estimated that between the ages of eighteen months and six years, the child adds an average of nine new words every day! Amazingly, it is suggested that the six-year-old child may have a comprehension vocabulary which reaches approximately 14,000 words (Carey, 1978). That becomes impressive when you consider how slowly vocabulary grows when the child creeps into adulthood. If you added just one word per day over the next year, you would add 365 words to your vocabulary. I doubt you have had that kind of vocabulary bonanza in more than a few years. The child at 24 months has about 200 to 300 words in his expressive vocabulary. The child in the latter months of Stage Two will probably have a productive vocabulary of about 400 words.

There are undoubtedly many factors that account for how the child apparently acquires so much information about words so quickly, and it will be many years before we identify all of them. Part of the explanation may be inherent in a process called **fast mapping** (Carey and Bartlett, 1978). The foundation for fast mapping is laid when the child first encounters a new word. Even if he does not understand the word completely, he is able to quickly gather information about the word from the context in which it is introduced. There might be information in the surrounding language, for example, that provides the child some insights about what the word means. There may be clues in the discourse in which the word was used. The child stores this information, no matter how fragmented and incomplete it may be in the beginning, in long-term memory. When he encounters the same word in the future in a different context, he gathers additional information that makes his understanding of the word more complete. Keep in mind that the child is repeatedly exposed to communicative routines and that his caregivers are constantly providing him reviewed and new information, factors Crais (1992) believes contribute to word learning. If we put all of these factors together, we understand that what appears to be a rapid acquisition of word knowledge may be somewhat illusory. That is, the child apparently understands and uses a wide range of words quickly, but he may actually understand only bits and pieces of these words. He understands enough of the bits and pieces to decode them and to use them, but we should not assume that just because words are included in the child's receptive and productive vocabularies at a young age that he understands them in the same way that adults understand them. What may be so rapidly acquired, therefore, are pieces of information about many words, and that is very different from complete understandings of many words.

The increase in word knowledge that occurs during Stage Two impacts virtually all language components. As was true in Stage One, the Stage Two child talks about people, objects, actions, and events, and his multiple-word utterances reflect his understanding of relational meanings. In Stage Two, however, he is using longer and more elaborate sentences resulting in meanings that are more elaborate and increasingly refined.

One development of note in this stage is that the child's cognitive grasp of emotionality is reflected in his language. Some children as young as 18 months begin to talk about emotions (Bretherton, Fritz, Zahn-Waxler, & Ridgeway, 1986), and by 24 months most children are including references to emotion in their language. The Stage Two child identifies emotions, those he is feeling as well as those being

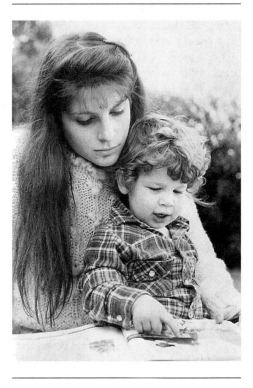

For the Stage Two child, communication is still heavily nonverbal.

experienced by others, and he talks about emotions experienced in the past. As he approaches the end of this stage, he understands that emotions are causative factors in human behavior. If he sees someone crying, for example, he might say, "She sad," reasoning that sadness causes crying. The time is rapidly approaching when the child will begin to use emotional language to manipulate the behavior of others. Is it difficult to imagine the late preschool child saying to his caregiver, "I love you," in the hope that this show of affection will translate into an ice-cream cone?

The child's general understanding of causality is reflected by the appropriate use of the words "because" and "so" as early as 30 months (McCabe & Peterson, 1985). It will be another year before the child is able to provide the language detail consistent with a complete understanding of how a causal factor produces a given circumstance. During Stage Two, for example, the child might say, "Milk allgone cause me," whereas in the next stage he might say, "I spilled milk Daddy shirt." Beyond the obvious language differences, we see a more precise understanding of the cause and the effect.

Because it is difficult to isolate the development of understanding within each stage, there is a general discussion of comprehension as it relates to cognitive development and language production at the close of this chapter. This section has provided a preview of the relationships we will examine. That is, as the child's understanding of things, people, and events increases, he acquires the vocabulary to name and describe these things, people, and events. As he develops the intellectual capacity to understand concepts, object permanence, causality, and means-ends, he acquires the language by which he can express these understandings. As we established earlier and as we have emphasized throughout this book, it is difficult to separate language and cognitive development. After we complete our examination of Stages Two through Five, we consider this critically important, interactive relationship once again, this time within the context of the child's language abilities as they have developed through the preschool years.

Pragmatics: Small Steps Toward Conversational Competence

We do not see dramatic changes in pragmatics in Stage Two, although in the stages that follow there are significant developments. In Stage Two, the child continues to use language to request objects from other people, to request that certain actions be taken, to obtain information by asking questions, and to respond to the questions or comments of others. One interesting development during this stage centers on the word "please." The child between the ages of 24 and 36 months uses "please" in his requests with some discretion. He is more likely to include "please" if he perceives his listener to be older, more dominant, and less familiar, or if his listener has something he really wants (Ervin-Tripp & Gordon, 1986).

Perhaps the most significant change in the child as a conversationalist in this stage is that he simply talks more. There are fewer nonverbal responses. His verbal responses are more frequent, and because of the other changes in his language we have already noted, his responses are more elaborate (Mueller, Bleier, Krakow, Hegedus, & Cournoyer, 1977). The Stage Two child is also more adept at gaining his listener's attention, and he is able to provide more complete and meaningful responses to his conversational partner's comments and questions (Wellman & Lempers, 1977). In this case, more is better!

In addition to increased verbal output, the child is showing greater skill in introducing new topics into the conversation, although he is still not able to sustain a topic for more than a turn or two. One of the problems the adult listener sometimes faces in conversations with a very young child is trying to figure out exactly what the topic is. Foster (1986) suggests that the child between 24 and 36 months is beginning to create understandable topics. Since the Stage Two child is still changing topics after only one or two turns, it is still a constant struggle for the adult partner to stay tuned to what the child is trying to say. This, however, is part of the magic of conversations between adults and toddlers. Some adult-to-adult conversations seem to never end. Adult-to-toddler conversations may be confusing and exasperating, but these exchanges have so many beginnings and quasi-endings they are never boring!

The child in this stage still has much to learn about turn-taking and the common courtesies of conversation. Although he is able to participate in conversations with one or two partners, the child does not always allow the speaker to complete his turn before he tries to speak. Ervin-Tripp (1979) has noted that most of these interruptions occur at syntactic junctures or when the speaker's prosody seems to signal conversational right-of-way. Whereas adults allow about one second between turns, the Stage Two child allows longer pauses. By the time he reaches his third birthday, however, he learns that these longer pauses can be interpreted to mean that no response will follow, so he shortens his response time to maintain his turn.

One of the skills all conversationalists must learn is **conversational repair.** If I say something to a listener which I believe the listener has not understood, I will revise or repair my message to increase the chances of successful communication. Gallagher (1977) studied conversational repairs in children between the ages of 20 and 30 months, a span that includes Stages One and Two. During conversations with these children, an adult listener indicated a lack of understanding by saying "What?" following a child's utterance. More than 75 percent of the requests for clarifications were followed by revised utterances from the children. Shatz and O'Reilly (1990) found that even though their subjects in this age range tried to repair, only about 38 percent of their repair attempts were successful. It is important to note that although children throughout this age range regularly try to repair when their listeners do not understand, how they revise changes as their language abilities become more sophisticated. According to Gallagher (1977), the younger child is most likely to repair by changing a speech sound. If the child says, "More cookie," and the adult does not understand, the child might say, "More tookie!" The child at 25 or 26 months tends to revise by deleting a word from his original statement. If his original utterance, "That little doggie," is not understood, he might say, "That doggie" or "Little doggie." By the end of Stage Two or the beginning of Stage Three, the child is more likely to repair by changing words. He might revise "She drink milk" to "She drink it" or "Mommy drink milk." It is important to note that a revision or repair is not necessarily more accurate or more correct. In the case of "tookie" for "cookie," for example, the revision is clearly incorrect.

The idea of conversational repair, however, for the child or even the adult is to try something different in order to make a communicative connection, and different is not always better. Listen carefully to the attempted repairs of adults and you will hear some fascinating attempts to clarify. Sometimes the harder we try to make something clear, the more confusing or embarrassing our communications become. Consider the following conversational exchange in an episode of the original Bob Newhart television series. Bob, a psychologist, is just leaving his apartment. He has been asked to lead a workshop for people whose marriages are in trouble because of sexual problems. The omnipresent next-door-neighbor, Howard, is entering the apartment just as Bob is leaving. Howard addresses Bob's wife: *Where's he going, Emily?* Emily answers, *Bob's going to a sex workshop.* Howard responds with a series of statements separated by startled, disbelieving looks from Emily. He says, *I'm sorry*

TABLE 5-1 Stage Two Highlights

Typical Age Range: 27 to 30 Months
MLU: 2.0 to 2.5 Morphemes

Grammatical Morphemes
- Brown's (1973) fourteen specified grammatical morphemes emerge during the latter months of Stage One and throughout Stage Two.
- As these morphemes develop, the child overextends their use, e.g., child → child*s*; go → go*ed.*

Pronouns
- Enters Stage Two using *I, it, this,* and *that.*
- Adds *my, me, mine,* and *you.*

Verbs
- Uses *have* and *do* as main verbs and as auxiliary verbs.
- Produces semi-auxiliary forms: *hafta, gonna, wanna.*

Noun Phrases
- Uses only determiners and adjectivals as modifiers.
- Elaborates in the object position of sentences.

Verb Phrases
- Uses present progressive forms of common verbs.

Sentences
- Understands that a sentence contains a noun phrase and a verb phrase.
- Produces negation by putting *no* or *not* at the beginning of a sentence.
- Produces a *yes/no* question by adding a rising intonation to the end of a sentence.
- Asks *what, where,* and *why* questions.
- Produces the imperative function but not the imperative form.

Pragmatics
- Continues to use language to request, to obtain information, and to respond.
- Fewer nonverbal responses than in Stage One.
- Sustains topic for one or two turns.
- Attempts conversational repairs when the listener does not understand.

---

to hear that Emily. I didn't know you were having those kinds of problems. Can I help . . .? I mean, can I be of any service . . .? I mean, can I function in any way as a friend . . .? I didn't mean any of those things . . . If you want me, I'll be in bed. . . ." These are conversational repairs based, not on lack of clarity in the words themselves, but a lack of clarity in the communicative intentions of the speaker, or more accurately, what the speaker perceives as possible lack of clarity from the viewpoint of his listener.

It is interesting that even though young children consistently respond to requests for clarification from their listeners, they make few requests for repairs when they listen to adult speakers (Gallagher, 1981). Perhaps these children are so accustomed to understanding only portions of the utterances of adults that they do not feel a need to request clarification, or perhaps as Gallagher suggests, they are reluctant to imply that adult speakers have not produced clear and effective messages.

Stage Three: Producing Longer, More Adult-like Sentences

The child is typically in this stage between the ages of 31 and 34 months and has an MLU of 2.5 to 3.0. By the time he reaches the end of this stage, the child knows that every sentence must have a verb or predicate, and within a few more months he understands that every sentence must also have a subject. Armed with this basic syntactic knowledge, the child can create complete simple declarative sentences, and he is acquiring knowledge of the rules for changing declarative sentences into negative and question forms. We saw the beginning of these forms in Stage Two, but they were primitive versions. In Stage Three, the child produces more advanced, adult-like negative, interrogative, and even imperative sentences.

Morphological Development Continues

Many of the morphological elements which emerged in Stage Two continue to develop in Stage Three, including the 14 grammatical morphemes we highlighted. In addition, the Stage Three child is more consistent in his use of personal pronouns such as "your," "yours," "she," "he," and "we." (Owens, 1996, p. 297), the demonstrative pronouns "this," "that," "these," and "those," as well as the articles "a" and "the" (Brown & Bellugi, 1964). Among the modifiers the child uses are a few quantifiers, including "two," "some," and "alot." The child is also using common adjectives such as "big," "little," "good," and "bad."

Although the Stage Two child was producing some auxiliary verbs, the Stage Three child is using these verbs, including "can," "will," and "do" more consistently. He is also using the verb "to be" as an auxiliary and as a copula, although in both cases, it may not correctly indicate person or number. He might say, "They is running," "She am my Mommy," or "We is here."

Phrases and Clauses: Construction Continues

The Stage Two child elaborated noun phrases when they were in the object position. The Stage Three child elaborates noun phrases in both the subjective and objective positions of sentences (Brown & Bellugi, 1964). He elaborates by adding the words we identified above. He adds demonstrative pronouns (*this, that, these, those*), possessive personal pronouns (*my, your*), quantifiers (*some, alot*), articles (*a, the*), and adjectives (*big, little, pretty*). He now produces noun phrases such as "My doggie," "Good cookies," and "Little boys."

The child is producing verb phrases that include auxiliary verbs such as "can," "do," and "will," and he is also including the auxiliary form of the verb "to be." As we noted earlier, however, the verb "to be" in both the auxiliary and copula forms may not correctly indicate person and number, and it may not be properly marked for tense. The child might say, "I *is*" for "I *am*" or he might say "She *is*" when he really means "She *was*." He will also overextend the regular past tense when he is using irregular verbs so that he will say "She runned away" or "I falled down" (Miller, 1981).

More Changes in Sentence Forms

The child was creating primitive forms of negative and question sentences in Stage Two. In this stage, he produces forms that are more adult-like in that he is including auxiliary verbs and the copula, and he is inverting words when they should be inverted.

In Stage Two, the child usually creates the negative form by adding "no" or "not" to the beginning of a simple declarative sentence. The negative version of "Go nite-nite" is "No go nite-nite." In Stage Three, the child places the negative element between the subject and predicate to produce an adult-like version. Instead of "No Daddy go bye-bye," for example, he says, "Daddy no go bye-bye." The child is also adding auxiliary verbs to negative forms as in "Doggie *don*'t bite." As indicated by this example, the child is producing contracted negative forms such as "can't," "don't," and "won't." Since he is also producing the affirmative forms of these verbs, we can assume that these contractions are based on the application of a rule and are not simply imitations of whole constructions. It is noteworthy that Brown (1973) considered the changes in the negative form to be one of the most important advances to occur in Stage Three.

The Stage Two child was creating questions by adding rising intonations to the ends of sentences. In Stage Three, he is including the auxiliary verbs we hear in adult speech, and he is inverting words according to adult production rules. Instead of "She go bye-bye?" with rising inflection, or even "She can go bye-bye?" (which includes the uninverted auxiliary verb), the Stage Three child says, "Can she go bye-bye?" The yes/no question is common in this stage, in sentences that include auxiliary verbs and in sentences that include copula verbs. Instead of the earlier question "I am good boy?", the child will ask, "Am I good boy?" with the subject and copula properly inverted.

The most frequent *wh-* words used in Stage Three are "what" and "where," but the child will also use "why," "who," and "how" (Tyack & Ingram, 1977). According to some researchers, the *wh-* questions during this stage are not inverted, but more recent evidence suggests that *most* of the child's *wh-* questions in Stage Three are inverted (Klee, 1985). The child might say, "Where the cookie is?", but he is more likely to produce the properly inverted form, "Where is the cookie?" He will also include some, though not all, of the required auxiliary verbs. He might say, "*Can* I go bye-bye?", but he might also say "Why Bobby kick me?" instead of "Why *did* Bobby kick me?"

In this stage we see the adult version of the imperative form. The child seems to enjoy this form and appreciates its power. In its proper form, the verb is not inflected and the subject is implied. The child says things like "Pick me up," "Give me a cookie," and "Turn on the light." As mentioned earlier, the child has been producing the imperative function from the beginning of his communicative life, long before the emergence of language, but in Stage Three, for the first time, he is using the syntactically correct form of imperative sentences.

Pragmatic Development: Slow Progress in the Art of Conversation

During Stage Three, the child's dialogues are still relatively brief. He continues to devote only about two turns per conversational topic, and he has difficulty conversing about things that are absent or events in the past. When the child does talk about things or events not in the present, his comments often catch the adult listener off guard because the comments do not seem to be connected to the immediate conversational context (Keenan & Schieffelin, 1976). The difficulty in talking about things and events that are not in the present is that the speaker and the listener must rely solely on language. With a limited vocabulary and limited language skills, the child can talk about things in the present because he can rely on nonverbal communications to fill his language gaps.

The child also has difficulty maintaining a conversational topic. Whereas adults maintain conversation by adding or seeking new information in each turn or by using one comment to prompt a new but related response, the child in Stage Three in not very adept at these skills. His primary strategy for maintaining conversation is to repeat. He will repeat part or all of the utterance just produced by his conversational partner. This strategy of exactly matching the topic of one's partner is called **topic collaborating** (Keenan & Schieffelin, 1976). The child in this stage will also maintain a conversational topic by responding to questions asked by the partner. Adults quickly learn that this is an effective way to keep a young child talking, so the conversational exchange consists of questions from the adult and answers from the child. The limiting factor in this kind of dialogue might be the adult's ability to keep asking questions about a relatively uninvolved topic. How many questions can you ask a child about a chocolate chip cookie? *What is that? Is it good? What are the brown things? Did it break? What do you suppose is the fat content of a single cookie, and how will that affect your eating habits for the rest of this day? If cookies are bad for you and spinach is good for you, why are wax beans yellow?*

The child in Stage Three continues to repair his conversational statements by changing words. As we noted in the previous stage, these changes do not always result in more correct statements, but the changes do indicate that the child knows his message was not clear, and he is trying to fix it. As his vocabulary grows and his understanding of how words are related increases, his repairs will be more effective. If I say, "He is morose," and I receive a quizzical look from my listener, I may repair my comment to "He's sad." The child's ability to make this kind of repair is obviously related to his language knowledge and skills so that conversational repair skills develop in a parallel manner with overall language development. In Stages Two and Three, the child repairs by using a different word, even if it is not a more appropriate word.

Although adults take into account what the child knows in adult-child conversations, the child's presuppositional skills remain relatively undeveloped. As long as the topic is immediately present, the adult will know the child's conversational

TABLE 5-2 Stage Three Highlights

Typical Age Range: 31 to 34 Months
MLU: 2.5 to 3.0 Morphemes

Grammatical Morphemes
• Continue to develop.

Pronouns
• More consistent in use of *you, your, yours, she, he, we, this, that, these,* and *those.*

Verbs
• Using the modal verbs *can, will,* and *do* more consistently.
• Using the verb *to be* as both copula and auxiliary, although there are mistakes in terms of person and number.

Noun Phrases
• Uses a few quantifiers: *two, some, alot.*
• Elaborates in the subject and object positions of sentences.

Verb Phrases
• Elaborates by using modals and the auxiliary forms of *to be.*
• Overextends the regular past tense form to irregular verbs, e.g., "He runn*ed* away."

Sentences
• Produces negation by putting *no* or *not* between the subject predicate to create an adult-like form. Also uses contracted negative forms: *can't, don't.*
• Questions include auxiliary verbs, and the elements are properly inverted, e.g., "She go bye-bye." → "Can she go bye-bye?"
• In addition to *what, where,* and *why,* he produces *who* and *how* questions, often properly inverted.
• Produces the imperative form of sentences.

Pragmatics
• Most exchanges are still limited to one or two turns per topic.
• Primary strategy for maintaining a topic is repeating part or all of the utterance produced by his partner.
• Continues to attempt conversational repairs, usually by using a different word even if it is not a more appropriate word.

focus, but the child often uses pronouns when their referents are not identifiable, and he provides little assistance to his listener except for supplying some details about the topic which might enhance understanding (Owens, 1996, p. 275).

Stage Four: Elaboration by Embedding

The child is typically in this stage between the ages of 35 and 40 months and has an MLU of 3.0 to 3.75. As the MLU increase from Stage Three to Stage Four indicates, the child continues to elaborate by adding words to his utterances, but in this stage we see elaboration take a new and exciting turn. In the previous stages, the child made phrases and clauses longer by adding modifiers or auxiliary verbs. In Stage Four, he places a phrase within a clause, and he combines two or more clauses into one clause. This combining process, called **embedding,** results in complex sentences, and it is one of the most important syntactic developments in this stage (Brown, 1973). An embedded phrase or clause becomes a grammatical element within a larger sentence. A phrase, for example, might function as a noun, an adjective, or an adverb.

Phrases: Embedding for Specific Grammatical Functions

There are essentially four kinds of phrases: (1) prepositional phrases, (2) participial phrases, (3) infinitive phrases, and (4) gerunds. You should not assume that when the child exits Stage Four, he is producing all of these phrases as embedded forms. Phrasal and clausal embedding are complex processes that develop over a long period of time. The child begins to develop prepositional phrases by using words like "in" and "on" as early as Stage Two, but he does not produce true infinitive forms until Stage Five and beyond (Bloom, Tackeff, & Lahey, 1984; Miller, 1981).

As the name suggests, a **prepositional phrase** contains a preposition like *in, on, under, over,* or *onto,* together with an object of the preposition and accompanying modifiers or articles. In the phrase, *under the old car, under* is the preposition and *car* is the object. The child will add prepositional phrases to the ends of his sentences early in Stage Four.

Verb forms, usually ending in *-ing, -ed, -en,* or *-t,* which function as adjectives are called **participles** in the following examples: *babbling* brook, **pickled** *egg,* **shaven** *head,* and *past* Wednesday. A **participial phrase** contains a participle and functions as an adjective. In the sentence *The woman calling my name is Aunt Bertha,* the participial phrase, *calling my name,* functions as an adjective describing *woman.*

Most of us are familiar with the term **infinitive** because we know we are not supposed to split infinitives when we speak and write. An infinitive is a verb form introduced by the word *to* or the phrase *in order to.* In the sentence, *I called to confirm my reservation,* the infinitive is *to confirm.* In the sentence, *I called to, after trying to remember the date, confirm my reservation,* the infinitive is split. An improved version of the same sentence would be, *After trying to remember the date, I called to confirm my reservation.* Infinitive phrases can function as nouns, adjectives, or adverbs. In the sentence, *Daddy wanted to go to the store,* the infinitive phrase *(to go to the store)* functions as a noun and is the object of the verb *wanted.* In the sentence, *Because of my job, I have little energy to devote to my hobbies,* the infinitive phrase *(to devote to my hobbies)* modifies *energy* and functions as an adjective. In the sentence, *My father exercises to increase his physical fitness,* the infinitive phrase *(to increase his physical fitness)* functions as an adverb in modifying the verb *exercises.*

The child is using forms such as "gotta" and "wanna" as early as 30 months, and these productions certainly sound like infinitive forms as in "I wanna (want to) go bye-bye." Many language experts refer to these productions as **semi-auxiliaries** and do not consider them to be true infinitives (James, 1990, p. 83). Simple infinitives in which the subjects are the same as the subjects of the main sentence emerge in Stage Four, and more difficult infinitives in which the subjects are different than the subjects of the main sentence emerge in Stage Five (Paul, 1981). In Stage Four, for example, the child might say, "Mommy want to eat cookie." The subject of the sentence and the infinitive ("to eat") is "Mommy." In Stage Five, the child might say, "I want the kitty to go outside." In this case, the subject of the sentence is "I," but the subject of the infinitive ("to go") is "kitty."

When a verb ending in "ing" functions as a noun, as either a subject or an object, it is called a **gerund.** In the sentence, "Sleeping is the most vigorous exercise of my day," "sleeping" is a gerund and the subject of the sentence. In the sentence, "Mary dislikes walking," "walking" is a gerund and the object of the verb, "dislikes." When a verb phrase operates as a noun, it is called a **gerund phrase.** In the sentence, "Compulsive eating is a serious health problem," "compulsive eating" is a gerund phrase and is the subject of the sentence. According to Paul (1981), gerund phrases tend to emerge later than infinitives. When her subjects has MLU's above 4.5, more than 90 percent were producing simple infinitive forms but only about 50 percent were producing sentences that included gerunds. Keep in mind that an MLU of 4.5 places the child within Stage Five.

Clauses Within Clauses: Complex Sentences

As we noted earlier in this chapter, a complex sentence is created when the speaker embeds one clause into another. A compound sentence is created when the speaker joins or conjoins two independent clauses. Even though the order might seem to violate common sense, the child engages in serious clausal embedding before he becomes proficient in clausal conjoining. There is evidence of some clausal conjoining in Stage Four, but Brown (1973) identifies clausal conjoining primarily with Stage Five.

According to Brown (1973), there are three types of embedded clauses; (1) object complement clause, (2) *wh-* question clause, and (3) relative clause. In a sentence with an object complement clause, there is an independent clause containing a verb like *think, hope, know, guess, mean,* or *need,* followed by a noun phrase that functions as an object. In the sentence, *I think you know what I mean,* the subordinate clause *(you know what I mean)* functions as the object of the verb *think.* The object complement clause emerges during Stage Four.

The embedded *wh-* clause also emerges during Stage Four, and these clauses also function as objects. Consider the following examples:

"I know what you did."

"He showed me where to get one."

"You probably know when he'll come back."

Since the child is learning to use these words in question sentences, it is not surprising that he sometimes produces sentences that seem to mix the inverted structure of the interrogative form and the embedded *wh-* clause. He might say, for example, "Show me where can I get one," instead of the more proper construction, "Show me where I can get one."

A relative clause is introduced by *who, whom, whoever, whomever, whose, which,* or *that,* and modifies the preceding noun. A problem for many speakers, including adults, is determining which relative pronoun should be used in a given sentence. Identifying and discussing the rules for selecting the proper pronoun is beyond the scope of this book, but a few examples may help you to understand some of what the child must learn about pronoun usage:

"He is the man who helped me last week."

"He's the boy whose finger was broken when he was hit in the nose."

"The ball that broke the window was thrown from a passing car."

Although we are introducing the concept of relative clauses as part of our explanation of clausal embedding, the reader should be aware that the child does not begin to use relative clauses until Stage Five and beyond.

As one might guess, the first conjunction used to link two or more independent clauses is "and." By the time the child is 25 to 27 months old, he is using "and" correctly to join words (Bloom, Lahey, Hood, Lifter, & Fiess, 1980). Even though he begins to conjoin clauses in Stage Four, the child does not consistently conjoin clauses with "and" and other conjunctions until late in Stage Five (Miller, 1981). It is interesting, though not surprising, that even after the child has acquired many conjunctions and is beyond his fifth birthday, he continues to favor "and" (Bennett-Kaster, 1986).

What's Happening on the Morphemic Front?

Although no dramatic developments in morphology are unique to Stage Four, the reader should keep in mind that overall growth in vocabulary is rapid throughout the five stages of language development we are describing. The fourteen grammatical morphemes we identified as emerging in Stage Two are continuing to develop.

The Stage Four child is consistently using the pronouns "they," "us," "her," "hers," "his," and "them" (Owens, 1996, p. 297). He is also using modifiers such as "some," "something," "other," "more," "one," "two," and "another" (Miller, 1981). The child's sentences are likely to include some past tense forms of common modals such as "could," "should," and "would" (Chapman, 1978), and he is putting "be" and the "-ing" form of verbs together to create sentences such as "He is running" (Chapman, Paul, & Wanska, 1981). As the child acquires more words, he incorporates them into his sentences to make them longer and more elaborate.

Elaboration of Noun Phrases and Verb Phrases

The Stage Four child understands that a sentence must have a noun or a pronoun as a subject (Ingram, 1971). Keeping in mind that the child was elaborating noun phrases as subjects and objects in the previous stage, he continues to elaborate in much the same way in Stage Four. That is, he usually adds only one modifier in front of the noun. He will produce sentences such as, *"The* boy took *my* ball," or *"That* doggie ate *his* bone." In looking ahead to the inclusion of several modifiers in front of a noun, think about what the child must learn. If I use three modifiers to describe the noun, *house,* I do not arrange the modifiers in random order. There are rules for sequencing modifiers. Take a moment to think about this intriguing little puzzle: I want to say, *There are* _____ , _____ , _____ *houses on this street,* and I am going to insert the modifiers, *white, three,* and *big.* What is the proper order? The answer, of course, is *Three big white. . . ."* If you put them in any other order, the phrase does not make sense. At some point in the child's language development, he learns the rules for ordering modifiers. In this example, number modifiers precede size modifiers, which precede color modifiers. Learning these rules takes time, time that extends well beyond Stage Five.

The Stage Four child is expanding his verb phrases by including the auxiliary "do" in negative and question forms and by including modals such as "would," "could," "should," "might," and "must" (Chapman, 1978). Although the child has been using modals, since Stage Two, he is now using them more consistently and appropriately. Remember that a modal reflects the speaker's attitude about what is happening in the sentence (Broderick, 1975, p. 81). In this stage, the child demonstrates by use of modals that he understands the difference between using "might" to indicate that something is *possible* and using "must" to indicate that the something is *required* or *obligatory.* You will notice, however, that the meanings of some modals are troublesome for children, and even adults, for a long time. For example, "can" means *ability* and "may" signals *permission,* but many speakers ask a question such as *"Can* I throw the ball?" when what they really mean is *"May* I throw the ball?" This particular confusion occurs so commonly that "can" is now considered to be an acceptable modal to express permission in informal social contexts (Broderick, 1975, p. 82). Sorting out what modals mean and how they should be used begins in earnest in Stage Four, but like so many aspects of language development, the learning and sorting will continue for many years.

The child was overextending the regular past tense in Stage Three, and he continues this overextension in Stage Four. Since he is now using present and past tense modals, however, we see some interesting constructions in which past tense is marked twice. The child might say, for example, "She couldn't catched the ball." Compare this construction with the correct version, "She couldn't catch the ball." Since the modal is marked for past tense, the main verb is not inflected. These are tricky rules! The main verb must be inflected to mark past tense *except* when the modal is marked for past tense in which case the main verb remains in the present tense. . . . That's not a fair rule! The child must also learn, of course, that some verbs are marked for past tense in the *regular* manner, some verbs undergo complete changes such as *go—went* or *see—saw*, and some verbs do not change at all, *hit—hit*. These examples are provided to help you understand why the child overextends and why it takes so long to understand all the rules and at least most of the exceptions.

Progress on Negative and Interrogative Forms

Prior to Stage Four, the child indicates negation by using the words "no" and "not" and by using the contractions, "can't," "don't," and "won't." By the end of Stage Two or the beginning of Stage Three, the child is properly placing the negative element between the subject and predicate. Although he is using words like "can't" and "won't" as early as Stage Two, these are probably not true contractions until Stage Three when he begins to use the positive forms of the modals involved in these contractions. By the end of Stage Four, the child has added the following negative contractions: "didn't," "doesn't," "isn't," and "aren't" (Miller, 1981). Once again the progress is slow but true. From the caregiver's point of view, the progress may actually seem slower than it really is. When the child produces a form such as "can't" as early as 27 to 30 months, the caregiver may assume the child understands the modal "can," the negative element "not," and the rule for producing the contraction. In fact, the child at this point is producing the word "can't" as a whole unit, without understanding its parts and the rule that makes the parts a new whole. He uses "can't" when he should use "won't" and vice versa. In fact, he often does not differentiate among any of the terms he uses to indicate negation. Over the next 10 to 12 months, he is learning a great deal that is not apparent to the caregiver. He learns what a modal is, and he learns which modal works in which context. He learns that modals can be contracted with negative elements to produce "can't," "won't," etc. He learns to place the negative form between the subject and predicate. Over the course of Stages Two, Three, and Four, therefore, he learns a great deal about creating negative forms, but the caregiver still hears only "can't" and "won't," and may have no idea that the "can't" of Stage Two is very different from the "can't" of Stage Four.

We see similar progress with interrogative forms. In Stage Two, the child signals a question by using a rising intonation at the end of a declarative statement. In Stage Three, he is including some auxiliary verbs, and he is learning to properly invert words to move from the declarative form of a sentence to the interrogative form of the same sentence. By the time the child reaches the end of Stage Four, he is producing adult-like questions in their inverted forms and with the appropriate auxiliary verbs. Prior to this stage, most of his *wh-* questions were introduced by "what" or "where." By the end of Stage Four, he is consistently creating questions initiated by "why," "who," and "how" which were used sparingly in the preceding stage, and he is using "when." The order in which *wh-* questions emerge may be explained according to how the words are used in sentences (Wootten, Merkin, Hood, & Bloom, 1979). Questions introduced by "what," "where," and "who" are among the earliest to emerge, perhaps because these words are **interrogative pronouns.** If the child says, "What is that?", the "what" is a pronoun representing a specific thing. "Who" represents a specific person, and "where" represents a specific location. Throughout his language and cognitive development, the child has managed to deal more effectively with things, people, and events in his immediate environment than with abstract concepts or with things, people, and events that are remote in time and space. Consider the problems created by words like "why," "how," and "when" which are acquired later than "what," "where," and "who." There are no easy and specific referents for these words. Even as adults, we may have trouble responding to some "why" and "how" questions. If someone asks, *Is the sky blue?*, we can provide a simple and direct answer, but the question *Why is the sky blue?* is much more difficult. Economists make a living trying to answer *why* and *how* questions like *Why does the value of the dollar affect the balance of trade?* or *How do the Dow-Jones averages measure the strength of the American economy?* What substitutes for the *why* and *how* in these questions can fill books. *When* questions are fairly easy for adults because we have a sense of the present in the relative context of past and future, but the child at two, three, or four years is still grappling with the concept of time in its past and future dimensions.

Pragmatic Development: Becoming a Better Conversationalist

Early in Stage Four, at about three years, the child learns a simple but important lesson about time in the art of conversation. He recognizes that there is a difference between a pause of less than one second and a pause greater than one second. Think about this for a moment. In your conversations with other adults, when there is a pause of several seconds, what does that mean? It could mean, of course, that the other person is thinking about his response, but if there is no nonverbal evidence of pondering, you are likely to conclude that no response is forthcoming. The Stage Four child has learned this lesson, that a pause greater than one second means that the conversational partner is probably not going to respond (Craig & Gallagher, 1983). Short pauses, those less than one second in duration, mean that exchanges on this topic will continue. As adults, we are so sensitive to this time factor that long pauses in conversations, especially with people we do not know well, are very uncomfortable. In fact, as we become skilled conversationalists, we learn to overlap our responses so that there are no pauses.

By the end of Stage Four or the beginning of Stage Five, at about 42 months, the child is able to maintain a topic for more than two turns (Bloom, Rocissano, & Hood, 1976). Not surprisingly, based on everything we know about children, the child is more likely to maintain a topic for several turns if the conversation centers on something in his immediate environment and if the topic interests him. Most adults respond in a similar way. When someone tries to engage me in a conversation about opera, there is usually only one exchange because my response is, *Don't like it,* but if someone wants to talk to me about baseball, football, or basketball, there is the potential for many turns. Part of the art of conversation, therefore, is finding a topic that interests your partner, and a good conversationalist is not necessarily someone who has a great deal to say but someone who knows how to get others to talk about what interests them. The lesson to be emphasized at this point, with the Stage Four child, is that the adult, by choosing topics that interest or fail to interest the child, usually determines how long child-adult conversations will last.

Before the child's third birthday, his presuppositional skills have been limited. Unless the topic of conversation is immediate, the adult often has difficulty following shifts in the conversation because the child does not provide the information the listener needs to keep abreast of the changes. During Stage Four, following his third birthday, the child begins to make some meaningful and helpful presuppositions in his conversations. The Stage Four child understands what the listener needs to know about the topic, and he can determine how much information he needs to provide (Shatz, Wellman, & Silber, 1983; Wellman & Estes, 1987). The child adjusts the amount of information he provides depending on whether or not the listener can directly observe the topic of conversation. That is, if the listener is looking at the object of the conversation, the child knows that little additional information is needed, but if the child is talking about something not present, he provides more information. The child also adjusts his speech according to the age of his listener. He uses very basic syntax and vocabulary when he is talking to a younger child and uses more sophisticated language when he is talking to adults or to children his own age.

The reader should keep in mind that presuppositional skills depend not only on the speaker's sensitivity to what the listener may need to know but on the speaker's cognitive and linguistic abilities to convey information the listener needs. Although the Stage Four child's presuppositional skills have improved, he is still limited in these skills by what he knows and what he is able to express. If the child has a firm cognitive grasp of the topic and if he has the vocabulary and language ability to talk about the topic, he is likely to provide the information necessary. If the topic is beyond his understanding and language abilities, he will have trouble providing the information the listener needs. Even adults run into this problem. If I were talking to someone about the operation of the engine in my Toyota, I might be very sensitive to my listener's informational needs, but beyond identifying what I think are spark plugs, the air filter, and the oil dip stick, I would probably use the word *thing* quite often, and my listener would never have adequate information. Presuppositional skills, you see, depend on knowledge, insight, understanding, vocabulary, syntax, and all the other elements of communication. As a conversationalist, the Stage Four child is perfectly willing to help, and he wants to help, but he will help only to the extent that he can help. Otherwise, he can only say, "Help!"

As mentioned earlier, *pragmatics* is concerned with using language to get things done. Adult speakers are often very direct in making requests or demands. If I say, for example, *Close the door,* there is no question about what is meant and the language is unequivocal. This is a *direct* request. I might say, *Can you close the door?* On the surface, this seems to be a question about the ability of the listener to close the door, but it is really an *indirect* request to close the door. I assume the listener has the ability, but I choose this manner to make my request because it is more polite and does not have the edge of a direct order. I can give the request an even softer edge if I say, *There seems to be a little breeze in here,* or I can give it a harder, sarcastic edge if I say, *Were you raised in a barn?!* These examples are even less direct, but the request is still being made. The child's ability to use language to make requests and demands, and to change the manner in which the requests are made, must evolve. This evolution is not rapid.

Prior to the emergence of language, the child indicates needs and makes requests by gesturing, crying, and by producing speech-like noises. By the time he is two years old, he is able to accompany these nonverbal communications with some words, but his efforts to gain attention and have his requests met often fail (Ervin-Tripp, O'Connor, & Rosenberg, 1987). He will use words like "mine," "want," and "more" (Newcombe & Zaslow, 1981), and when he begins to combine words, he will make requests such as "I want cookie," "I need blankie," or "Give me ball" (Ervin-Tripp, 1977). At this point, virtually all requests are direct.

Keeping in mind that the Stage Four child has developed an understanding of the meanings of most common modals, he is now using these modals to make *indirect* requests. He might say, for example, "Could you give me a cookie?" or "Can you pick me up?" Just as he has learned the power of "please" with adults (Ervin-Tripp & Gordon, 1986), so has he learned that these indirect and more polite requests are often more effective, or at least more warmly received, than their direct equivalents. This is a small but important example of how pragmatic skills advance as a direct result of greater language ability. The child cannot make an indirect request until he has the language required for such a request, and we witness only the first step in indirect requests in this stage. As the child matures and as his language becomes more sophisticated, he will be able to make requests so subtly and indirectly that he will make his listener believe the satisfaction of the request is the listener's idea, not the child's. We all know a few people, children and adults, whose talents in this area of pragmatics are amazingly effective!

TABLE 5-3 Stage Four Highlights

Typical Age Range: 35 to 40 Months
MLU: 3.0 to 3.75 Morphemes

Grammatical Morphemes
• Still developing . . . slowly but surely.

Pronouns
• More consistent in use of *they, us, his, her, hers,* and *them.*

Verbs
• Using past tense of common modals: *could, should, would.*

Noun Phrases
• Continues to elaborate by adding only one element in front of the noun.

Verb Phrase
• Elaborates by including *do* in negative and question forms and by including modals such as *could, would, might,* and *must.*
• Continues to overextend the regular past tense form to irregular verbs.

Sentences
• Adds the following contractions in his productions of negative sentences: *didn't, doesn't, isn't,* and *aren't.*
• More consistent in use of *why, who,* and *how* questions. Also asking *when* questions.

Pragmatics
• Learns that short pauses mean that exchanges will continue; long pauses mean that responses are not forthcoming.
• By the end of Stage Four, is able to sustain conversation for more than two turns.
• Developing primitive presuppositional skills, i.e., understanding what the listener needs to know and proving appropriate information.
• Beginning to make indirect requests, e.g., "Can you pick me up?"

Stage Five: Polishing the Act

As we have suggested throughout this chapter and the preceding chapter, these five stages do not finish the acquisition of speech and language. The child still has much to learn when he completes Stage Five, but he has certainly learned all that can be considered basic in speech and language by the end of this stage. The child is typically in this stage between the ages of 41 and 46 months and has an MLU range of 3.75 to 4.5. During Stage Five, the child reaches closure on some language behaviors, elaborates upon others, and is still struggling with other aspects of language. The process of acquiring and learning about speech and language will continue throughout childhood and adolescence, and even into adulthood. It is certainly a reasonable hope that five years from the day you read these words you will know more about language than you do now, that you will use language more skillfully in writing and speaking, and that you will be more sophisticated in the art of conversation. The Stage Five child has come a long way in his quest for communicative competence, but beyond his fourth birthday, he still has miles and miles to go.

Morphemic Development: The Acquisition Continues

If we consider the aggregate findings of Brown (1973) and Miller (1981), we can conclude that nine of the fourteen specified grammatical morphemes are mastered by the close of Stage Five. The remaining five are mastered by 50 months, just 4 months beyond the upper age limit we have used to mark Stage Five. More specifically, the Stage Five child masters or is close to mastering the irregular past form of common verbs, the contractible copula, the uncontractible auxiliary, and the regular and irregular markers for third person singular.

The regular past tense of verbs is created by adding *-ed*. Verbs that are made past tense by some other change are considered **irregular.** Although there are relatively few irregular past tense verbs in English, they are used frequently and pose an immediate problem for the child learning English. In Stages Three and Four, the child manages this problem by overextending the regular past tense form to these irregular verbs. He says, "catched" instead of "caught" and "throwed" instead of "threw." Early in language development, the child might give the appearance of understanding some irregular past tense forms. He might say, for example, "Daddy went work," but a few months later he might say, "Daddy wented work." This might seem like a regression to the caregiver, but it is actually a step forward in the child's understanding of past tense. He continues to have a problem, however, knowing the difference between regular and irregular past tense forms, so he uses the regular form on all verbs. By the end of Stage Five, he understands the difference, at least for commonly used irregular past tense forms such as "sat," "went," "broke," "ate," "ran," and "fell." He may continue to have problems with verbs like "hit" and "put" that do not change when they move from present to past tense. He might also try to find regularity where there is none. For example, he might reason that if the past tense of "sing" is "sang" and the past tense of "ring" is "rang," then the past tense of "bring" must be "brang." He would, of course, be wrong, but eventually he will get most of the exceptions and irregularities figured out.

To this point we have used the terms contractible and uncontractible in reference to the copula and auxiliary forms of the verb *to be* with little explanation. Although these terms seem to be self-explanatory, the issue of contractibility may be more complex than you imagine. The speaker must learn that sometimes it is permissible to contract and sometimes it is not, and the rules for contractibility are not always clear. I can say *He is tall,* or I can contract this copula form to *He's tall.* This is a **contractible** copula form. If the same copula form is in an answer to a question, adult usage suggests that a contraction is not acceptable. If you ask, *Is he tall?*, I will respond *He is,* or *Yes, he is tall,* but the answer, *He's,* does not sound right because it violates a rule of contractibility based on usage. In this case, the copula is **uncontractible.** Consider contractibility in a question such as, *Do you know how tall he is?* It would not be acceptable to say, *Do you know how tall he's?* although you could say, *He's tall, isn't he?* You can say, *He's tall,* or *He isn't tall,* but you cannot say, *He'sn't tall,* because it is not acceptable to contract a form that is already contracted, although the slang form *tisn't* meaning *it is not* is an exception of sorts. Notice, however, that the *i* and *t* in *it* are inverted. It is also not permissible to contract the copula when it is in the past tense. I can say, *He's tall,* but in the past tense, I must say, *He was tall.* The child must learn when it is permissible to contract and when it is not. It is not surprising that he is still struggling with contractible and uncontractible forms of the copula and auxiliary versions of *to be* as he enters Stage Five.

Although the child is producing some uncontractible copula forms as early as Stage Two or Three, he does not master the uncontractible copula until Stage Five (Miller, 1981). The child masters the contractible copula even later, toward the end of Stage Five or beyond (Miller, 1981). According to Brown (1973), a copula is contractible even if it is not actually contracted in a given production. I might say, *He's tall,* or *He is tall.* In both cases, I have used a contractible copula. The child must not only learn when the copula is contractible and when it is not, he must learn the forms of the copula that reflect **person** ("I *am.*" "She *is.*"), **number** ("I *am.* "We *are.*"), and **tense** ("I *am.*" "I *was.*") and the various combinations of these. If there are several people, not including me, and I am referring to the past, I will say, *They were.* If there are several people, including me, and I am referring to the future, I will say, *We will.* It takes the child considerable time to learn all the copula's variations, how they combine with nouns and pronouns, and to determine when it is acceptable to contract and when it is not.

The child must also learn when it is permissible to contract the auxiliary forms of *to be.* As with the copula, the child uses the uncontractible form of the auxiliary before the contractible form. The auxiliary form is uncontractible when it is past tense. The sentence, *He was running away,* cannot be contracted to *He's running away,* because *He's* is interpreted in the present tense. If someone asks, *Who is running away?,* the contraction *He's* would not be an acceptable answer whereas *He is* would be acceptable. In response to the question, *Is he running away?,* I might respond, *He isn't running away,* or *He's not running away,* but I cannot combine the contractions into *He'sn't.* The child masters the uncontractible auxiliary during Stage Five. The contractible auxiliary is mastered beyond Stage Five, and as with the copula, the child masters the "is" and "are" forms before he masters the "am" form. That is, he will say, "He's running," or "They're running," before he says, "I'm running."

In English, the **person(s)** performing the action of the verb is indicated by the person and the number of the noun or pronoun. Using the verb *eat,* I can create sentences like *I eat, We eat, You eat,* and *They eat.* The verb stays the same regardless of the person or number of the subject, but notice what happens when I have a third person singular subject. I now produce sentences such as *He eats, She eats,* and *John eats.* The only marker I use to indicate **third person singular** on the present tense forms of regular verbs is the addition of *s: He sings, She jumps, Mary writes, John stands.* A few verbs require irregular adjustments to reflect third person singular. I say, *I do, You do,* and *They do,* but I add *-es* to say, *He **does.*** I say, *I have, You have,* and *They have,* but I say, *He **has.*** The regular and irregular forms of third person singular markers on verbs emerge in Stage Two, but they are not mastered until Stage Five and beyond (Trantham & Pederson, 1976).

The Stage Five child is producing the personal pronouns "its," "our," "ours," "him," "their," "theirs," "myself," and "yourself" in sentences such as:

"The dog has something in *its* ear."

"It's *our* house."

"Do you have a doggie like *ours?*"

"I like *him.*"

"*Their* Mommy is nice."

"We have a tree like *theirs.*"

"I can do it *myself.*"

"You can watch TV by *yourself.*"

During the late preschool years and into the early elementary years, the child learns how to change the meanings of words by adding suffixes. Certain adjectives can be changed to **comparative** or **superlative** forms by adding *-er* and *-est* respectively. The comparative form of *big* is *bigger,* and the superlative form is *biggest.* The Stage Five child understands the superlative forms of common adjectives, but he does not understand the comparative form until he is about 60 months, well beyond the end of Stage Five (Carrow, 1973). It should also be emphasized that the child *understands* these forms before he *uses* them. Even after he understands the comparative and superlative concepts, he may struggle for many years with some adjectives because he does not know or remember whether comparative is marked with *-er* or with *more* and superlative is marked with *-est* or *most.* Does this sound like a familiar problem? The general rule is that if the descriptive adjective is one syllable, use *-er* and *-est.* Two-syllable adjectives often require *more* and *most,* and adjectives of three or more syllables usually require *more* and *most.* The comparative and superlative forms of single-syllable adjectives like *tall* and *cold* are *taller—tallest* and *colder—coldest,* but consider the following:

Beautiful—More beautiful—Most beautiful.

Ridiculous—More ridiculous—Most ridiculous.

Using *-er* and *-est* on these words would be awkward. Some children, and even adults, get so carried away with the comparative and superlative concepts that they say things like, "It was the most ugliest dog I have ever seen," or "She is more shorter than I am." When my youngest daughter was five years old, she loved the word "ridiculous" and used it often, but she had trouble with the comparative and superlative forms. She produced delightfully entertaining sentences such as, "It was the most ridiculousest thing I ever saw," and that's not easy to say! The Stage Five child is just beginning this struggle. It will be years before he uses the comparative and superlative forms of some adjectives correctly, and he may continue into adulthood with doubts about some. He must learn, for example, that it is not proper to produce comparative and superlative forms of *absolute adjectives.* There are no degrees of *dead* or *perfect,* so it is improper to say, *He was the most perfect man I ever met.* Likewise, it makes no sense to say, *Max the goldfish is deader than Xanadu the mouse,* and there is no such thing as *more pregnant.* Let's see now, is it *more lucky* or *luckier?*

During the same preschool period, the child learns to produce the noun versions of certain verbs by adding *-er.* A person who runs, for example, is a *runner,* and a person who plays is a *player.* These are called **agentive** forms. When the child is two or three years old, he usually creates this form by adding "man" to the verb to produce words like "runman," or "runningman." He understands and uses the regular agentive form when he is about five years old.

Noun and Verb Phrases: Still Adjusting the Pieces of the Puzzle

Not much happens in Stage Five relative to the elaboration of noun and verb phrases, nothing at least that is unique to this stage. The child's sentences are a little longer, on average, as indicated by the increase in MLU from Stage Four to Stage Five. Nevertheless, the construction of his noun phrases is much the same as in Stage Four. That is, he continues to use only one element in front of the noun. This element might be a demonstrative pronoun (*"That* cat . . ."), a possessive pronoun (*"My* Mommy . . ."), an article (*"The* doggie . . ."), or an adjective ("I saw a *big* car"). The child continues to have difficulty matching the number of the subject and the verb in this stage and well beyond this stage (Miller, 1981). He will produce sentences such as "The doggies is eating my sandwich," and "Joey and Billy is playing baseball." It may seem a simple task to establish subject-verb agreement in terms of number, but the reader should be reminded that many adults struggle with this requirement in certain situations. When the subject of a sentence is conjoined, one might assume the verb should be plural, and in most cases the verb should be plural, but not always. It is correct to say, *The pitcher and catcher* **are** *important members of the team,* but in the sentence, *The director and star of the movie* **is** *Rock Hunk,* the verb is singular because *director* and *star* refer to one person. When *or* or *nor* conjoin singular words, the verb should be singular as in *Neither George nor Ralph* **needs** *the job.* When *or* or *nor* conjoin plural words, the verb must be plural as in *Forks or spoons* **are** *stored in this drawer.* When a gerund phrase containing a plural noun is the subject of a sentence, the verb is singular as in the sentence, *Collecting baseball cards* **is** *my favorite hobby.* Some nouns are plural in form but singular in meaning, and they require a singular verb—*Politics* **is** *a dirty business.* In some cases, a sum of money or a unit of time requires a singular verb. I would say, *Three dollars* **were** *found on the sidewalk,* but I would also say, *Forty thousand dollars* **is** *too much to spend for that car,* or *"Four months* **is** *plenty of time to paint the house.* Indefinite pronouns like *all* or *few* can require singular or plural verbs depending on how they are used. I would say, *A few of these* **are** *spoiled,* but I would also say, *A few is all he could eat at* *one time.* These are just a few examples of the problems that face the speaker on the single issue of subject-verb agreement. The Stage Five child is still struggling with the most basic of these problems. As he moves through his school years and into adulthood, he will have many opportunities to wrestle with the more difficult challenges of subject-verb agreement.

The changes we see in verb phrases in Stage Five occur as a result of the child's acquisition of the grammatical morphemes we identified earlier. As the child progressively masters irregular past tense forms, the contractible copula, the uncontractible auxiliary, and the markers for regular and irregular third person singular, his verb phrases become more adult-like. His verb phrases are not necessarily longer, but they are more correct according to adult language standards.

Sentence Construction: Negatives, Questions, Embedding, and Conjoining

By the close of Stage Five, the child is using negative past tense forms of the verb "to be," as in the sentence, "He wasn't a good boy." Although they do not appear often, he also produces the negative past tense of common modals, including "wouldn't," "couldn't," and "shouldn't" (Miller, 1981), resulting in sentences such as the following:

"Mommy couldn't open the can."

"She wouldn't eat her soup."

"Bobbie shouldn't do that."

Progress in the creation of negative sentences in Stage Five centers on the use of past tense and appropriate modals, and we see the same adjustments as the child continues to develop the interrogative form of sentences. The child is producing correctly inverted question forms in Stage Four, but he is somewhat inconsistent in making the required inversions. In this stage, he is much more consistent in moving from a declarative statement such as "He is playing baseball," to the interrogative version, "Is he playing baseball?" We also see the appearance of the **tag question** in Stage Five, an interrogative form not frequently used in American English (Klee, 1985). The easiest and most common form of tag question is acquired in Stage Five. In this version, the speaker adds a tag like "huh" or "okay" to the end of a sentence as in "I'm going to leave now, okay?" or "You're going to buy me some ice-cream, huh?" Beyond Stage Five, the child learns a somewhat more difficult form of tag question, not including a negative element, as represented in the sentence, "You're going to buy me some ice-cream, are you?" Within the next few years, he is producing the adult form of tag questions, complete with a negative element, as in the sentence, "You're going to buy me some ice-cream, aren't you?" The progression from "huh" to "are you" to "aren't you" sounds subtle, but each step reflects a more sophisticated use of language (Reich, 1986).

During Stage Five, the child begins to embed relative clauses in the object position of sentences. He will not embed relative clauses into subjects until he is beyond the age of five years (Menyuk, 1977). As indicated earlier in this chapter, a relative clause is introduced by a relative pronoun such as *who, which, what,* or *that.* In the sentence, *The man who came to dinner with Sally is my brother,* the clause *who came to dinner* is embedded into the subject to describe or modify *man.* The child's earliest relative clauses are used to describe **empty nouns.** These are nonspecific nouns such as "thing" or "one." Using these nouns, the Stage Five child produces sentences containing object-embedded relative clauses such as "She's the one *that I kissed,*" or "That's the thing *that I broke.*" By the end of this stage, the child will produce a few sentences in which the relative pronoun is omitted and understood, but still only in the object position. Without the relative pronouns, our example sentences would be produced as follows: "She's the one I kissed," and "That's the thing I broke." Perhaps because the relative pronoun helps to preserve the meaning of the sentence, preschool children are less likely to delete it than adults (Menyuk, 1977). The first relative pronoun the child is likely to use in all circumstances is "that." Whereas the adult would say, "She's the one *who* came to the party," the child in Stage Five will probably say, "She's the one *that* came to the party." Even when the child adds other relative pronouns to his repertoire, he often uses them incorrectly. He might continue to use "that" for "who" for some time, and he might use "what" for "who" or even for "that," resulting in sentences such as the following:

"George is the one *what* broke the window."

"The glass is the thing *what* spilled."

By the close of Stage Five, the child is producing multiple embeddings (Miller, 1981). He might produce a sentence that embeds an infinitive into a subordinate clause which serves as the object of the sentence: "I think I want to eat all the cake." The clause, "I want to eat all the cake," is the object of the verb "think." The infinitive "to eat" is embedded in this clause, so we have a sentence that contains an embedded subordinate clause which, in turn, contains an embedded infinitive. This is only the beginning of the possibilities. As the child moves into the school years, he will produce sentences with even more elaborate embeddings, and he will learn to embed and conjoin at the same time. That sounds illegal, doesn't it?

Although the child uses the conjunction "and" as early as the end of Stage One and adds other conjunctions such as "but," "so," "if," and "or" in Stage Three, he does not conjoin clauses until Stage Four, and he does not really get serious about clausal conjoining until Stage Five (Brown, 1973). The child's favorite conjunction is "and," and he continues to favor it in combining clauses well beyond Stage Five (Bennett-Kaster, 1986).

According to Bloom, Lahey, Hood, Lifter, and Fiess (1980), the semantic relations conveyed in conjoined sentences emerge in an identifiable sequence. In the beginning, the child uses "and" to express all of these semantic relations. The first conjunctive relation to emerge is **additive,** a relation we are most likely to associate with "and." In an additive sentence, the child combines two clauses that are independent of one another. He might say, "I went to Billy's house, and I'm a big boy." In this sentence, the combined meaning is the same as the added meanings of the separate clauses. The child then uses "and" to express **temporal** relations. In the sentence, "I went to Billy's house, and I played with his toys," the child is talking about one event that follows another in time. The child then expresses the **causal** relation. One clause expresses an action or state of being, and the other clause provides a reason or describes the effect. The child might say, "I ate all the cake, and my tummy is full." The combined meaning in this sentence is clearly greater than the sum of the meanings of the separate clauses. The child then expresses the **adversative** relation in his conjoined sentences. In this case, the two parts of the sentence represent a contrast. The child says, "This doggie big, and this one little." The children in this study also used "and" to connect a clause that described or elaborated upon the subject of the preceding clause. The child might say, "I got a baseball bat, and you play baseball with it." The authors called this semantic relation **object specification.** They conclude that the child is using "and" to appropriately link subjects and objects in a listing sense by the end of Stage One or the beginning of Stage Two.

As already noted, some children conjoin clauses with "and" as early as Stage Four, but we usually do not see clausal conjoining until the end of Stage Five (Miller, 1981). Although the dominant conjunction continues to be "and" for some time, the child is using "if" to conjoin clauses by the close of Stage Five. Other conjunctions, including "because," "but," "so," and "when" do not emerge until after Stage Five when the child's MLU is about 5.0 (Owens, 1996, p. 334).

Pragmatic Development: The Conversational Fine Tuning Continues

We generally think of the child's becoming a social creature between the ages of three and four. This maturity seems to be reflected in the Stage Five child's conversation, which is becoming increasingly social. When he speaks to others, his utterances are appropriately structured, understandable, and designed to meet his listeners' conversational needs (Mueller, 1972).

In Stage Four, we observed that the child develops a sensitivity to the time factor in conversational exchanges. That is, when there is a time delay of less than one second, he concludes that exchanges will continue, but if the delay is longer than one second, he concludes that no response is forthcoming (Craig & Gallagher, 1983). In Stage Five, the child's turn-taking continues to be affected by his interpretations of short and long pauses. As is true of the adult in conversation, the child uses the pause as a cue for initiating his turn (Garvey & Berninger, 1981). Perhaps of even greater significance, he takes into consideration what is likely to be included in the next turn. That is, he shows an awareness of what is being discussed in the present turn, and he anticipates how this topic will be completed in

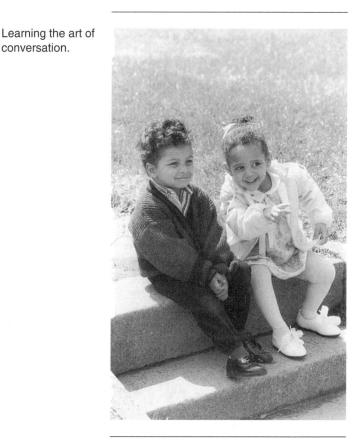

Learning the art of conversation.

succeeding turns (McTear, 1985). He is sensitive to problems his partner may have in finishing his or her turn, and when he senses his partner is having difficulty, he will attempt to help by completing what he perceives to be his partner's thought. In addition, he is developing a sensitivity to the problems created by simultaneous talking. When he senses that information will be lost when he and his partner are talking at the same time, he is willing to give up his turn in order to preserve the conversational topic. By the time the child is ready for school, he has developed considerable turn-taking skills, but conversational inadequacies remain.

Some preschool children are able to handle conversations involving two partners, but struggle with three-party conversations (Ervin-Tripp, 1979). Interruptions remain a problem for young communicators for some time. Remember that interruptions are sometimes necessary to capture one's turn in a conversation. The child must learn how and when to interrupt according to the "rules" of conversational etiquette. Sachs (1982) found that the preschool child typically does not use polite verbal or nonverbal strategies for gaining the attention of his listener. That is, he does not say, "Excuse me," or he does not gently tap his listener's shoulder or lean forward or gesture in a manner that suggests he wants to say something. He simply yells at his listener. Only 36 percent of the utterances produced by Sachs's subjects, who ranged from 40 to 66 months, were at a conversational loudness level. Not surprisingly, only the oldest subjects in this study were sensitive to their proximity to their listeners. The older children did not try to initiate conversation until they were within an appropriate range. Even then, they yelled. The younger children just yelled. If you have spent much time around children in this age range, you are probably saying, "Yep, that just about captures it!"

Over the course of the preschool years, the child improves his ability to imitate and sustain a conversation. As we have mentioned, the child does not maintain a topic for more than two turns until he is about 42 months, which marks the beginning of Stage Five (Bloom et al., 1976). By the time the child is five years old and well beyond Stage Five, he maintains a topic for an average of five turns compared to the eleven turns on average by adult speakers (Brinton & Fujiki, 1984). Even when the preschool child is maintaining a topic through three or four turns, he is not contributing much new information. He maintains the conversation primarily through repeating part of what his partner has already said or by asking questions about his partner's comments. Even when the child is in the early elementary school years, he seldom adds significant information to a conversation (Brinton & Fujiki, 1984). In this sense, he remains a conversational follower.

We see no radical changes in conversational repairs during Stage Five, although as the child's overall language skills improve, he is better able to respond to requests for clarification. As early as Stage One or Two, the child has shown an awareness of the need for conversational repairs. Throughout the five stages of language development, he tries, within the limits of his intellectual and linguistic abilities, to provide the information his conversational partner finds lacking or confused. Even as Stage Five closes, however, he sometimes has difficulty identifying the part of the message that needs to be repaired (Brinton & Fujiki, 1989, p. 92), and he still responds more readily to requests for repairs than he makes requests for repairs from his conversational partners.

In Stage Four, we noted that the child's presuppositional skills depend on his knowledge of the topic and his language skills. Nothing has changed in this regard as he moves into Stage Five. Naturally, his presuppositional skills improve as he moves toward his fourth birthday, but the limitations are the same. Several studies requiring young children to describe stimuli to listeners have demonstrated these limitations. When preschool children and even kindergarten children have tried to describe blocks of varying sizes, colors, and geometric shapes to listeners so that the listeners could choose the correct blocks, they did not perform well. They were not able to provide the information the listeners needed. In their study, Krauss and Glucksberg (1977) had two four-year-old children sitting at a table and separated by a screen so they could not see one another. Each child had an identical set of blocks of unfamiliar geometric shapes. The speaker's task was to describe one of the blocks so that the listener could successfully select it. The following exchange occurred:

CHILD ONE: It's a bird."
CHILD TWO: "Is this it?"
CHILD ONE: "No."

One could conclude, of course, that the speaker in this situation simply had inadequate presuppositional skills, but there is another and perhaps more reasonable interpretation. This task was beyond the cognitive abilities of these children. They did not know these shapes, and the speaker was unable to retrieve an image from his mental bank that was a close enough match to the block he was trying to describe to help his partner who was also unfamiliar with these shapes. Two adults, unfamiliar with the Chinese alphabet, might have similar problems if one were trying to describe a Chinese character to the other. The adults would have the advantage of larger vocabularies, more sophisticated language abilities, and greater experience with a wider range of stimuli that might be similar in important respects to the Chinese character, but it would still be a difficult task. The point is, the Stage Five child might appear to have inadequate presuppositional skills when the real problem is a lack of knowledge. When he is talking about things he knows and understands, he is much more adept at providing the information his listener needs.

The Stage Five child continues to increase his use of indirect requests, although indirect requests are still far less frequent than direct requests. Between 42 and 52 months, less than 10 percent of children's requests are indirect, but we see a dramatic increase in use of the indirect form beyond Stage Five at about 54 months (James & Seebach, 1982; Wilkinson, Calculator, & Dollaghan, 1982). The child will make requests such as "Don't forget to get my cookie," or "Why don't you get me some candy?" These are clearly requests, but they are more subtle and more polite than "Give me a cookie," or "Get me some candy." When the child increases his use of indirect requests, he will also include rationalizations for his requests. He might say, for example, "I ate all my peas. . . . Don't forget to get my cookie," a polite and indirect way of saying that he has been a good boy, has fulfilled the obligations of his dinner-eating contract, and now wants his reward. As early as four years, the child's requests are shaped by his sensitivity to the roles and viewpoints of his listeners and the need to be polite (Gordon & Ervin-Tripp, 1984), and he responds appropriately to indirect requests made to him (Carrell, 1981). He has been using "please" since he was 24 to 36 months old, but in the beginning, he uses it mostly with people who are older or more dominant (Ervin-Tripp & Gordon, 1986). By the time he is four years old, "please" has become the magic word that can be used with almost anyone to get almost anything, and over the next few years, he will learn to use the magic word even more effectively.

Pragmatic Development: The Beginnings of Narrative Discourse

In addition to learning the technical skills and artistic nuances of conversation, the child is soon confronted with a new discourse challenge: He must learn how to tell a story, a common narrative form. As is true of a conversation, a narrative consists of a series of sentences, not juxtaposed randomly, but in an orderly and interconnected sequence. The sequence of sentences allows the speaker to convey information about events or experiences in a systematic manner, each sentence building upon the preceding sentence. Unlike a conversation in which the communicative responsibility is shared by all participants who take turns as speakers and listeners, the narrative form is essentially a monologue in which the responsibility for conveying the message belongs almost exclusively to the speaker. Just as there are rules governing conversation, so are there rules, or principles, for structuring a narrative so that it is a cohesive and effective community entity.

We will address narrative skills in their more fully developed form in Chapter Six. In this section, we will consider the basic constructs of narratives that develop during the preschool years. These narrative fundamentals will form the foundation for the more complete and complex narrative skills that develop during the school years.

If you listen carefully to a child who is two to three-and-a-half years old, you will hear what are called **protonarratives.** A protonarrative is a primitive story about something that has happened to the child. As we have already noted, the child at this age has been repeatedly exposed to familiar routines or scripts in the common events of his life. While the child at this age cannot accurately and completely describe what happened during an event, he will often produce a series of utterances that, taken together, have a story-like quality. Visualize a very common routine, mealtime. The child is eating one of his least favorite foods, and he and his caregiver go through their usual tortuous exchange of words and actions related to his consumption of this food. That evening, his Aunt Mary comes over for a visit, and she asks him about dinner. He says to his Aunt Mary, "It made me sick. I throwed it away. It was lumpy. I don't like oatmeal!" I suspect that the caregiver's version of this event would be quite different and certainly more detailed than the child's version, but the child does convey a message that bears some resemblance to a story, even if it is a little short on detail and even if his description is not exactly on target. Miller and Sperry (1988) note that between the ages of 24 and 30 months, children use protonarratives with increasing frequency, and they improve their ability to put events into simple sequences.

When the child develops his first narratives, he uses two basic strategies to provide their organizational structure. One strategy, called **chaining,** involves ordering events that share one or more features in common. Each event in the chain logically follows the preceding event. The second strategy, called **centering,** involves building a story around a central theme. Each item or action in the narrative is connected to the central theme by an attribute that is related to the theme, however marginal that relationship might seem to an adult observer.

According to Sutton-Smith (1986), the child will begin to produce his own stories sometime between the ages of 24 and 36 months, and if he is a typical child, most of his earliest narratives will be built around central themes. The central themes of these early stories tend to focus on unusual or upsetting events that have had a significant impact on the child's life (Ames, 1966). An adult, listening to this kind of story, may want to understand exactly what happened to the child, when it happened, and why it happened. The adult listener is likely to be disappointed. In his earliest stories, the child does not take into consideration the listener's need for background information. In fact, even at 42 months, he does not provide much information about the participants in his narratives (Peterson, 1990). Even if the adult listener is struggling to make sense of it all, the child remains excited about telling his story, and it does not seem to matter much if the listener has a complete grasp of what happened or not. As we mentioned, the child's earliest narratives tend to be centered, or central theme, stories, but by the time he is three years old, he may be using the chaining strategy as often as he uses the centering strategy (Owens, 1996, p. 286).

The child's narrative skills noticeably improve during the preschool years. When he is two years old, the child organizes a narrative by generating a series of brief, unrelated statements connected only by a common originating stimulus. The process the child uses to get from one utterance to the next is something like the free association used by psychotherapists. The critical difference, of course, is that the child is prompting himself and the therapist is prompting a client, but the prompting principle is the same. The therapist instructs the client to say the first thing that comes to his mind, resulting in an exchange such as the following:

THERAPIST: "Dog"
    CLIENT: "Animal"
THERAPIST: "Animal"
    CLIENT: "Linebacker"
THERAPIST: "Linebacker"
    CLIENT: "Overpaid"
THERAPIST: "Overpaid"
    CLIENT: "Therapist"
THERAPIST: "Our time's up. That'll be $100."
    CLIENT: "Dog!"

Despite the silliness of the example, the reader should be able to sense that these responses are connected, but not in a categorical or cause-effect sense. They are connected, very loosely, in that one response prompts another. A set of unrelated statements connected by a common originating stimulus produced by the two-year-old child is called a **heap.** When he creates a heap, the child uses a basic sentence structure and simply adds or chains one bit of information onto another, prompted by his own observations. In the following example of a heap, you will not find a meaningful organization, even though you should be able to figure out the association that prompts each succeeding utterance. Notice too that you could rearrange these utterances into any order without affecting the overall meaning of the heap. Why is the overall meaning of the heap not affected by a reorganization of the utterances? And the answer is . . . there is no overall meaning. This narrative is like an abstract Swedish movie from the 1960s. It's going nowhere.

> Mommy sit here. Baby go "Waa!" Kitty go "meow." Doggie play ball.

At the next level of narrative development, the child's stories have a little more cohesion and a bit more focus. That is, the child's statements reflect a characteristic that several things have in common, or they reflect several events that were juxtaposed by time. Even though he may talk about several things that took place within the same general timeframe, the child's statements are not organized in a temporal manner in the sense that the first statement refers to the first thing that happened, the second statement refers to the second thing that happened, etc. Neither is there the suggestion of a cause-effect organization. The child's statements are simply chained, or added together, which means that they can still be reorganized into any pattern of presentation without affecting the integrity of the story. An example of this kind of narrative follows:

> Daddy threw a straw. Suzie ate ice cream. I had a Pepsi.

Sometime between the ages of three and five years, the child is producing narratives that have at least a rudimentary temporal organization (Owens, 1996, p. 287), but the glue that holds this kind of narrative together is still the central theme. The child's story statements convey what happened and in what order, but the emphasis is clearly on the essence of the event itself. That this is still a primitive form of narrative is made clear by the absence of a plot and by the absence of cause-effect references. An example of this kind of narrative follows:

> Mommy took me to the zoo. There was a lion. He made a noise. There was a monkey. And I got some popcorn. And we drived home.

The child's narratives will not typically include causality organization until he is five to seven years old (Owens, 1996, p. 288). When he adds this dimension to his stories, his narratives will change dramatically. We will consider these changes and the continued maturation of the child's narrative skills in Chapter Six.

Understanding Language: Cognition, Comprehension, and Production

As has been noted at a number of junctures in this book, it is not possible to separate intellectual growth from language development, and it is not possible to separate the comprehension of language from the production of language. These processes are inextricably connected, and they have interactive relationships. The child thinks before he has language, but language eventually facilitates and shapes thought. As common sense suggests, comprehension generally precedes

TABLE 5-4 Stage Five Highlights

Typical Age Range: 41 to 46 Months
MLU: 3.75 to 4.5 Morphemes

Grammatical Morphemes
- Nine of the fourteen specified morphemes ar mastered by the close of Stage Five.
- The remaining five morphemes (irregular past tense, contractible copula, uncontractible auxiliary, regular third person, and irregular third person) are mastered by 50 months.

Pronouns
- More consistent in use of *its, our, ours, him, their, theirs, myself, yourself.*

Adjectives
- Understands the superlative forms of common adjectives but does not understand comparative forms until he is about 60 months.

Noun Phrases
- Continues to elaborate by adding only one element in front of the noun.

Verb Phrases
- Continues to have difficulty matching the number of the subject and the verb.
- Verb phrases become more adult-like as the child masters verb-related grammatical morphemes.

Sentences
- Using negative past tense forms of *to be*, e.g., *weren't, wasn't*
- Occasionally uses negative past tense modals , e.g., *wouldn't, couldn't*
- More consistent in creating questions by properly inverting words, e.g., "He is playing baseball." → "Is he playing baseball?"
- Produces primitive tag questions, e.g., "I'm going now, OK?"
- Embeds relative clauses into the object position of sentences, e.g., "That's the plate *that I broke.*"
- Conjoins clauses, usually with *and.*

Pragmatics
- Conversational skills improve as a direct result of more sophisticated language.
- Increases his use of indirect requests, although direct requests are still far more common.

production, but production can also assist understanding. That is, sometimes we learn lessons about how language works by producing the language behaviors that illustrate the lessons. As we observe children acquiring language, it appears that some lessons are learned in a dramatic flash of illumination while others are learned more slowly, in an evolution of understanding that is steady but progresses in small steps. We should also keep in mind that language often reflects what one understands about the things, people, and events in reality, and language production often reflects what one is able to comprehend in language. Even college students are inclined to say, *I know what I mean, but I just can't express it,* when the truth is probably closer to *I wish I knew what I mean, but since I don't know, I'll use words that clearly express my confusion and benign ignorance.* Although there are exceptions, it is generally true that clear thinking results in clear speaking or writing, and muddled communications reflect muddled or incomplete thinking. If adults struggle with the interactions among cognition, comprehension, and production, imagine how the relationships among these processes affect the child between the ages of two years and four years, the approximate age span between Stages Two and Five. The child must know the words that represent the things, people, places, and events in his environment, of course, but he must also know how to change nouns to reflect plurality and possession, how to replace nouns with pronouns, how to mark verbs to indicate present, past, and future, how and when it is appropriate to contract, how to embed phrases and clauses to elaborate or indicate relationships, etc., etc., etc. There is much to understand about the world, much to understand about language, and much to know about producing language. Much of this understanding and producing occurs within the first four or five years of the child's life, and it is all connected. Let's examine a few examples of the language components the child must unravel to comprehend what he hears and what he produces.

Cognitive Development: Paving the Way for Understanding and Production

Common sense would certainly suggest that the child cannot receive or produce language that reflects understanding he does not have at the cognitive level. Before the child can embed phrases or clauses to reflect the manipulation of two or more linguistic units, he must be able to cognitively manipulate two or more objects (Ingram, 1975).

The words used in *wh-* questions emerge in the following order: *what, where, who,* and then *when, how,* and *why.* What does this order suggest to you about the order of acquisition of concepts that underlie these words? Why are words like *when, how,* and *why* acquired late? These last three words relate to the concepts of time and causality, and these concepts are acquired relatively late in cognitive development (Piaget, 1926). Very simply, the child must understand *time* before he can understand or produce "when" questions, and he must understand *cause-effect* before he can comprehend or produce "how" or "why" questions. Before the child has these later *wh-* words, he often responds to *when, how,* and *why* questions as though they are *what, where,* or *who* questions. Tyack and Ingram (1977) suggest that the child with a limited understanding of *wh-* terms uses two strategies in answering *wh-* questions: (a) Answer the question as though the *wh-* word is one I already know, or (b) Answer the question in a manner consistent with my understanding of the verb. Using the first strategy in responding to the question, *When did Susie eat?*, the child might assume it is a *what* question and respond, "Cracker." Using the second strategy, he might respond in the same way because he associates "cracker" with the verb "eat."

Piaget (1966) suggests that the child understands the sequencing of events before he understands duration. This too is reflected in his understanding and use of language. The child understands and produces words such as "before" and "after" which indicate *order* before he uses words such as "until" or "since" which indicate *duration.*

These are just a few examples of the obvious connections between what a child understands about his world at a cognitive level and what he is able to understand and produce in language. Look for the cognitive-language connections in the examples that follow. Some are obvious, and others are more subtle, but it may be impossible to find any aspect of receptive or expressive language development that is not directly or indirectly tied to a corresponding development in cognition.

Understanding Active and Passive Sentences

Consider the problems the child encounters as he tries to sort out active and passive sentences. An active sentence is considered **reversible** if either noun can be either the agent or the object. For example, I can say *The dog chased the cat,* or *The cat chased the dog.* These are reversible active sentences. The child understands the reversible active sentence in Stage One or Two (Chapman & Miller, 1975), but he has trouble interpreting reversible passive sentences until he is five years old or older. Why is this a problem? To interpret an active sentence, the child must learn that the first noun is the agent and the second noun is the object. He encounters an entirely different word order in passive sentences. In the passive sentence, *The cat was chased by the dog,* the first noun *(cat)* is the object of the verb *chased,* and the second noun *(dog)* is the agent. The child in Stage One or Two interprets this sentence in the same way as he interprets active sentences. If he were asked to point to one of two pictures, one showing a dog chasing a cat and the other a cat chasing a dog, he would point to the picture of the cat chasing the dog because he interprets the first noun as the subject and the second noun as the object. The child does not correctly interpret reversible passive sentences until he is beyond Stage Five. During the child's early struggles with passive forms, between the ages of three and four years, he will understand passive sentences that include animate objects better than sentences including inanimate objects (Lempert, 1990). Even at five, the child is more likely to correctly interpret reversible passive sentences containing active verbs than those which contain nonactive verbs. That is, *The boy was bitten by the girl,* would be interpreted more easily than *The boy was loved by the girl.* The child will probably not completely sort out passive sentences until he is in elementary school.

We should add a cautionary note at this point. The conclusions about understanding active and passive sentences are based on research that required children to act out the sentences they heard. A more recent technique requires that children only look at paired videos, one showing the agent-object relationship reflected in the sentence and the other showing the opposite agent-object relationship (Golinkoff,

Hirsh-Pasek, Cauley, & Gordon, 1987). Since acting out sentences is a more intense exercise requiring greater cooperation from the child, it may appear that children gain an understanding of passive and active sentences later than they really do. This new approach, which requires little effort, may eventually demonstrate that this understanding is acquired earlier.

Word Order: Which Comes First, Comprehension or Production?

Because word order is very important in English, experts who study English-speaking children are interested in the word order portion of the acquisition puzzle. Does the child comprehend word order before he produces language containing appropriate word order? The answer is temptingly obvious. There seems little doubt that comprehension of word order would precede production, and early research supported this assumption, but there have been some interesting and contradictory findings.

Chapman and Miller (1975) studied the comprehension and production of reversible active sentences in Stage One, Two, and Three children. In the comprehension task, the children were instructed to act out sentences produced by an adult. In the production task, the children were instructed to describe an action produced by an adult. The children in all three stages performed better in the production task than in the comprehension task, leading the authors to conclude that for word order at least, production precedes comprehension. Their conclusions were supported by later research (Gleitman & Wanner, 1982). How can this be?

It may be that we have oversimplified the comprehension-production equation. When the child in normal circumstances responds to the utterances of others, he is responding to more than linguistic information. He interprets the situation and reads all the nonverbal messages he is receiving from the speaker as well as comprehending the language forms he hears. If his caregiver says, *Put your toys in the toy box,* while pointing to the toys strewn all over the floor and to the empty toy-box, the child sees the toys and the box, hears the tone of his caregiver's voice, observes the caregiver's gestures and facial expression, *and* hears the words of the imperative sentence. He has been through this routine before and knows that the routine calls for him to pick up the toys and put them in the box. He puts all the information, linguistic and nonlinguistic, together to arrive at a correct interpretation of the total message. Now consider what occurred in the Chapman and Miller (1975) exercise. The child is instructed to act out a sentence, not unlike the one we have used here, but he is given no other information. He must rely on linguistic information alone. It may be, therefore, that the child first comprehends linguistic messages within situational and nonverbal contexts, then produces language, then understands language without the supporting situational and nonverbal contexts. Once again, we must be careful not to draw unwarranted conclusions. It may be that the kinds of responses required of children in some of these studies obscure what they really know and what they can really do. Acting out sentences and interpreting sentences being acted out may add levels of complexity that mask the child's true receptive and expressive abilities. Techniques that place fewer demands on the child's attention and that require less physical cooperation, such as the video technique developed by Golinkoff et al. (1987), may lead us to different conclusions about how and when the child comprehends and produces word order.

Words Expressing Relations: From Concepts to Production

A **relational** word, as the name suggests, identifies relationships among people, objects, and events. Relational words are used to identify spatial, temporal, quantity, and dimensional relationships. The child's understanding of the concepts that underlie these words and his comprehension of the words that describe the concepts develop during the preschool years. These are difficult concepts, however, and they are not acquired quickly or easily.

Spatial terms include prepositions such as "in," "on," "under," "over," "beside," "behind," and "in front of." By the time the child is two years old, he is using "in" and "on," but he may be applying a very simple strategy in deciding how to use these prepositions. In general, if he is describing an object in relation to a container, he will use "in." If he is describing an object in relation to a surface, he will use "on," but he does not fully understand that "on" can be used to describe an object in relation to a container, and he does not understand "under" until he is about three years old (Clark & Clark, 1977). He continues to have problems with terms such as "beside," "next to," "behind," and "in front of" until he is four or five years old (Johnston, 1984). The difficulty with these later developing prepositions is that the child must consider the object he is describing in relation to the spatial orientation of another object. In order to use the term "behind," for example, he must know which is the front and which is the back of the referent object. As common sense would suggest, he will use these prepositions most accurately with referent objects that have clearly defined fronts and backs. He will understand, for example, "Your sock is behind Mommy," more easily than "Your sock is behind the ball," because Mommy has an obvious front and an equally obvious back, but where is the "back" of the ball? When the referent object has no obvious front or back, the adult listener interprets "behind" or "in front of" on the basis of his position in relation to the object. That is, the surface of the ball nearest the listener is the "front," and the opposite surface is the "back." Children first understand these prepositions in relation to their own bodies, then in relation to referent objects with clearly defined fronts and backs, and finally in relation to objects without clearly defined fronts and backs (Conner & Chapman, 1985). This means, therefore, that in the earliest stage of understanding, the child who is directly facing a ball upon hearing the sentence, "Your sock is behind the ball," is likely to turn around and look for his sock behind his own back.

Temporal terms are used to describe relationships based on time. As we mentioned earlier in this section, the child understands terms based on *order* such as "before" and "after" earlier than he understands terms based on *duration* such as "since" and "until." Although the research has not provided a clear order of acquisition for temporal terms, it does seem clear that the child understands "before" and "after" by the time he is five years old.

Words such as "more" and "less" are **quantity** terms. These terms are used to identify the amount of something or the number of things in a group. These words are troublesome for the preschooler. When the preschool child is asked to point to the one with "more" or the one with "less," he points to the one with more. When he is asked to point to one of them, he points to the one with more. Some experts have concluded that these undifferentiated responses mean that the child believes "more" and "less" mean the same thing. According to Clark and Clark (1977), the child understands both words to mean "amount." Using this understanding, the child points to the one with the greater "amount" which is, of course, the one with more. Whatever the child's interpretation, he does not understand the difference between "more" and "less" until he moves into the elementary school years, and then he becomes confused about the meanings of words such as "few" and "couple." Someone asks the child, "Do you understand the difference between 'less' and 'few'" and he responds, "More or less!" Someone asks the child, "What is the difference between 'couple' and 'few'?" He answers, "When there are more than a couple, use 'few'. When there is more than one but less than a few, use 'couple'." Although there might be a few disagreements about whether "few" is less than "less" or whether some people use "less" when they should use "few," the child's response is more or less correct. The point of this hypothetical banter is to remind the reader that these are difficult terms and difficult concepts. It is not surprising that the preschooler does not yet have a solid understanding of quantity concepts and words.

Dimensional terms are used to identify the opposite ends of the limits of a person or object. They include words such as "big/little," "tall/short," and "thick/thin." More general dimensional terms such as "big/little" are understood before more specific terms such as "tall/short" (Clark & Clark, 1977). That is, the child will first understand that "big" is used to describe something exceptionally tall, wide, or deep. As his understanding of size is refined, he will understand and use more specific terms. If I simply described someone as *big,* you would probably request more specific information. You might ask, *Is he tall or fat?* I might then reply, *Oh, he's not fat. He's tall with broad shoulders and a thick chest.* Words like "tall," "broad," and "thick," which are more specific dimensional terms, are acquired after the more general term, "big." Within each dimensional pair, the child understands the positive term first. That is, he will understand "big," "tall," "thick," "broad," and "deep," before he understands their native counterparts: "little," "short," "thin," "narrow," and "shallow" (Brewer & Stone, 1975). The positive term in each pair is used to specify the dimension. When we ask about someone's height, we tend to say, *How **tall** is he?* not *How short is he?* When we ask the waiter about the size of a steak, we are likely to say, *How **thick** is the steak?* not *How **thin** is* *the steak?* We also say, *Bill is six feet **tall**,* not *Bill is six feet **short**.* We say, *The lake is 25 feet **deep**,* not *The lake is 25 feet **shallow**.* Why does the child learn the positive terms in these pairs before the negative terms? It may be that because the positive terms are used more often in the speech of adults, the child uses them earlier simply because he hears them more often, but there is probably a cognitive connection as well. That is, the child understands the concepts that underlie the positive terms before he understands the concepts that underlie the negative terms (Klatsky, Clark, & Macken, 1973).

This discussion has certainly not included all we now know about the development of comprehension during the preschool years. We have provided examples of concepts, words, and structures that must be understood, and we have tried to emphasize the complex relationships that exist among cognitive development, the comprehension of language, and the production of language. There is much we still do not know about the interactions of cognition, language comprehension, and language production, but we can declare with certainty that the simplistic notion that comprehension always precedes production is not valid. The relationship of thinking, understanding language, and the production of language cannot be represented on a linear graph with three colored lines. These three phenomena intersect and interact to such an extent that the lines which seem to separate them are blurred and rendered meaningless. Even as an adult thinker and speaker, you must surely sense that these processes do not work independently. Sometimes in talking aloud about a difficult concept, you suddenly understand the meaning of your own words, and your cognitive grasp of the concept is enhanced. In this case, you have actually operated in a manner that appears backward. The production of language facilitates the comprehension of language, which facilitates cognitive understanding.

And That's Not All, Folks!

The child has been a busy language activist during his preschool years, but he still has more work to do. As he moves into his elementary school years, adolescence, and even into adulthood, his vocabulary will continue to grow, he will refine and elaborate the language structures he has acquired, and he will become a more sophisticated conversationalist. These changes do not occur as quickly as in previous years, and they are not as dramatic, but they are important changes that will make him a more effective language receiver and producer. In the next chapter, we trace language development beyond Stage Five.

Review Questions

1. What is meant by obligatory context in relation to grammatical morphemes? What determines obligatory context?

2. What does it mean to say that a child overextends or overgeneralizes a grammatical morpheme? Cite examples.

3. What is the general order of pronoun acquisition? How would you explain this order?

4. In the use of pronouns, what is an *anaphoric* reference? Give three examples of anaphoric references.

5. Define the following terms and provide an example of each: phrase, noun phrase, verb phrase, clause, independent clause, subordinate clause, compound sentence, and complex sentence.

6. What language forms does the Stage Two child use to express negation, ask questions, and make demands or requests?

7. What does it mean to repair in conversation? How does the Stage Two child try to make conversational repairs?

8. How does *fast mapping* contribute to the child's acquisition of word knowledge, and how does the child's acquisition of word knowledge affect overall language competence in Stage Two?

9. How does the Stage Three child express negation and questions?

10. Define prepositional, participial, infinitive, and gerund phrases as embedded forms. Provide an example of each.

11. Define the following types of embedded clauses: object complement, *wh*-question, and relative.

12. How does the Stage Four child express negation and questions?

13. What lessons has the Stage Four child learned about the art of conversation?

14. Which grammatical morphemes are mastered by the close of Stage Five?

15. Differentiate between contractible and uncontractible forms of the verb *to be*. Why is the Stage Five child still struggling with the issue of contractibility?

16. What problems does the Stage Five child encounter in understanding and using the comparative and superlative forms of adjectives?

17. What is meant by multiple embedding and conjoining? Provide several examples of each.

18. Describe the conversational strengths and weaknesses of the Stage Five child.

19. Compare and contrast *narrative* and *conversation* as forms of communication.

20. What is a *protonarrative*? From what kinds of life experiences are protonarratives drawn?

21. In reference to building narratives, what is *chaining*? What is *centering*?

22. What significant changes occur in the child's narratives between the ages of two and five years?

23. How are cognition, comprehension, and production related?

24. What problems does the child encounter in understanding active and passive sentences?

25. What do you believe is a reasonable answer to the question: *Which comes first in mastering word order, comprehension or production?* Justify your answer.

26. What relationships among people, objects, and events are identified by the use of *relational* words? Discuss common problems the child may encounter in mastering relational words.

References and Suggested Readings

Ames, L. (1966). Children's stories. *Genetic Psychological Monographs, 73,* 307–311.

Applebee, A. (1978). *The child's concept of story.* Chicago: University of Chicago Press.

Au, T. (1990). Children's use of information in word learning. *Journal of Child Language, 17,* 393–416.

Bellugi, U. (1965). The development of interrogative structures in children's speech. In K. Riegel (Ed.), *The development of language functions* (Report No. 8), Ann Arbor: University of Michigan Language Development Program.

Bennett-Kaster, T. (1986). Cohesion and predication in child narrative. *Journal of Child Language, 13,* 353–370.

Berko-Gleason, J. (Ed.) (1989). *The development of language.* (2nd ed.) Columbus, OH: Merrill/Macmillan.

Bernstein, D. (1989). Language development: The preschool years. In D. Bernstein & E. Tiegerman (Eds.), *Language and communication disorders in children.* (2nd ed.). Columbus, OH: Merrill/Macmillan.

Beveridge, M., & Marsh, L. (1991). The influence of linguistic context on young children's understanding of homophonic words. *Journal of Child Language, 18,* 459–467.

Bloom, L. (1970). *Language development: Form and function of emerging grammars.* Cambridge, MA: MIT Press.

Bloom, L., Lahey, P., Hood, L., Lifter, K., & Fiess, K. (1980). Complex sentences: Acquisition of syntactic connectors and the semantic relations they encode. *Journal of Child Language, 7,* 235–262.

Bloom, L., Rocissano, L., & Hood, L. (1976). Adult-child discourse: Developmental interaction between information processing and linguistic interaction. *Cognitive Psychology, 8,* 521–552.

Bloom, L., Tackeff, J., & Lahey, M. (1984). Learning "to" in complement constructions. *Journal of Child Language, 11,* 391–406.

Bretherton, I., Fritz, J., Zahn-Waxler, C., & Ridgeway, D. (1986). Learning to talk about emotions: A functionalist perspective. *Child Development, 57,* 529–548.

Brewer, W., & Stone, J. (1975). Acquisition of spatial antonym pairs. *Journal of Experimental Child Psychology, 19,* 299–307.

Brinton, B., & Fujiki, M. (1984). Development of topic manipulation skills in discourse. *Journal of Speech and Hearing Research, 27,* 350–358.

Brinton, B., & Fujiki, M. (1989). *Conversational management with language-impaired children: Pragmatic assessment and intervention.* Rockville, MD: Aspen Publishing Company.

Broderick, J. (1975). *Modern English linguistics*. New York: Thomas Y. Crowell Company.

Brown, R. (1973). *A first language: The early years*. Cambridge MA: Harvard University Press.

Brown, R., & Bellugi, U. (1964). Three processes in the child's acquisition of syntax. *Harvard Educational Review, 34*, 133–151.

Brown, R., Cazden, C., & Bellugi, U. (1969). The child's grammar from I to III. In J. Hill (Ed.), *Minnesota symposia on child psychology*, (Vol. 2). Minneapolis: University of Minnesota Press.

Carey, S. (1978). The child as word learner. In M. Halle, J. Bresnan, & G. Miller (Eds.), *Linguistic theory and psychological reality*. Cambridge, MA: MIT Press.

Carey, S., & Bartlett, E. (1978). Acquiring a single new word. *Papers and Reports on Child Language Development, 15*, 17–29.

Carrell, P. (1981). Children's understanding of indirect requests: Comparing child and adult comprehension. *Journal of Child Language, 8*, 329–345.

Carrow, E. (1973). *Test of auditory comprehension of language*. Austin, TX: Urban Research Group.

Cazden, C. (1968). The acquisition of noun and verb inflection. *Child Development, 39*, 433–438.

Chapman, R. (1978). Comprehension strategies in children. In J. Kavanaugh & W. Strange (Eds.), *Speech and language in the laboratory school and clinic*. Cambridge, MA: MIT Press.

Chapman, R., & Miller, J. (1975). Word order in early two- and three-word utterances: Does production precede comprehension? *Journal of Speech and Hearing Research, 18*, 355–371.

Chapman, R., Paul, R., & Wanska, S. (1981). Syntactic structures in simple sentences. In J. Miller (Ed.), *Assessing language production in children: Experimental procedures*. Baltimore: University Park Press.

Chapman, R., Streim, N., Crais, E., Salmon, D., Strand, E., & Negri, N. (1992). Child talk: Assumptions of a developmental process model for early language learning. In R. Chapman (Ed.), *Processes in language acquisition and disorders*. St. Louis, MO: Mosby-Year Book, Inc.

Chiat, S. (1986). Personal pronouns. In P. Fletcher & M. Garman (Eds.), *Language acquisition* (2nd ed.). New York: Cambridge University Press.

Clark, H., & Clark, E. (1977). *Psychology and language: An introduction to psycholinguistics*. New York: Harcourt Brace Jovanovich.

Conner, P., & Chapman, R. (1985). The development of locative comprehension in Spanish. *Journal of Child Language, 12*, 109–123.

Craig, H., & Gallagher, T. (1983). Adult-child discourse: The conversational relevance of pauses. *Journal of Pragmatics, 7*, 347–360.

Crais, E. (1992). Fast mapping: A new look at word learning. In R. Chapman (Ed.), *Processes in language acquisition and disorders*. St. Louis, MO: Mosby-Year Book, Inc.

Dale, P. S., & Crain-Thoreson, C. (1993). Pronoun reversals: Who, when, & why? *Journal of Child Language, 20,* 573–589.

de Villiers, J., & de Villiers, P. (1973). A cross-sectional study of the acquisition of grammatical morphemes in child speech. *Journal of Psycholinguistic Research, 2,* 267–278.

Edmonsten, N., & Thane, N. (1992). Children's use of comprehension strategies in response to relational words: Implications for assessment. *American Journal of Speech-Language Pathology, 1,* 30–35.

Ervin-Tripp, S. (1977). Wait for me roller-skate. In S. Ervin-Tripp & C. Mitchell-Kernan (Eds.), *Child discourse.* New York: Academic Press.

Ervin-Tripp, S. (1979). Children's verbal turn-taking. In E. Ochs & B. Schieffelin (Eds.), *Developmental pragmatics.* New York: Academic Press.

Ervin-Tripp, S., & Gordon, D. (1986). The development of requests. In R. Schiefelbusch (Ed.), *Language competence: Assessment and intervention.* San Diego, CA: College-Hill Press.

Ervin-Tripp, S., O'Connor, M., & Rosenberg, J. (1987). Language and power in the family. In C. Kramerae & M. Schulz (Eds.), *Language and power.* Urbana: University of Illinois Press.

Foster, S. (1986). Learning topic management in the preschool years. *Journal of Child Language, 13,* 231–250.

Gallagher, T. (1977). Revision behaviors in the speech of normal children developing language. *Journal of Speech and Hearing Research, 20,* 303–318.

Gallagher, T. (1981). Contingent query sequences within adult-child discourse. *Journal of Child Language, 8,* 51–62.

Garvey, C., & Berninger, G. (1981). Timing and turn taking in children's conversations. *Discourse Processes, 4,* 27–57.

Gertner, B. L., Rice, M. L., & Hadley, P. A. (1994). Influence of communicative competence on peer preferences in a preschool classroom. *Journal of Speech and Hearing Research, 37,* 913–923.

Gleitman, L., & Wanner, E. (1982). Language acquisition: The state of the state of the art. In E. Wanner & L. Gleitman (Eds.), *Language acquisition: The state of the art.* Cambridge, MA: Cambridge University Press.

Golinkoff, R., Hirsh-Pasek, K., Cauley, K., & Gordon, L. (1987). The eyes have it: Lexical and syntactic comprehension in a new paradigm. *Journal of Child Language, 14,* 23–45.

Gordon, D., & Ervin-Tripp, S. (1984). The structure of children's requests. In R. Schiefelbusch & J. Pickar (Eds.), *The acquisition of communicative competence.* Baltimore: University Park Press.

Gropen, J., Pinker, S., Hollander, M., & Goldberg, R. (1991). Syntax and semantics in the acquisition of locative verbs. *Journal of Child Language, 19,* 115–151.

Haas, A., & Owens, R. (1985). *Preschoolers' pronoun strategies: You and me make us.* Paper presented at the annual convention of the American Speech-Language-Hearing Association.

Hoff-Ginsberg, E. (1990). Maternal speech and the child's development of syntax: A further look. *Journal of Child Language, 17,* 85–89.

Huxley, R. (1970). The development of the correct use of subject personal pronouns in two children. In G. Flores d'Arcais & W. Levelt (Eds.), *Advances in psycholinguistics.* Amsterdam: North-Holland.

Ingram, D. (1971). Transitivity in child language. *Language, 47,* 888–910.

Ingram, D. (1975). The acquisition of fricatives and affricatives in normal and linguistically deviant children. In A. Carramazza & E. Zuriff (Eds.), *The acquisition and breakdown of language.* Baltimore: Johns Hopkins University Press.

James, S. (1990). *Normal language acquisition.* Austin, TX: Pro-Ed.

James, S., & Kahn, L. (1982). Grammatical morpheme acquisition: An approximately invariant order? *Journal of Psycholinguistic Research, 11,* 381–388.

James, S., & Seebach, M. (1982). The pragmatic function of children's questions. *Journal of Speech and Hearing Research, 25,* 2–11.

Johnston, J. (1984). Acquisition of locative meanings: "behind" and "in front of." *Journal of Child Language, 11,* 407–422.

Keenan, E., & Schieffelin, B. (1976). Topic as a discourse notion: A study of topic in the conversation of children and adults. In C. Li (Ed.), *Subject and topic: A new typology of language.* New York: Academic Press.

Klatsky, R., Clark, E., & Macken, M. (1973). Asymmetries in the acquisition of polar adjectives: Linguistic conceptual? *Journal of Experimental Child Psychology, 16,* 32–46.

Klee, T. (1985). Role of inversion in children's question development. *Journal of Speech and Hearing Research, 28,* 225–232.

Klima E. S., and Bellugi-Klima, U. (1971). Syntactic regularities in the speech of children. In A. Bar-Adon & W. Leopold (Eds.), *Child language: A book of readings.* Englewood Cliffs, NJ: Prentice-Hall, Inc.

Klima, E., & Bellugi, U. (1966). Syntactic regularities in the speech of children. In J. Lyons & R. Wales (Eds.), *Psycholinguistic papers.* Edinburgh: Edinburgh University Press.

Krauss, R., & Glucksberg, S. (1977). Social and nonsocial speech. *Scientific American, 236,* 100–105.

Lemish, D., & Rice, M. (1986). Television as a talking picture book: A prop for language acquisition. *Journal of Child Language, 13,* 251–274.

Lempert, H. (1990). Acquisition of passives: The role of patient animacy, salience, and lexical accessibility. *Journal of Child Language, 17,* 677–696.

McCabe, A., & Peterson, C. (1985). A naturalistic study of the production of causal connectives by children. *Journal of Child Language, 12,* 145–159.

McCormick, L. (1990). Sequences of language and communication development. In L. McCormick & R. Schiefelbusch (Eds.), *Early language intervention: An introduction* (2nd ed.). Columbus, OH: Merrill/Macmillan.

McTear, M. (1985). *Children's conversation.* Oxford, England: Basil Blackwell.

Menyuk, P. (1977). *Language and maturation.* Cambridge, MA: MIT Press.

Miller, J. (1981). *Assessing language production in children: Experimental procedures.* Baltimore: University Park Press.

Miller, P., & Sperry, L. (1988). Early talk about the past: The origins of conversational stories of personal experience. *Journal of Child Language, 15,* 293–315.

Milosky, L. M. (1990). The role of world knowledge in language comprehension and language intervention. *Topics in Language Disorders, 10,* 1–13.

Morgan, J., & Travis, L. (1989). Limits on negative information in language input. *Journal of Child Language, 16,* 531–552.

Mueller, E. (1972). The maintenance of verbal exchanges between young children. *Child Development, 43,* 930–938.

Mueller, E., Bleier, M., Krakow, J., Hegedus, K., & Cournoyer, P. (1977). The development of peer verbal interaction among two-year-old boys. *Child Development, 48,* 284–287.

Naigles, L. (1990). Children use syntax to learn verb meanings. *Journal of Child Language, 17,* 357–374.

Newcombe, N., & Zaslow, M. (1981). Do 2 ½-year-olds hint? A study of directive forms in the speech of 2 ½-year-old children to adults. *Discourse Processes, 4,* 239–252.

Owens, R. (1996). *Language development: An introduction* (4th ed.). Needham, MA: Allyn & Bacon.

Owens, R. (1995). *Language disorders: A functional approach to assessment and intervention* (2nd ed.). Boston, MA: Allyn & Bacon.

Owens, R. (1990). Development of communication, language, and speech. In G. Shames, & E. Wiig, (Eds.), *Human communication disorders: An Introduction* (3rd ed.). Columbus, OH: Merrill/Macmillan.

Paul, R. (1981). Analyzing complex sentence development. In J. Miller (Ed.), *Assessing language production in children: Experimental procedures.* Baltimore: University Park Press.

Peterson, C. (1990). The who, when and where of early narratives. *Journal of Child Language, 17,* 433–455.

Piaget, J. (1926). *Language and thought of the child.* London: Routledge & Kegan Paul.

Piaget, J. (1966). Time perception in children. In J. Frazer (Ed.), *The voices of time.* New York: Braziller.

Reich, P. (1986). *Language development.* Englewood Cliffs, NJ: Prentice-Hall.

Resnick, J. S., & Goldfield, B. A. (1994). Diary vs. representative checklist assessment of productive vocabulary. *Journal of Child Language, 21,* 465–472.

Rice, M., Buhr, J., & Nemeth, C. (1990). Fast mapping word-learning abilities of language-delayed preschoolers. *Journal of Speech and Hearing Disorders, 55,* 33–42.

Roth, F., & Spekman, N. (1985, June). *Story grammar analysis of narratives produced by learning disabled and normally achieving students.* Paper presented at the Symposium on Research in Child Language Disorders, Madison, WI.

Sachs, J. (1982). "Don't interrupt!": Preschoolers' entry into ongoing conversations. In C. Johnson & C. Thew (Eds.), *Proceedings of the Second International Congress for the Study of Child Language,* Vol. 1 (pp. 344–356). Washington, DC: University Press of America.

Schober-Peterson, D., & Johnson, C. (1989). Conversational topics of four-year olds. *Journal of Speech and Hearing Research, 32,* 857–870.

Schober-Peterson, D., & Johnson, C. (1991). Non-dialogue speech during preschool interactions. *Journal of Child Language, 18,* 153–170.

Shatz, M., Wellman, H., & Silber, F. (1983). The acquisition of mental verbs: A systematic investigation of the first reference to mental state. *Cognition, 14,* 301–321.

Shatz, M., & O'Reilly, A. (1990). Conversational or communicative skill? A reassessment of two-year-olds' behavior in miscommunication episodes. *Journal of Child Language, 17,* 131–146.

Shipley, K., Maddox, M., & Driver, J. (1991). Children's development of irregular past tense verb forms. *Language, Speech, and Hearing Services in Schools, 22,* 115–122.

Stemberger, J. P. (1993). Vowel dominance in overregularizations. *Journal of Child Language, 20,* 503–521.

Sutton-Smith, B. (1986). The development of fictional narrative performances. *Topics in Language Disorders, 7*(1), 1–10.

Trantham, C., & Pedersen, J. (1976). *Normal language development.* Baltimore: Williams & Wilkins.

Tyack, D., & Ingram, D. (1977). Children's production and comprehension of questions. *Journal of Child Language, 4,* 211–224.

Waterman, P., & Schatz, M. (1982). The acquisition of personal pronouns and proper names by an identical twin pair. *Journal of Speech and Hearing Research, 25,* 149–154.

Weist, R., Wysocka, H., & Lyytinen, P. (1991). A cross-linguistic perspective on the development of temporal systems. *Journal of Child Language, 18,* 67–92.

Wellman, H., & Estes, D. (1987). Children's early use of mental verbs and what they mean. *Discourse Processes, 16,* 141–156.

Wellman, H., & Lempers, J. (1977). The naturalistic communicative abilities of two-year-olds. *Child Development, 48,* 1052–1057.

Wells, G. (1985). *Language development in the preschool years.* New York: Cambridge University Press.

Wells, G. (1979). Learning and using the auxiliary verb in English. In V. Lee (Ed.), *Language development.* New York: Wiley.

Wilkinson, L., Calculator, S., & Dollaghan, C. (1982). Ya wanna trade—just for awhile: Children's requests and responses to peers. *Discourse Processes, 5,* 161–176.

Wootten, J., Merkin, S., Hood, L., & Bloom, L. (1979, March). *Wh- questions: Linguistic evidence to explain the sequence of acquisition.* Paper presented at the biennial meeting of the Society for Research in Child Development, San Francisco.

SIX

Taking Language
to School

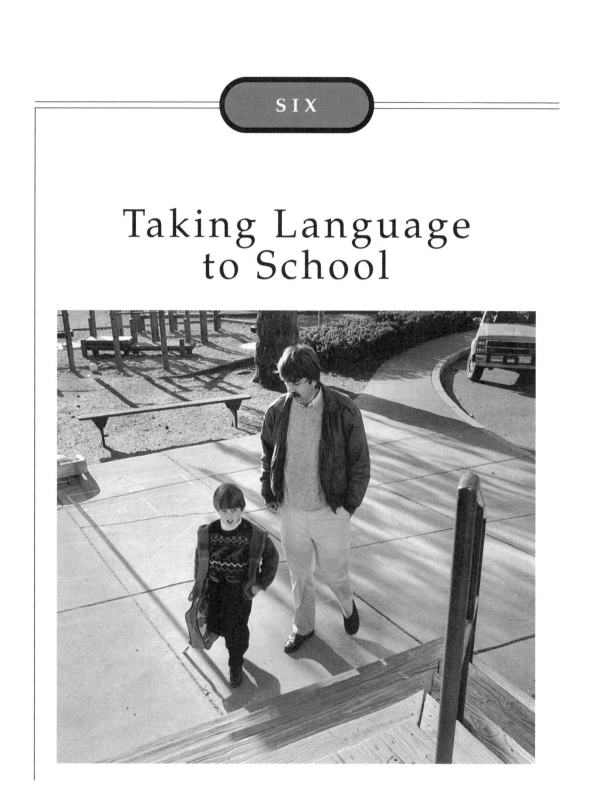

Chapter Objectives

Although much of language acquisition occurs from birth through the preschool years, development continues throughout the school years, especially during the primary grades. It is also true that people continue to add to their language knowledge and their communication competencies into their adult years, perhaps all their lives. In this chapter, we consider the continuation of language acquisition as the child enters school, including the interactive growth of vocabulary and cognition, and developmental changes in syntax, morphology, and pragmatics. We examine the emergence of gender differences in communication, metalinguistic development, and the application of language knowledge to the learning of reading and writing. Specifically, this chapter is designed to facilitate understanding of the following topics:

- A profile of the five-year-old as a communicator.
- The interactive development of cognition and vocabulary, including changes in how words are defined and understood, and the emergence of figurative language forms.
- Further developments in syntax, including refinement of passive forms, determining when the principle of minimal distance applies and when it does not apply in the interpretation of sentences, conjoining with conjunctions expressing complex clausal relationships, and creating longer, more elaborate sentences.
- Learning that words can function in more than one grammatical category.

- Fine tuning the art of conversation, including responding to stacked repair sequences, more subtle forms of indirect request, and becoming more sensitive to the listener's communication needs.
- Narratives: Improving storytelling abilities.
- The emergence of gender differences in communication.
- Dealing with communication demands in the classroom.
- Developing metalinguistic skills that enable the child to analyze and understand the language he uses.
- Reading and writing: New applications of language.

The first few years of the child's communicative life have been extraordinarily busy and exciting. Even before he is born, the child is connected to his primary caregivers, literally and figuratively. During the months of his fetal development, his caregivers may sense, or believe they sense, communications from the womb. The child's caregivers may attempt to interpret the meaning of each movement, each kick. His first communications after birth come in the form of cries and gaze-couplings, but it is not long before he expands his communication system to include coos, giggles, touches, grabs, and first-rate wet kisses. By the end of his first year, he is producing words. Before the end of his second year, he is putting words together. Once he begins combining words, his language development proceeds at a pace that challenges our best efforts to understand and describe what is happening. In the preceding two chapters we have traced the explosion of language development that occurs from birth through the preschool years. In this chapter, we consider the further development of language during the child's school years and beyond.

Bringing My Stuff to School: Pencils, Crayons, and Language

We begin with a profile of the five-year-old child as a communicator. What kind of language and what kind of communication skills does he bring with him to that first day in school, and what do these abilities suggest about what he still needs to learn about language and the use of language? In considering our hypothetical child, it is important to remember that language and language use are both universal and idiosyncratic. That is, there are aspects of language shared by all five-year-old children who speak English, and there are aspects of language shared by all five-year-old children who speak all the languages of the world. At the same time, each child's communication experiences coming into school have been unique, and these experiences have shaped the child's language and his communication skills.

Based on universal aspects of language acquisition, we would expect our five-year-old child to have well-developed receptive and expressive vocabularies, an almost intact speech sound system, fairly sophisticated syntactic abilities, and developing conversational skills. By the time the child enters school, he knows virtually all the words we might consider basic in his language. Although his understandings of words are not fully developed, he has a good idea about what words mean and how they should be used. He is producing complete sentences and is able to transform declarative sentences into question and negative forms, even though he is still learning the nuances of these transformations and still has difficulty with passive sentences. He is able to understand and produce imperative sentences, and although he is still learning to produce indirect requests, he responds appropriately to indirect requests made of him, assuming they are not too subtle or obscure. The child is still oriented primarily to present time and place, but he is able to use language to talk about something in the past or future, and he is able to talk about things and people that are not in sight. The adult must keep in mind, of course, that *past* and *future* do not mean the same thing to a five-year-old as to an adult, but the child has no difficulty talking about something that happened yesterday, and he may be eager to talk about something exciting that will happen tomorrow or in a few days. If you try to talk to this child about what his life will be like in twenty years, however, be prepared for the blank stare of utter indifference.

If the child's caregivers have included singing, nursery rhymes, and speech-related games like patty-cake and peekaboo in his early communication experiences, he will come to school ready to engage in language play. If his caregivers have read books to him, he will recognize the difference between writing and drawing, and he will understand that reading and writing are forms of communication related to speech and language. The foundations for teaching the five-year-old child to read and write, therefore, have been laid during the preschool years. Some five-year-old children already know how to read, of course, but they remain exceptions, at least for now. Personally, I anticipate the day when parents will buy their child a subscription to the *Wall Street Journal* during the second trimester of his fetal development. Somehow they will arrange to fax the contents into the womb, and the child will be born ready to read and ready to deal!

And what differences do the differences make? Consider the obvious differences. A five-year-old reared in Dallas, Texas, will not sound like a five-year-old reared in Boston, Massachusetts, and neither of these children will sound like a five-year-old reared in Tokyo, Japan. The child who grows up in a home full of talkative older siblings and adults who constantly engage the child in communicative exchanges is likely to talk more, and perhaps be more interested in language, than the child who is reared by reticent parents who make little effort to facilitate speech and language production. The child who is exposed to vulgar words will use vulgar words. The child who is exposed to complete, correct models of language is more likely to use complete, correct sentences than the child who is exposed to models that are syntactically deficient. We must be careful not to extend this too far because few children are exposed to only inadequate speech and language models, but as a general rule, we would not expect a child's speech and language abilities to be better than the models to which he is predominantly exposed.

Language Development During the School Years

How and where does language development proceed as the child moves through his school years? As we have already noted, the advances in language development after Stage Five are not as dramatic as the changes that occurred through the preschool years, but the changes in language during the school years are of no less importance. Some of the changes are universal and shared by all children. Other changes are the product of the child's unique experiences and often reflect the child's unique interest in language itself. Throughout the school years and throughout the remainder of the child's life, he acquires vocabulary. During the first few years of school, he puts the finishing touches on his speech sound system. The child continues to develop his syntactic and semantic abilities, primarily by expanding and refining the skills he developed during the preschool years. He develops considerably more sophistication in the use of language. He becomes a better conversationalist, and learns how to use language more effectively to get things done. He develops an interest in language itself and learns how to use language to analyze and understand language, an ability called **metalinguistic awareness.** During the school years, he also learns how to read and write, language abilities that will give the child virtually limitless intellectual and creative freedoms. Reading will open vistas absolutely devoid of space and time restrictions. Through the reading of books, the child will be introduced to the thoughts, opinions, and wisdom of the greatest, most influential minds of human history. In writing his own prose and poetry, he may discover means of intellectual and personal expression that are not available to him in speech alone.

The advances in language development we examine in this chapter may not be as explosive as those we observed in the preschool years, but they are important and they are exciting. The changes in language closely parallel other changes the child is experiencing. He is growing up. He is becoming his own person. He is expanding his interests into the greater world beyond his house, beyond his school, beyond his community. It is not an exaggeration to assert that this personal growth depends to a large extent on the child's developing language and communication knowledge and skills.

The Miracle Worker is the story of Helen Keller's struggle to overcome blindness and deafness. In her early years, Helen Keller was a prisoner in a noncommunicative world. Only as she learned to express herself through sign language and to read and write, did she grow into the complete, creative, and productive person she was destined to become. The hearing and sighted child does not have to break the bonds of deafness and blindness, but he must still discover how to be a whole person as he grows up, and communication is just as important to him in this discovery process as it was to Helen Keller.

Vocabulary and Cognition: Still Growing Together

One of the most obvious changes in language that continues throughout the rest of the child's life is the acquisition of new vocabulary. The child not only learns new words, he learns to use old words in new ways. The young child understands "crack" as a small fissure in the driveway. As he develops more sophistication with language, he will understand that a person might be referred to as a "crack reporter," and he will understand that "crack" also refers to the sound made by a whip. He will develop more precise definitions for the words he uses, and he will choose from among words with similar meanings the word which best fits the intended communication. As a young child, he uses "big" to describe anything of unusual size. As he matures, he uses words that more precisely differentiate "bigness" such as "tall," "deep," "wide," and "broad," and if he wants to describe someone who is "big" and "tough," he might use words like "burly" or "husky."

The preschool child uses words in a very literal sense. As he matures, he learns to use words figuratively. At three or four years, he might be confused by sentences such as "He's a real animal," or "He comes at you like a Mack Truck," but he eventually learns how words are used to create mental images to enhance the specificity or strength of a message. He also comes to understand puns, jokes based upon words that sound like or remind the listener of other words which do not fit the immediate context. Here is one of my favorite puns: "Did you hear about the guru who went to the dentist but refused novacaine? He wanted to transcend dental medication."

Obviously, vocabulary growth does not continue at the same furious rate we observe during the preschool years, but vocabulary growth does continue throughout a person's life. In fact, the common myth that older people lose vocabulary is simply not true, except in cases of failing health. After the age of seventy, some people are not able to retrieve words as quickly as they once did, but they do not lose words from their vocabularies (Obler, 1989).

Vocabulary Growth: Acquiring, Understanding and Categorizing New Words

To appreciate vocabulary growth during the school years, one must understand that vocabulary *growth* involves more than the acquisition of new words, although new words are certainly acquired. Beyond adding words to his vocabulary, however, the child is developing new ways to use words, and he is refining the meanings of the established and new words in his vocabulary. The changes we observe in the child's semantic competencies during his school years can almost certainly be attributed to corresponding maturational changes in his cognitive processing abilities (Emerson & Gekoski, 1976).

As a child moves through the preschool and school years, his vocabulary and word usage tend to mirror his cognitive shift from concrete to more abstract levels of thinking. He learns that words can be placed in categories just as things can be

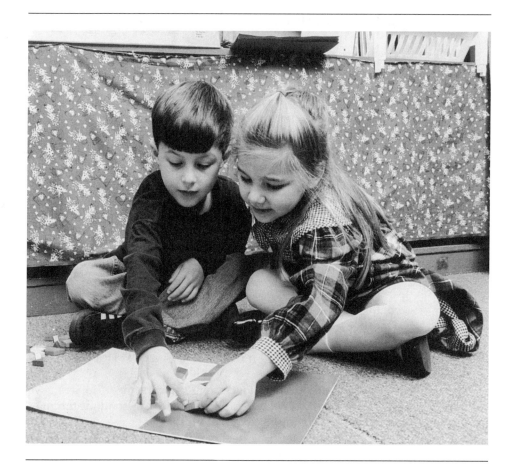

Using language to help solve problems and get things done.

placed in categories. He learns that words can be used in a hierarchical manner such as "big," "bigger," "biggest." He learns that words can be used to recall things, people, and events that are not immediate. He learns that words can be used to facilitate the solving of problems.

The process of placing words into categories based on their semantic relationships is called **chunking.** The child has a cognitive category for animals, for example, and he also has a vocabulary category for animal words, which includes *horse, dog, fish,* and *elephant.* As he matures, he chunks in a more differentiated manner. He retains a category for animals, but he develops subcategories, so that farm animals includes words such as *horse, cow, chicken,* and *pig,* and jungle animals includes words such as *elephant, monkey,* and *lion.* These vocabulary chunks facilitate remembering. There is evidence that chunking is a more commonly used strategy for recalling words by seventh-grade children than by children in the first grade (Vanevery & Rosenberg, 1970), a change in vocabulary categorization that is consistent with changes Piaget (1963) identified in cognitive development.

An example of language knowledge shaping thinking can be observed in the child's efforts to cope with ambiguities among words in his vocabulary. How does the child differentiate among words that sound the same, such as *dear-deer, bye-by-buy, not-knot*, and *right-write?* Perfetti and Goodman (1970) suggest that he addresses the potential ambiguities among these words by sorting them according to their semantic functions. That is, *dear* functions as a modifier, and *deer* functions as a noun. *Not* is a negative element, and *knot* is a noun. As the child develops knowledge about the semantic functions of words, therefore, he is able to use this language knowledge to cognitively sort and categorize words and their referents according to the semantic roles they fill.

Another change we see in the child's processing and organization of words occurs in what is called the **syntagmatic-paradigmatic shift** (Ervin, 1961). In a word-association task, the preschool child is likely to respond to a word according to its syntactic role. In responding to "Mommy," for example, he might say "kiss." He processes and organizes the stimulus word according to the word that is likely to follow it in a sentence. As he changes his cognitive processing strategies (Emerson & Gekoski, 1976), he responds to words in a paradigmatic manner, based on the semantic features of the word he hears. If he hears "Mommy," he says "girl," "woman," or perhaps "Daddy" as the opposite of "Mommy." The shift from syntagmatic to paradigmatic processing occurs slowly, but the most rapid change is observed between five and nine years (Muma & Zwycewicz-Emory, 1979), and the shift is not complete until adulthood.

These and other changes in cognitive processing account for the growth in vocabulary we observe during the school years and beyond, and they account for the changes we observe in the meanings of the child's words. We are most likely to notice that the child's vocabulary is growing in size, but he also understands words differently as he matures. His first definitions of words are developed quickly and are superficial, but over the years these definitions are progressively refined (Carey & Bartlett, 1978). As the child moves through school into adulthood, his definitions become increasingly specific and precise until they resemble the kinds of definitions one finds in the dictionary (Wehren, DeLisi, & Arnold, 1981). The child's initial understandings of words are concrete and are related to immediate contexts. These understandings gradually become more abstract until the child has stable, consistent meanings for words which are not dependent on specific contexts.

The Expansion of Meanings: Wider and Deeper

The child's definitions become more specific and precise as he expands his understandings of words **horizontally** and **vertically** (McNeil, 1970). The horizontal expansion occurs as he adds semantic features to his definitions. When the child first uses the word "doggie," it might have only two features: animal and four legs.

This is why the two-year-old child uses the word "doggie" to name a horse, pig, elephant, and giraffe. These objects are all animals, and they all have four legs. As the child matures, he adds more semantic features to his understanding of "doggie," such as wagging tail, wet nose, domestic pet, barking sounds, and canine. This horizontal expansion makes the child's definition of "doggie" or "dog" more specific, and it helps him to recognize the similarities and differences between dogs and other animals. A definition expands vertically as the child learns the various meanings a given word may have. As mentioned earlier, the child will first understand that the word "crack" refers to a fissure or slit, but he gradually adds other meanings for "crack" including smash, sever, chip, fracture, bang, insult, hit, leak, and puncture. Each of these meanings adds to the vertical dimension of the definition of "crack," and unfortunately as a sign of the present day, the child is likely to add "cocaine" to his definition of "crack." Horizontal and vertical expansions of definitions occur throughout the preschool years, of course, but they are most noticeable during the school years when the child is using and understanding words in a progressively more adult-like manner.

A Shift from Personal to Shared Definitions

The child's earliest definitions are personal and based on his own unique experiences. His initial definition of "dog," for example, may be strongly influenced by his first experiences with a dog. A child whose first dog experiences are with a small, friendly, playful poodle will have a very different definition of "dog" than a child whose first encounters involve a larger, more ferocious dog. As the child matures through the early school years, his definitions progress from personal, experience-based understandings to more socially shared understandings (Litowitz, 1977). He might still be afraid of dogs if his first experiences with dogs were frightening, but he will develop a definition of "dog" that will be independent of his personal fear or distrust of dogs.

A Shift from Single-Word to More Elaborate Definitions

Another change noted by Litowitz (1977), is the shift from single-word definitions to definitions based on sentences providing appropriate detail and explanation. The child begins this shift when he is about seven years old and in the second grade (Wehren, DeLisi, & Arnold, 1981), but it continues throughout the school years and during adulthood. Adult definitions are descriptive and explanatory and typically include restrictions, synonyms, antonyms, and even the word's grammatical category or categories. Obviously, the shift from single-word definitions to comprehensive, detailed definitions occurs gradually in an evolutionary manner. Even the adult has more complete and accurate definitions for some words than others. The less knowledge the adult has about a particular word and its referent, the more childlike will be his definition of that word. Quick, make a list of words you might define in three words or fewer! Make another list of words you use all the time for which you have no cogent definitions. How about *cogent?* The point to be made here is that our definitions are always evolving, constantly reflecting more elaborate and complete understandings.

From Literal to Figurative: Having Fun with Words

It might seem reasonable to assume that the preschool child uses language only in literal ways, an assumption that would not be true. Young children often use language creatively but their creativity is usually not intentional. The cute and unusual expressions of the preschool child are often the products of incomplete language knowledge. That is, the child will use the language he has to describe things, people, and events in the absence of more appropriate language he has not yet acquired. When my oldest daughter was about three years old, she ran out of our apartment without benefit of clothing. When I called for her to return, she yelled, "Look, Daddy, my bottom is barefootin'!" She understood that a foot without a shoe is a "barefoot," so she applied this language to other parts of her anatomy including her naked tush! This was not, strictly speaking, figurative language. It was my daughter's honest and direct attempt to describe her public nudity, using the language available to her. There were no arrests.

There is evidence that the child as young as five years is able to understand sentences that include figurative language (Nippold & Sullivan, 1987), but he cannot explain these sentences until he is about ten or eleven years old. The most significant developments in the child's understanding and production of figurative language occur during the school years. **Figurative language forms** include metaphors, similies, idioms, and proverbs.

A **metaphor** is a figure of speech involving an implied comparison between two dissimilar things. A **simile** is an explicit comparison. In describing the unseemly eating habits of someone, I might say, *He eats like a pig,* which is a simile. The metaphor version would be *He's a pig.* The preschool child might produce many utterances that sound like metaphors. He might call a man's cap a "head sock," or he might refer to a barn as a "horsie house." The child is using language creatively to describe the cap and the barn because he does not have the words *cap* and *barn* in his vocabulary. The preschool child does not have enough language knowledge to know how to use language figuratively (Hakes, 1982). Interestingly, as the child's language develops and his vocabulary increases, these apparent metaphors decrease in frequency, especially after the age of six years, probably because he gains enough vocabulary that he does not have to overextend his words to similar but inappropriate referents (Gardner & Winner, 1979). Metaphors increase in frequency again only when the child's vocabulary, his language knowledge, and his cognitive insights develop enough to allow him to understand the commonalities among dissimilar things that make metaphors and similes effective elements of figurative language. In describing a curious child, I could simply say, *John is a very curious child* but if I say, *John is as curious as a hyperactive kitten,* the image is much stronger. Keeping in mind that Piaget (1963) describes the child's thinking as "concrete" throughout the elementary school years, we would not expect him to produce and process metaphors and similies frequently and effectively until he moves into the formal operations stage of cognitive development, which takes him from the sixth grade through his sophomore year in high school. That is, during his preschool and elementary school years, the child thinks and talks about what is real and immediate. As he moves into his junior high and high school years, he begins to think and talk more abstractly. If he should falter, there is always that helpful English teacher who insists that he identify and understand the "symbolism" in great pieces of literature. Surely, you remember this kind of challenge: *"The Old Man and the Sea* is about an old man who fishes, but what does the fish represent and who is the old man?"

An **idiom** is a figurative expression peculiar to a particular language or group of people. Idioms cannot be understood literally, and that is why they are so troublesome for people learning the language to which they are indigenous. If someone just learning to speak English requested a favor I could not grant because of institutional rules, I might say, *I'm sorry but my hands are tied.* As you might imagine, this would create some confusion for my listener because, under normal circumstances, my hands are rarely tied. The idiom means that there is nothing I can do. The person learning English must learn not only the vocabulary of the language and the rules, but he must also learn the idioms. Consider the problems one might have trying to literally interpret the following American English idioms in simple sentences:

He was beating around the bush.	It takes two to tango.
I beat you to the punch.	I lost my shirt in that deal.
I'll fix your wagon.	Just keep your pants on.
I put my foot in my mouth.	Did the cat get your tongue?
The cat's out of the bag.	She'll have to face the music.
He'll have to toe the line.	He's still wet behind the ears.
She made money hand over fist.	My back is to the wall.
His nose is out of joint.	I bent over backward for you.
He really flew off the handle.	She's just spitting in the wind.
I'll fly by the seat of my pants.	We'll play it by ear.

The child learning English as his native language does not encounter the problems associated with translating idioms from English into another language, which creates extraordinary and sometimes humorous confusion, but he must still learn how to use and understand idioms.

During his preschool and early elementary school years, the child's interpretations of idioms tend to be literal. When the child in this age range is shown pictures depicting literal and figurative interpretations of idioms, he chooses the literal interpretation first. Given the same choices, adolescents and adults are more likely to choose the figurative interpretation first. The child as young as five or six will understand some idioms, but he does not handle all the common idioms of his language until he is about twelve or thirteen years old. Beyond adolescence, he learns some of the more unusual idioms, and he gradually understands the derivations of at least some idioms.

A **proverb, adage,** or **maxim** is a popular, wise saying or a precise statement of truth. Proverbs often provide common sense advice or cautions. See if you can interpret the meanings of the following proverbs commonly used by American English-speaking adults:

You can lead a horse to water, but you can't make him drink.

An ounce of prevention is worth a pound of cure.

A penny saved is a penny earned.

A rolling stone gathers no moss.

The grass is always greener on the other side of the fence.

The squeaky wheel gets the oil.

Time is money.

Haste makes waste.

Don't put the cart before the horse.

You can't have your cake and eat it too.

A bird in the hand is worth two in the bush.

People who live in glass houses shouldn't throw stones.

A stitch in time saves nine.

There is none so blind as he who will not see.

Now try to imagine how the preschool child would interpret these statements. As with idioms, the young child initially interprets proverbs literally. Proverbs are more difficult for the child to understand than other forms of figurative language, including idioms and metaphors. There are some fairly logical reasons for this difficulty. The syntactic structures of proverbs are often unusual. They sometimes contain unfamiliar words, or familiar words are used in unfamiliar ways. The concepts that underlie proverbs are often difficult for the young child to comprehend. Even if you can help the preschool child unravel the language meaning of *There is none so blind as he who will not see,* you will probably find it difficult to teach him the proverb's lesson. Truth and wisdom, no matter how precisely or eloquently stated, are difficult matters for mature adults. We should not expect the child to easily grasp the truths in proverbs or understand the language in which they are packaged. Although some common proverbs may be understood by the child during his early elementary school years, he will typically not understand proverbs until he is an adolescent (Billow, 1975). Even in adulthood, the understanding of some proverbs may be murky and incomplete. I still struggle with *You can't have your cake and eat it too.* If I ingest the cake, do I not still have it? Is having the cake in its decorated, uneaten form any more satisfying than having the cake in my stomach? I think not, unless of course, *My eyes are bigger than my stomach,* which creates another confusion that is as much anatomic as philosophic. And then there are proverbs well known to children that turn out not to be true at all. We all grow up hearing that *Sticks and stones may break your bones, but words can never hurt you,* but we all know that some words from some people in some circumstances hurt far more than sticks.

Figurative language plays an important role in **humor,** and we see the same growth in the child's understanding of the language of humor as we see in his understanding of metaphors, idioms, and proverbs. A joke can be a physical prank, but we normally think of a joke as a brief humorous narrative, a funny language form. Humans typically laugh at actions or words that are unexpected or incongruous. Consider the following common riddle: *"What is it that a man does standing up, a woman does sitting down and a dog does with one leg in the air? Shake hands."* Sometimes the humor in language is not by design, especially when children are involved, but the humor is still evoked because what is said is unexpected. When a Sunday school teacher asked a child about the "epistles," he said, "The epistles were the wives of the apostles." Another child in talking about Mount Vesuvius said, "Vesuvius is a volcano. You can see the creator smoking there day and night." Another child, a nine-year-old girl, came home from school on the Monday before Easter. She was terribly excited as she told her mother that this was going to be the last week of school. Her mother, knowing that school would be in session for several more months told her daughter that she must be mistaken. The little girl said, "But, Mommy, it's true. The teacher sent home a note about it. It says that all Brownsburg schools will be closed for Good Friday."

In order to appreciate the humor in each of these examples, one must understand the incongruities. As we have already established, preschool children tend to interpret language literally, and because they do not understand multiple meanings of words or appreciate that some words that sound alike have different meanings, they are likely to miss the humor in common jokes. Research (Lund & Duchan, 1988; Schultz & Horibe, 1974) indicates that as the child matures and comes to appreciate and understand figurative language, he responds to progressively more sophisticated forms of humor. Prior to his sixth birthday, for example, the child will laugh at slapstick actions, the physical pratfalls and pies-in-the-face antics of circus clowns, but he will not understand language-based jokes. Between the ages of six and nine years, he will laugh at jokes based on words that are phonologically similar to other words he knows, as in this example provided by Lund & Duchan (1988):

A diner says, "What is this?"

The waiter responds, "It's *bean* soup."

The diner says, "I don't care what it's *been.* What is it now?"

Between the ages of nine and twelve years, the child appreciates the humor in jokes that rely on words with multiple meanings. You may remember this oldie from your own childhood: "What's big and white, has four wheels and *flies?* A garbage truck." When the child passes his twelfth birthday, he understands humor based on two or more possible meanings within a single sentence, as in this classroom classic:

A teacher asks, "Where was the Declaration of Independence signed?"

The student answers, "At the bottom."

The essence of this joke has been repeated thousands of times in movies and television programs when one character says, "Johnny kissed Susan," and another character, usually overwrought by this development, asks, "Where did he kiss her?" The first character answers, "Right in the living room!" Most jokes adults find funny are based on words with multiple meanings, or on sentence structures that can be interpreted in two or more ways. What makes them funny is that the listener anticipates the most obvious meaning and is caught off guard by a different meaning or by an unexpected twist in the way a word is used. It should be easy to understand, therefore, that the child will understand language-based jokes only to the extent that he knows and understands all the possible meanings of the words contained in these jokes and only to the extent that he understands that a single sentence might have two or more possible underlying meanings. These understandings develop throughout the school years and even into adulthood. We all know a few adults we think of as naive, innocent, or gullible because they do not seem to know all the possible meanings of the words in punch lines, especially unsavory or potentially offensive meanings.

Syntax and Morphology: Still Expanding and Acquiring

There is so much to understand about the pieces of language and about how to put the pieces together in grammatically acceptable ways that the business of acquiring syntax and morphology is never really complete. One of the fascinations of language is that it is a creative process. Creative processes are never complete because there are always innovations and new adaptations of old productions. This is true in art and music, and in a very real sense, it is true of language. From birth through the preschool years, the child has learned the rudiments of language. During the school years, he improves his language skills by expanding the forms he has already acquired, by increasing his language knowledge, and by learning how to use language creatively.

Figuring Out Passive Sentences

As mentioned in the preceding chapter, the child has considerable difficulty with passive sentences. In active sentences, the first noun is the agent, and the second noun is the object. In passive sentences, the order changes, and this apparently causes the child to be confused. The preschool child understands "The dog chased the cat" but has trouble interpreting "The cat was chased by the dog." Passive sentences remain troublesome throughout most of the child's elementary school years.

Even though the five-year-old child understands some passive sentences, especially those that include action verbs such as "hit" or "eat," he produces very few passive forms. The passive sentences he does produce tend to be abbreviated forms that exclude the agent. He might say "Billy was pushed," or "The ball was kicked," rather than "Billy was pushed by Tom," and "The ball was kicked by Sally."

Horgan (1978) studied the development of **reversible** and **nonreversible passive** sentences in preschool and school-age children. You may recall that a passive sentence is considered reversible if either noun can act as the agent. For example, "The dog was chased by the cat" is a reversible passive because it is also possible to say, "The cat was chased by the dog." The passive sentence, "The candy was eaten by the boy," is nonreversible because its opposite version, "The boy was eaten by the candy," is not a viable alternative. Horgan found that her preschool subjects under the age of four years produced more reversible passive sentences than nonreversible forms. Although reversible and nonreversible passive forms were produced by her preschool and school-age subjects, no child produced both forms until about eleven years, and even among the children between eleven and thirteen years, only 50 percent produced both forms.

There is no question that the development of passive sentences is slow. Although preschool children produce some abbreviated passive forms, most children are not producing full passive sentences until the late elementary school ages. Baldie (1976) found that about 80 percent of eight-year-old children produce full passive sentences, and Horgan's (1978) findings suggest that some passive forms do not emerge in productive language until about eleven years.

The Principle of Minimal Distance: Dealing with an Exception

As noted by Slobin (1978) and others who study the development of language, the young child goes out of his way to avoid exceptions. He learns general rules first, and then over time he gradually sorts out and masters the exceptions to the rules. We have noted examples of this strategy in the preceding two chapters. The child learns the rule for regular past tense first and overextends the rule to verbs that require different past tense markers. That is, he says "bak*ed*," "kiss*ed*," and "play*ed*," which require regular past tense, but he also says "go*ed*," "sitt*ed*," and "hitt*ed*," which should be "went," "sat," and "hit." Many of the exceptions to the rules of language are discovered and mastered during the school years.

One intriguing example of learning an exception was studied by Carol Chomsky (1969), who analyzed the problems children have in interpreting sentences that violate the principle of minimal distance. She was specifically interested in sentences containing the verbs *ask, tell,* and *promise.* According to the principle of minimal distance, the preceding noun closest to the verb is treated as the subject of the sentence. This principle certainly holds in most basic sentences such as the following:

The boy hit the ball.

Sally jumped over the fence.

Mom picks me up after school.

The dog ate my birthday cake.

In each of these sentences and countless others that we all produce every day, the subject immediately precedes the verb. When there is a separation, it is typically only one word as in "Mom *always* picks me up after school." Chomsky found that the principle of minimal distance, and exceptions to the principle, are demonstrated in sentences that include the verbs *ask, tell,* and *promise.* If the verb *tell* is used, the principle of minimal distance can be consistently applied in sentences such as "Mary told Joe to cook dinner." In this sentence, *Mary* and *Joe* precede the infinitive verb *to cook,* but *Joe* is closer to the infinitive verb, and according to the principle of minimal distance, is the subject of this verb. In this sentence the principle works because Mary is the one doing the telling and Joe is the one doing the cooking.

Consider what happens, however, when we use a verb that violates the principle of minimal distance as in the sentence, "Mary promised Joe to cook dinner." Even though the surface structure of this sentence is the same as in the earlier example, the principle of minimal distance cannot be used in the interpretation. In this sentence Mary is doing the promising, but she is also the one who will be doing the cooking, even though *Joe* is closer to the infinitive verb *to cook.*

The verb *tell* consistently adheres to the principle of minimal distance, and the verb *promise* consistently violates the principle. The verb *ask* is especially troublesome because it sometimes adheres to the principle and sometimes violates it. If I say, "Mary asked Joe to cook dinner," application of the principle of minimal distance will result in a correct interpretation, but if I say, "Mary asked Joe what to cook for dinner," the principle will not work. In the first case, Joe will be doing the cooking, but in the second case, Mary will be doing the cooking. What really matters here, of course, is that someone will be cooking dinner, because Mary and Joe are getting hungry!

The child uses the principle of minimal distance by the time he is about five years old, but learning the exceptions takes time. In reference to the verbs in Chomsky's (1969) study, he will have little trouble with *tell* because it consistently adheres to the principle. He will have only somewhat more trouble with *promise* because, although it violates the principle of minimal distance, it violates the principle consistently. Chomsky found that the child correctly interprets *tell* and *promise* by the time he is nine years old, but he does not master his interpretation of the pesky, inconsistent *ask* until he is about ten.

The child's struggle with the principle of minimal distance relative to *tell, promise,* and *ask* is a revealing example of his overall struggle with rules and their exceptions. He learns general rules relatively early and tends to overapply them. He then learns the exceptions. The greater the inconsistencies and the further the exceptions deviate from the general rules, the longer it takes the child to understand and produce these forms that are the square pegs of language trying to fit into round holes.

Conjoining with More Complex Conjunctions

The child begins to conjoin clauses during the preschool years, usually with the conjunction "and." During the school years, he not only conjoins more often, but he uses a wider range of conjunctions expressing more complex relationships among the clauses of his sentences. Menyuk (1969) identified the conjunctions the child will eventually acquire to express these more complex clausal relationships: *conditional* (if), *causal* (so, because, therefore), *disjunctive* (but, or, therefore), and *temporal* (before, after, when, then). There is evidence that the child may use some of these conjunctions before he fully understands them (Hood & Bloom, 1979), although his comprehension of most conjunctions will be relatively complete by the end of his elementary school years.

The conjunction "because" is troublesome for the child because he must understand the underlying cause-effect relationship expressed in the conjoined clauses, and he must understand the temporal relationship between the events described. In the normal thought process, a cause is identified before its effect is considered. For example, if I stand in the rain (cause), I will get wet (effect). If I prick my finger with a pin (cause), my finger will bleed (effect). The preschool child understands cause-effect relationships, and he is able to express them in conjoined sentences such as "I fell down the stairs, and I hurt my knee." Notice the difference, however, between this sentence and a version using the conjunction "because": "I hurt my knee because I fell down the stairs." The cause and effect are now reversed. "I hurt my knee" is the *effect,* but it is mentioned before the *cause* ("I fell down the stairs"). The child who is accustomed to interpreting cause-effect on the basis of order of mention is likely to be confused. Prior to his seventh birthday, the child will use "because," "and," and "then" as though they mean the same thing (Corrigan, 1975). He might say, for example, "I fell down the stairs, *and* I hurt my knee," but he might also say, "I fell down the stairs *because* I hurt my knee." Apparently, the child has less difficulty when he is describing two events that are occurring simultaneously or that overlap in time than when he is describing related but distinctly successive events. That is, he can produce and understand sentences such as "I'm eating ice-cream because it tastes good" (simultaneous events), and "I throw the ball because we're playing baseball" (overlapping events), but he has trouble interpreting sentences such as "I have to stay in my room because I told a lie" (distinctly successive events). Not until he is about ten or eleven years old does he fully and consistently comprehend the ordering and causal meanings of "because" (Emerson, 1979).

Other conjunctions pose similar problems for the child. He must understand *contrast* before he can use "but" correctly. He must understand *consequence* before he can use "therefore" appropriately. He must understand *condition* before he can use "if " properly. Wing and Scholnick (1981) have noted that the child at ten years may still have problems with the conjunction "unless" because he does not fully understand disbelief and uncertainty. Conjunctions may seem to be simple words, but the concepts and relationships they denote are clearly not simple. The child must have a cognitive understanding of the concepts underlying conjunctions before he is able to comprehend and produce conjoined sentences that include these conjunctions. As the child moves through his school-age years, his understanding of the concepts and his ability to apply this knowledge to language interpretation and production improve steadily.

Embedding in All Parts of the Sentence

The preschool child embeds infinitive phrases, object complements, and relative clauses modifying noun phrases in the object position but not in the subject position. After he passes his seventh birthday, the child will produce sentences in which the relative pronoun is deleted but understood as in "I just saw a movie [that] you would really like," and he will embed in the subject position or center of a sentence as in "The man *who bought our car* is a teacher" (Menyuk, 1971). Sentences involving subject position or center embedding are initially difficult for young children to interpret because they violate the subject-verb-object order. If the child hears, "The dog that bit the cat ran away" and applies the subject-verb-object rule, he might conclude that the cat ran away. The semantic roles of the words in the sentence may help the child avoid confusion even if the subject-verb-object rule is violated. If the object of the center embedding is inanimate, for example, he is not likely to misinterpret the sentence (Maratsos, 1974). That is, hearing the sentence, "The dog that chewed the shoe ran away," the child will correctly conclude that the dog ran away, not the shoe, because dogs can run and shoes cannot. By the time the child is about twelve years old, he will correctly interpret embedded sentences no matter where the embeddings occur, and he will base his interpretations on his grammatical knowledge, not simply on word order or semantic roles (Abrahamsen & Rigrodsky, 1984).

Noun and Verb Phrases: Still Expanding

Do you remember the first time a teacher asked you to write a 500-word essay? I remember this experience vividly and those that followed. I can remember thinking that it must be almost impossible to write 500 words about any topic. I remember counting the words. If there were not enough words, I rarely considered elaborating my thoughts. My first instinct was to simply add words to the sentences I had already created. Surely you remember how this works:

The man walked. (3 words)

The man walked across the street. (6 words)

The haggard, gray-bearded man whose last meal must have been consumed about three weeks before the birth of the new world, walked with short, labored, arthritic steps across the windswept, deserted street to the dark and desolate hole in the wall that 20 years ago was the most exquisite restaurant in the city. (53 words . . . only 447 to go!)

As this example suggests, a sentence can be made longer by adding adjectives and adverbs, and by embedding prepositional phrases and subordinate clauses into the original sentence, which consisted of a basic noun phrase (*The man*) and simple verb phrase (*walked*). The child has been elaborating these phrases throughout the preschool years. As he moves through the school years, he produces longer and more elaborate noun and verb phrases. He refines forms he has been producing.

He adds new forms. He learns which language forms must be retained and which forms can be eliminated because they are redundant.

During the early school years, when the child is about five to seven years old, he may still be omitting articles (*a, an, the*) even though he adds other redundant information, such as the infamous double negative. The child might say, for example, "I don't got (the) ball no more." This same child is likely to have problems with some prepositions, with marking verbs appropriately for tense, and with marking plurality (Menyuk, 1971). As one would expect, cases of plurality and tense changes that violate the regular rules are the most troublesome for school-age children. As the child moves through elementary school, he addresses each of these problems. He learns to retain function words, including the articles. He eliminates redundant negative terms, and he gradually learns the exceptions for verb tense, plurality, and other language forms.

During the school years, the child completes his sorting of pronouns. He learns to separate subject pronouns (*I, we, he, she, they*) from object pronouns (*me, us, him, her, them*), and he learns to use reflexive pronouns such as *myself, herself,* and *themselves*. The school-age child learns to recognize the antecedents of pronouns even when the nouns and pronouns are in different sentences, as in the following example: "Joe's brother was badly hurt in an automobile accident. He [Joe] goes to see him [Joe's brother] in the hospital every day."

As demonstrated in the example in the opening of this section, one of the ways to elaborate noun phrases is to add adjectives. When the child begins to string adjectives together, he must learn the rules for ordering adjectives. Each adjective in a sequence refers to a specific attribute of the noun being modified or described. There are rules for how adjectives are ordered (Whorf, 1956), although we do not have a complete understanding of these rules. We do know, however, that "three, hyperactive, preschool children" *sounds right,* whereas "hyperactive, preschool, three children" does not even sound close. We also know that children as young as three years demonstrate some of the same sequencing rules used by adults (Richards, 1980). During the school years, the child will develop a more complete understanding of the attributes reflected in adjectives and a more complete understanding of how these attributes are related to one another. As these understandings mature, he will learn the remaining rules for sequencing adjectives, even if he is never able to express the rules. Can you explain why *four, wild-eyed, ice-cream lovers* is "correct," and *ice-cream, four, wild-eyed lovers* is kinky but "incorrect"? I think not!

You are probably familiar with the differentiation between a **common noun,** which refers to a general class of people, places, or things and a **proper noun,** which refers to a specific member of a class. Nouns are also classified as **concrete** (names of real, tangible objects), **abstract** (names of ideas, emotions, concepts), **collective** (names of groups of people or things), **count** (nouns that can be counted or tallied), and **mass** (names of homogeneous, aggregate substances). The child learning language must understand all these categories of nouns, of course, but the distinction between count and mass nouns is especially difficult. During the school years, the child gradually comprehends the difference between these categories and learns which quantifying adjectives can be used with each category (Gathercole, 1985). Count nouns can be modified by numbers, of course, but they can also be modified by adjectives such as *many* and *few,* as in the following examples:

> There are *few* students in class today.
>
> John keeps *many* pencils in his desk.

Mass nouns require different modifiers, such as *little* and *much,* as in the following examples:

> There was *little* meat left on his plate.
>
> You put too *much* sugar in my coffee.

Now mix these adjectives by using *few* for *little, many* for *much,* and vice versa. You will quickly discover that you know which adjectives should be used with count nouns and which should be used with mass nouns. The child has usually mastered this understanding by the time he approaches adolescence, although he might still use *much* when *many* is appropriate as in "Can you believe how much girls were at that party?" While he is trying to figure out which adjectives should be used with which category of nouns, he might use *lots of* in reference to both categories. In fact, if you listen carefully to the speech of adults, you may hear sentences such as the following:

> John keeps *lots of* pencils in his desk. (count)
>
> You put *lots of* sugar in my coffee. (mass)

Since one can get lots of mileage out of *lots of,* one may tend to use *lots of* lots of the time!

During the school years, the child learns what adverbs mean and how to use them. As with other categories of words, some adverbs are easier to understand than others. Adverbs of likelihood such as *definitely, probably,* and *possibly* are especially difficult because, although they can be used in the same contexts, they express varying degrees of likelihood. The differences may seem small or nonexistent to the young child, but they are critical. Assume that you are standing with your back to me, and I tell you to fall straight backward. You ask, "Will you catch me?" You will listen very carefully to the adverb of likelihood in my answer because you know there is a bodily risk difference between "I will *probably* catch you," and "I will *definitely* catch you." During the preschool years, the child does not understand the subtle but vital differences among adverbs of likelihood, but he has a fairly good grasp of the differences by the time he is in the fourth grade. He does not learn these adverbs at the same time, and as you might guess, he tends to understand *definitely* before he understands *probably* and *possibly* (Hoffner, Cantor, & Badzinski, 1990).

Morphological Modifications

Early in the elementary school years, at about seven, the child understands how to produce gerunds. A gerund, you may recall from earlier discussions, is a noun form of a verb created by adding *-ing* to the verb. *Running* is the gerund form of *run*, for example, and *fishing* is the gerund form of *fish*. The seven-year-old child also understands the agentive forms of common verbs (Carrow, 1973). The agentive form identifies the person who performs the action of a verb. Someone who *runs*, for example, is a *runner*, and someone who *sings* is a *singer*, but as with other language forms, there are many exceptions. Someone who *cooks* is a *cook*, not a *cooker*, although *cooker* refers to a certain kind of cooking pot. Someone who fishes is a *fisherman*, not a *fisher*. A person who *types* is a *typist*, not a *typer*, but a person who sets type is a *typesetter*.

When the child is seven years old, he also understands and is able to produce the adverb forms of common adjectives by adding the bound morpheme, *-ly*. By adding this morpheme, the adjective *slow* becomes the adverb *slowly*. The adjective and adverb forms of *slow* are included in the following sentence: "The train moved *slowly* [adverb] down the tracks on a *slow* [adjective] day in August." Many adverbs are created by adding *-ly*, including *quickly, rapidly*, and *swiftly*, but notice that the child must learn exceptions here too. The adjective *fast*, for example, does not have an adverbial form, *fastly*. The adverb form of *fast* is *fast*, and sometimes nouns can function as adverbs as in the following examples:

After watching the movie, John went *home.*

Mary moved *yesterday.*

In the first sentence *home* modifies the verb *went* by specifying *where* John went. In the second sentence, *yesterday* specifies *when* Mary moved. Still other adverbs, which always function as adverbs, do not end in *-ly*, such as *again, often, now*, and *never*.

Pragmatic Development: Conversational Skills Continue to Improve

The most dramatic changes in language development during the school years are in the area of pragmatics or the use of language. The child comes to school understanding and producing virtually all basic language forms, but his conversational skills are still pretty rudimentary. As the child moves through the school years and into his adult years, he masters the art of conversation. He becomes more sophisticated in using language to manipulate the behaviors, feelings, and attitudes of other people. He learns how to manipulate people so indirectly with his words that they scarcely know they are being manipulated. He learns the art of narration or the telling of stories. He learns how to adjust his vocabulary and modify his language style to accommodate listeners of varying ages, backgrounds, and genders. Some people make greater progress in pragmatic development than others, of course. Some become effective communicators at an early age, and some adults never become adept conversationalists or storytellers. Some people have excellent pragmatic skills in some speaking situations, but are inept in others. Whatever pragmatic competence one ultimately achieves, however, he begins to seriously hone these skills during the school years.

Building Conversational Competence

As the child matures through the preschool and school-age years, he becomes more capable of maintaining a conversational topic, moving from one topic to a related topic, and introducing new topics, but this progress is slow. At three years, the child typically sustains a topic only if he is interested and only if his partner responds directly to the child's utterances. Even at four years, the child has difficulty sustaining a true dialogue (Gelman & Shatz, 1977). As the child grows older, he becomes increasingly sensitive to the issue of **relevance,** which guides the conversations of adults. That is, the more pertinent, useful or timely a topic, the more likely the older conversationalist will sustain that topic. The preschool child tends to move from one fairly discrete topic to another, sometimes without warning. As he matures, he learns how to **shade** conversations by moving from one topic to a different but related topic. In adult conversations, shading occurs so subtly that it is often difficult to determine, based on the final topic, how the conversational partners got there. The preschool child talks about concrete topics, about things, people, and events in the here and now. By the time the child is eleven or twelve years old, he is able to discuss abstract topics. If you ask a four-year-old to talk about *love,* you are likely to be greeted by a blank stare, but a twelve-year-old would be able to discuss questions such as *What does love mean to you?* or *How does love affect a person's happiness?*

How a topic is maintained changes as the child develops. The preschool child typically maintains a topic by repeating some or all of his partner's utterance. The elementary school-age child maintains a conversation by adding new information to the established topic. Adolescents and adults maintain their conversations, not only by adding information during their turns, but also by shading one topic into another.

In the preceding chapter, we traced the preschool child's attempts at conversational repair. If the listener does not understand what the speaker has said and asks for clarification, the speaker tries to repair the conversational breakdown. The preschool child, even as young as 20 to 30 months (Gallagher, 1977) will respond to requests for clarification, but these early repairs are crude and rarely helpful. At 20 months, the child tries to repair by changing a speech sound in an important word. At 25 months, he typically deletes a word. By 30 months, he changes words. The point is, he tries to repair the broken conversation even if he does not know exactly where the failure has occurred. If the preschool child's first attempt to make a repair does not succeed, he will try again, but he finds the process increasingly difficult and will eventually give up (Brinton, Fujiki, Loeb, & Winkler, 1986).

A series of requests and attempted repairs are called **stacked repair sequences.** The following example illustrates a typical sequence:

SPEAKER: "I just bought a Sony HQ VHS VCR with editing capacity."
LISTENER: "You bought what?"

SPEAKER: "I bought a Sony VCR in the VHS format. It is the latest HQ model and it has standard editing features."

LISTENER: "What does all that mean?"

SPEAKER: "Well, Sony makes both Beta and VHS formats, and this one is VHS and it has advanced high quality video. I can also use this machine to delete or rearrange portions of tape when I copy."

LISTENER: "I still don't understand what you're talking about."

SPEAKER: "I just blew $1,500 on a video tape recorder!"

The preschool child typically makes a valiant effort to respond to the first request for clarification, but he has trouble with additional requests. The five-year-old will usually respond to two requests, but if he is asked for a third repair, he will either give an inappropriate response, or he will simply give up. As the child matures through the elementary school years, he is more likely to respond to repeated requests for clarification, but he also learns how to use information in the requests to shape his attempted repairs. In other words, he becomes more skilled at determining exactly where and why the breakdown has occurred, and he responds to that problem. We can expect to see evidence of this pragmatic ability when the child is about nine years old (Owens, 1996, p. 345). Keep in mind, however, as the example above suggests, that all speakers have their limits in the area of conversational repair. Sometimes the listener is so entirely disconnected from the message the speaker is attempting to convey that all efforts to make the message clear are futile. Listen sometime to conversations between parents and teenage children, and you will hear some classic examples of failed conversational repairs!

Indirect Requests: The Delicate Art of Hinting

As indicated in the preceding chapter, an indirect request is a subtle, more polite form of request than a direct request. If the room is cool because a window is open, I might make a direct request or demand by saying, *Shut the window,* or *Please, shut the window,* but I can accomplish the same request indirectly by saying *It's a little too cool in here for me,* or *Don't you think it's cool in here?* Children learn to understand and use indirect requests gradually over the preschool and school years.

The preschool child tends to be very direct in his expressive language, and he has difficulty understanding subtle language, including indirect requests (Ervin-Tripp, 1977). The four-year-old might respond to *Don't you think it's cool in here?* by saying, "Yes," but he would probably not understand the question as an indirect request to close the window. He needs the more direct, *Please, shut the window.* By the time the child is six years old, he is responding to many forms of indirect requests, including a form as subtle as a loud sigh (Cherry-Wilkinson & Dollaghan, 1979). If, for example, a parent tells the child to pick up his coat, and the child does not respond immediately, the parent might look the child in the eye and produce a clearly audible sigh which nonverbally and indirectly restates the request and signals impatience. The six-year-old child will correctly interpret this kind of indirect request.

As would be expected, some forms of indirect request are more difficult for the preschool and early school-age child to comprehend than others (Carrell, 1981). He understands declarative terms such as *you should, you shouldn't*, or *you must* more easily than he understands their interrogative versions, *should you?, shouldn't you?*, and *must you?* He understands positive forms more easily than negative forms. One of the obvious problems with negative forms in indirect requests is that what appears on the surface does not match the intention of the message. Assume, for example, that an adult says to a child on a rainy day, *Shouldn't you put on your boots?* This indirect request includes a negative form, but it is calling for positive action. Even the words contained in indirect requests can be troublesome. The child at four and five years has more difficulty understanding indirect requests which include *should* and *must* than requests containing *can* and *will* (Leonard, Wilcox, Fulmer, & Davis, 1978). By the time the child reaches adolescence, he responds to indirect requests as well as adults, although even adults become confused at times by negative and interrogative forms of indirect request (Clark & Chase, 1972).

The child first produces indirect requests during his preschool years, and the number of his indirect requests compared to direct requests increases between three and five years (Garvey, 1975). Throughout this time, however, direct requests are far more frequent than indirect requests, and the child is seven years old before he is fairly proficient in producing indirect requests (Grimm, 1975).

When the child enters school, he becomes increasingly adept at using nonstandard or creative forms of indirect request based on two simple rules: (1) be brief, and (2) be clever enough to avoid appearing demanding (Ervin-Tripp & Gordon, 1986). As the child applies these rules to his use of indirect requests, he begins to shape the manipulative behaviors that bring joy and delight to the lives of all who know and love him through his school years. Even at the tender age of eight years, the child understands the importance of being more polite to adults than to his peers and to people whose favor he is trying to win than to people whose favor he already possesses (Corsaro, 1979; Parsons, 1980). After the age of eight years, the child's indirect requests are more likely to be influenced by his sensitivity to his listener's situation (Ervin-Tripp & Gordon, 1986). He will no longer assume that a request will be filled, but will ask in a manner that suggests the listener has a right to exercise a real option. Whereas a younger child might say, "Take me home," or "Can you take me home?" the older child might say, "If it's not too much trouble or too far out of your way, could you take me home?" The older child will also recognize that the need to be polite in making requests increases when he is interrupting his listener or when he is asking the listener to do something that is difficult or inconvenient (Mitchell-Kernan & Keman, 1977). There is a difference, you see, between "Would you mind opening that door for me?" and "Excuse me, I know you're busy, but when you finish painting your house, you wouldn't mind painting mine . . . would you . . . perchance?"

Presuppositional Skills: Considering the Listener's Perspective

As we noted in Chapter Five, the preschool child may appear to be deficient in pre-suppositional skills when the real problem is a lack of knowledge about the conversational topic. It is difficult for any speaker to provide information to his listener if his own understanding is lacking. The school-age child is not only continuing to improve his language abilities, but he is also learning more about the things, people, places, and events in his world. The combination of general knowledge, improved cognitive abilities, and greater language competence leads directly to improved presuppositional skills.

Whereas the four-year-old child has difficulty describing blocks of unfamiliar geometric shapes to another four-year-old child when they are separated by a screen (Krauss & Glucksberg, 1977), the school-age child is much more successful in the same task. The school-age child has learned the names for geometric shapes, and he has acquired other words that he can use to describe shapes he does not know. His knowledge of shapes and his increased vocabulary allow him to provide more specific and helpful information to his conversational partner. The school-age child understands the importance of organizing and sequencing information for his conversational partner as evidenced by his ability to explain how a game is played. He first describes the purpose of the game and clarifies what is required to win. He then delineates the rules and explains the mechanics of playing the game, step-by-step. The preschool child is unable to structure his explanations in a manner that facilitates his listener's understanding, and he does not grasp the importance of moving from general to more specific information.

Narratives: The Continuing Evolution of Storytelling Skills

As the reader will recall from the preceding chapter, the child began to develop narrative abilities during his preschool years. In the beginning, the child's narratives were not true stories, but they had "story-like" qualities. More importantly, his first narrative attempts laid a solid foundation for the narrative discourse skills he will develop during his school years. To appreciate what happens relative to narrative discourse development during the school years, we should briefly review the child's narrative attempts between the ages of two and five years.

At the age of two years, the child's narrative-like productions were sets of brief unrelated statements called *heaps*. There was no discernible organization in these primitive narratives. They were, in the most elemental sense, stories about things the child found frightening, upsetting, or shocking in his own life (Ames, 1966). Style was more important than substance (Sutton-Smith, 1986) in these early narrative attempts, and the child relied more on prosody than on information to make his stories work (Scollon & Scollon, 1981).

Between the ages of three and five years, the child began to take the temporal factor into account, so that his narratives had beginnings, middles, and endings, but his stories lacked identifiable plots, and he did not develop cause-effect relationships. Even though the child at the age of three years understood cause-effect and expressed this understanding in his language, he was not able to incorporate causal sequences in his narratives (Kemper & Edwards, 1986).

Obviously, there is a considerable gap between the primitive narratives produced by the preschool child and the kinds of narratives produced by older children and adults. A primitive narrative lacks the elements we typically associate with a story. There is no plot. There is little or no organization. There are no characters, and there is certainly no character development. The story is not pushed from one event to another by causality, by what one person does or says to another or by how one act prompts another act. During the school years, we see all of these story elements emerge in the child's narratives. The single factor that is essential to making more mature narratives possible is *organization,* and that is where we pick up our story about storytelling.

Researchers have studied common stories to discover how they are organized. According to Stein and Glenn (1979), a story consists of a setting and one or more episodes. The **setting** provides information about the main character, and about the time and place in which the story occurs. Each **episode** contains the following elements: (1) an initiating event that causes the main character to do something, (2) an internal response in the form of thoughts or feelings the character has about the initiating event, (3) the main character's plan of action, (4) the main character's attempt to carry out his plan, (5) the consequence of the main character's implemented plan, and (6) the main character's reaction to the end result. You will recognize many of these elements in the stories adults tell about the events in their own lives. Mature speakers understand the importance of the information contained in these elements, and they understand the necessity of framing this information into appropriate narrative structure. When you listen to a narrative and complain about not being able to follow the story, you are almost certainly responding to an organizational problem or to the fact that important information has not been included. At the very least, we must know why the main character is motivated to do what he is going to do. We must know what he is going to do, and we must know the consequences of his actions (Stein, 1979).

By the time the child is seven years old, his stories have plots, even if they are not fully developed plots. A problem, the plan of action for resolving the problem, and the results of the actions implemented are included. There is still not much focus on motives and feelings, and there is not much detail, but the essential elements of the narrative are present. As is true of the adult, the child prefers narratives in which there is a clearly established goal (Stein & Policastro, 1984). That is, a story about a child who struggles to make the baseball team and ends up hitting the winning homerun in the championship game is more intriguing to a child than a story titled, "A Day in the Life of a Bookkeeper."

After the child passes his eighth birthday, he begins to create narratives with more clearly defined plots (Peterson & McCabe, 1983; Sutton-Smith, 1986). As the child moves through the remainder of the elementary school years and into junior and senior high school, his narratives mature in a number of important ways (Johnston, 1982). Problems are more clearly identified and more neatly resolved. He includes important detail but eliminates superfluous information. He is more careful about establishing the time and place settings of his narratives. He introduces his characters with greater care. He attends to the feelings, thoughts, and motives of his characters, and he includes the organizational elements required of complete narratives.

According to Stein (1982), there are four basic types of narrative discourse: recounts, eventcasts, accounts, and fictionalized stories of people or other animate beings who are trying to reach a goal. In a **recount,** the speaker talks about a past personal experience or about an event he has seen or read about. Recounts are common in the homes of middle- and upper-middle socioeconomic children whose parents often ask the question, *What did you do in school today?* or *Tell us about your trip to the zoo,* and they are common in school. The age-old assignment, "What I Did During My Summer Vacation," calls for a recount narrative. An **eventcast** is a narrative that describes a future event or something happening now. The child learns to use an eventcast to manipulate the behavior of other people with whom he is interacting. To get his way about what will happen tomorrow, for example, he might say, "Tomorrow, we'll all go to Billy's house after school. He has a big yard, so we can play football, and then Billy's Mom can give us some milk and cookies like she always does." An **account** is a narrative in which a child spontaneously shares his experiences, usually beginning with "You know what?" The crucial difference between an account and a recount is that an account is initiated by the child, and a recount is initiated by a request from someone else, usually an adult. As you might expect, most children prefer accounts to recounts! A story is the kind of narrative we have been describing above. Although it might be reality-based, Stein (1982) views a story as a **fictionalized narrative** that follows the story form we have already outlined. By the time the child begins school, he is usually well acquainted with all four types of narrative discourse.

Shifts in Style and Vocabulary: The Emergence of Gender Differences

Are there differences between men and women in terms of how they talk? There are. Are these differences genetically or environmentally determined? Although we do not know for sure, it seems likely that most, if not all, the communicative differences between men and women are the products of environment. That is, boys are probably socialized to talk like men, and girls are socialized to talk like women. As other gaps between the genders close, we may discover that the differences noted in this section will no longer exist. The reality today, however, is that there are vocabulary differences and conversational style differences between men and women.

Men and women do not include different words in their vocabularies so much as they use different words with greater frequency (Thorne, Kramerae, & Henely, 1983). Men are more likely than women, for example, to use coarse or crude language and to use profanity in their conversations, whereas women are more likely than men to use polite words such as *please, thank you,* and *you're welcome* (Greif & Berko-Gleason, 1980). Women use words such as *lovely, darling,* and *adorable* more

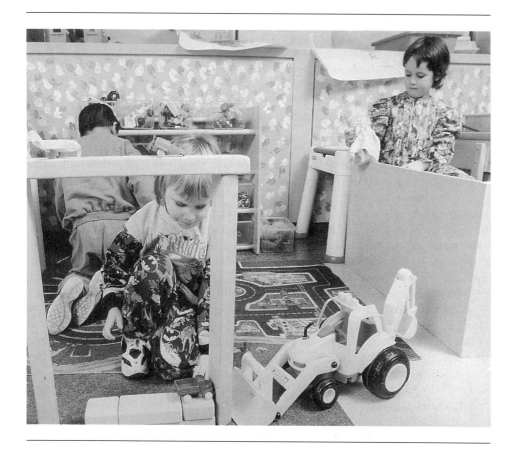

Gender differences in interests and in language emerge early.

often than men. Whereas a man might call all shades of a color *red,* a woman is more likely to name shades of red. When a woman breaks a plate, she is likely to use an expression such as *Oh, my goodness!* or *Dear me!* whereas a man is more likely to say, *#*##@*+=#%!!* Part of the perception that the female is the gentler sex is probably based on the fact that women use gentler language.

One of the oldest stereotypes about women is that they talk more than men. Wrong! Although there are wide individual variations, of course, men tend to talk more than women (Swacher, 1975). The conversations between men and other men are longer than women's conversations with men or with other women. Women are also more courteous in conversation than men. Men interrupt more often than women, and men are more likely to interrupt women than to interrupt other men (Parlee, 1979). It is interesting, and probably socially revealing, that both sexes are more likely to interrupt a woman than a man (Willis & Williams, 1976).

Women are more likely than men to surrender their conversational turns. Women introduce more new topics into conversation than men, but only about a third of the topics introduced by women are sustained in conversation, and nearly all topics introduced by men are sustained (Ehrenreich, 1981).

One of the common stereotypes about men and women in conversation is true. Whereas women tend to talk openly about their relationships and feelings, men avoid these topics and prefer to talk about impersonal subjects such as cars, politics, work, and sports.

When do children first become aware of gender differences in language, and when do listeners first notice these differences in the speech of children? By the time children are in the first grade, they are able to determine the gender of a speaker based on the vocabulary used in emotional expressions (Edelsky, 1977). At this same age, the early elementary school years, the language children use begins to reflect the same gender differences we have noted in the language of adult men and women (Craig & Evans, 1991; Haas, 1979). Even before adult-like gender differences are noted, boys and girls talk about different things. Boys as young as four years talk about sports (Haas, 1979). Kindergarten girls talk about subjects related to traditional female roles (Sause, 1976).

Although we do not know the full importance of these findings, research has demonstrated that parents talk differently to their sons and daughters. Mothers imitate their preschool daughters more often than their sons, and they spend more time talking to their daughters (Cherry & Lewis, 1976). Fathers attach nicknames such as *nutcake* and *ding-a-ling* to their sons, but call their daughters *sweetheart* and *honey* (Berko-Gleason & Greif, 1983). Consistent with gender differences noted among adults, fathers interrupt their daughters more often than their sons (Warren-Luebecker, 1982).

Gender differences in language are fascinating, not so much because of what they tell us about language, but because of what they tell us about differences between the sexes. We shall return to this topic in Chapter Eight, which includes an examination of a wide range of environmentally determined language differences.

The Classroom and Language: New Demands

The child learns most of his language in the comfort of his own home, in interaction with the most caring people in his world. The child acquiring language at home has the advantage of knowing the routine of his family life and knowing the nuances of the nonverbal communicative assists provided by his caregivers. If he does not understand all that is said to him, he can fill in the missing information by taking all the familiar nonverbal context into account. Most of his conversations at home are one-on-one, so if there is a breakdown and a repair is needed, his partner will usually recognize the need immediately. If not, he is comfortable enough with his partner to ask for help. Home is a safe and comfortable place for learning and using language, but what happens when the child begins school?

The classroom, no matter how nurturing and caring the teacher, does not provide an environment for language as supportive and secure as the child's home.

The young student must process not just the spoken language of the teacher and the varying language systems of his peers, but he must learn to process the written language of books. These can be heavy burdens for the young child. The child whose language abilities meet the language demands of the classroom will adjust to this new environment without difficulty, but the child with deficient language skills may have considerable difficulty in this new environment, and he will endure some emotional and social pains as a consequence (Gerber, 1981; Nelson, 1985). As he moves through the grade levels, the child must process the language of teachers who will use progressively longer and more complex structures, spoken at more rapid rates (Nelson, 1986). In many cases, there is little or no nonverbal context the child can use to fill in the gaps, and because the teacher is addressing a group rather than one student, the need for repairs is often not noticed. The child who does not understand, perhaps believing everyone else does understand or perhaps because he is embarrassed, will often not ask for the language help he needs. The child who lags behind in language, therefore, will quickly fall behind in school. Until the language deficit is addressed, academic maladjustment and failure are virtually assured.

Metalinguistic Development During the School Years

One of the most significant changes to occur in the child's use of language as he moves from the preschool to the school years is the rapid development of metalinguistic awareness. Before he begins school, the child uses language almost exclusively as a means of communication. Sometimes he talks for the sheer pleasure of hearing his own voice, and sometimes he just plays with sounds and words, but he mostly uses language to communicate. When he enters school, he learns to separate himself from language and to separate language from communication so that he can identify, analyze, study, and think about the elements of language.

Sometimes we have experiences in life that are so intense that we can almost see ourselves from a distance. We call these out-of-body experiences. During these experiences, we see ourselves more objectively and may understand our own behaviors more clearly. In much the same way, the child does not really know what he knows about language until he is able to examine and study language objectively, from a distance. The term, **metalinguistic ability,** refers to the capacity to use language to analyze, study, and understand language. Metalinguistic ability, or awareness, is the out-of-body experience of language. The most noticeable and dramatic increase in metalinguistic awareness occurs between the ages of five and eight years (Bernstein, 1989, p. 145). Beginning at this time, but continuing even into adulthood, the child notices and develops an understanding of each of the basic components of language, including phonology, semantics, syntax, and pragmatics. Not surprisingly, the development of metalinguistic awareness is related to cognitive development, intellectual capacity, scholastic achievement, reading skills, and environmental factors, including the child's play experiences and the kind of stimulation he receives from adults (Saywitz & Cherry-Wilkinson, 1982).

The typical adult may not have a sophisticated understanding of the components of language, but every adult has an awareness of each component and has at least a rudimentary understanding of the rules that govern the various dimensions of language. It is a speaker's metalinguistic ability that allows him to make judgments about whether or not a sentence sounds grammatical or about which marker for tense or plurality sounds correct. When a speaker produces language, he does so automatically with little or no conscious attention to the rules he is applying, but when he is asked to make a judgment about a language form, he must consciously attend to the form and apply his knowledge of the rules to determine whether or not the form is correct. The production of language is a linguistic function. The evaluation of language is a **metalinguistic** function.

Awareness of Speech Sounds

We can determine a person's awareness of phonology, or speech sound system, by asking him or her to count the number of sounds in a word or separate one or more sounds from the word. Some adults have difficulty with these tasks because they associate sounds with their corresponding alphabet symbols. Although our sound system and alphabet are related, there is not always a direct correspondence between what one sees and what one hears. We all know, for example, that some letters are silent. The pronunciation of *caught* does not include sounds for *g* or *h*. Sometimes sounds are present even when they are not directly represented by letters. The second *sound* in *quick,* for example is *w,* and the last sound in *fox* is *s.* There are five letters in the word *watch,* but there are only three sounds. Can you identify them? If you cannot identify the sounds now, you should be able to do so after you read the next chapter in this book. Although the child will probably not correctly count the sounds in all words, he does show awareness of phonology by separating and counting speech sounds by the time he is six or seven years old.

Awareness of Semantics

We typically think of meaning in relation to words, but there is also meaning in sentences that goes beyond the additive meanings of the individual words in sentences. In considering the child's developing awareness of semantics, researchers have considered word meanings and sentence meanings. The child's awareness of word meanings can be evaluated by asking him to define words, to judge words as hard or easy, or as big or little. If the child is asked, for example, if the word *whale* is big or little, he might say it is big because he is not able to separate the referent from the word. The child who is aware of semantics at the word level understands that the connections between words and the things they represent are arbitrary. Sometimes a little word represents a little thing (e.g. *ant*), but sometimes a big word represents a little thing (e.g. *microorganism*) and sometimes a little word represents a big thing (e.g. *ship*). The fact that words are arbitrary labels might also mean that one word can have two or more very different meanings. The word *down,* for example, is most commonly understood to mean *in a lower position,* but the word *down* also refers to soft, fluffy feathers. Researchers have used riddles to determine if children understand the multiple meanings of key words. Consider the following riddle: *Why did the man throw his clock out the window? Because he wanted to see time fly.* To understand this riddle, the child must understand that the word *fly* has at least two possible meanings: (1) to move through the air, and (2) to pass quickly. By the time the child is six or seven years old, he is able to separate words from their referents as evidenced by his ability to understand multiple meanings of words and his ability to recognize the arbitrary connection between words and the things they represent.

As one might suspect, practice makes a difference in developing definitional skills. Snow (1990) found that the ability of elementary school children to create correct formal definitions was associated with their experience with language, and specifically with their experience in using language to talk about what words mean. That is, definitional skills depend upon the opportunity to practice definitions. In this case, practice does not necessarily make perfect, but practice does make better.

Researchers have evaluated awareness of sentence meaning by asking children to evaluate the acceptability of sentences based on their semantic appropriateness. A child who is aware of the rules governing sentence meaning will be able to judge whether or not a sentence makes sense. For example, he will recognize that the sentence *The dog ate the cookie* is meaningful, whereas the sentence *The paper ate the cookie* is not meaningful because a *dog* is an animal capable of eating, and *paper* is an inanimate object not capable of eating. The child can typically make judgments about the semantic appropriateness of sentences as early as five years, and he can often point out the problem. In the example cited, he might say, " 'The paper ate the cookie' is wrong because paper can't eat."

Awareness of Syntax

The child's metalinguistic awareness of syntax can be assessed by asking him to decide whether sentences are grammatically correct or incorrect. To ensure that the child is making a judgment about a sentence based on a grammatical error, we can ask him to correct the mistake. If he determines that a sentence is incorrect and is able to make the grammatical correction, we may assume he has developed syntactic awareness. By the time the child is six years old, he would be able to determine that the sentence, *The dog chased the cat tree up the,* is incorrect, and he would be able to produce the correction. A somewhat more difficult judgment involves the identification of syntactic ambiguities in sentences. For example, *"Visiting relatives can be a pain"* can be interpreted in two ways: (1) Going to visit relatives can be a pain, or (2) Having relatives visit can be a pain. The child may be eleven or twelve years old before he has enough metalinguistic awareness to recognize this kind of ambiguity.

Awareness of Pragmatics

Less attention has been given to the development of pragmatic awareness than to other metalinguistic skills. We do know that by the time the child is five or six he is able to make judgments about whether enough information is contained in a message or not. That is, if the child listens to a set of instructions, he will know if the instructions are adequate or if more information is needed. At about this same age, the child will recognize glaring contradictions or inconsistencies. He will recognize, for example, that a character in a story cannot be the hero and the villain at the same time. He will understand that a man's saying, *When I was a little girl . . .* does not make sense even if the sentence is correct according to all the rules of syntax. As early as three years, the child understands that the inclusion of the word *please* makes requests more polite, and by the time he is five years old, he understands that indirect requests are more polite than direct commands. Some pragmatic awareness, therefore, develops before the child enters school.

Reading and Writing: New Applications of Language

Even though we do not need to immerse ourselves again in all the arguments about the contributions of nature and nurture to the development of language, it is important to emphasize one more time that language expressed through speech is common to all human beings. There is convincing evidence that human beings are born to speak. But are they genetically predisposed to read and write? The answer to this question lies, to some extent, in two basic facts about human beings as communicators. Anthropologists have never discovered a group of people, no matter how primitive their lifestyle, without a highly developed spoken language. They have found, however, groups of people whose languages have no written forms. In addition, there are many people who speak languages that do have written forms but who are unable to read and write. It is reasonable to conclude, therefore, that a more powerful biological drive exists for humans to speak than to read and write. Although humans are innately endowed with the sensory, perceptual, and cognitive abilities to learn to read and write, environmental factors are more crucial in the emergence of these language capabilities than in the emergence of speech.

Extensive language research conducted over the past several decades has changed our views about how language is acquired, even if this research has not provided closure to all the questions we have posed about how the acquisition process occurs. At the same time that language people have tried to understand how language is acquired by human children, other researchers have tried to understand how reading and writing are learned. They have used their findings to suggest more effective strategies for facilitating literacy development in children, both in their homes and in their schools.

It is often helpful to examine old views in order to appreciate why new understandings emerge from current research findings. A brochure entitled *Current*

Research on Language Learning, published by the National Council of Teachers of English in 1993, includes summaries of previous and current thinking about the emergence of reading and writing. According to the previous view, the child must learn the smallest parts of language before he can learn to read and write whole texts, a view commonly referred to as "part-to-whole." The teaching/learning strategy that emerged from the "part-to-whole" view involved a progression from teaching and learning the letters of the alphabet, the sounds letters make, simple words, and then the production of short sentences. This strategy invested considerable time in teaching skills that were considered prerequisite to reading and writing. In truth, many children did learn to read and write using the "part-to-whole" approach, but many other children struggled and failed. The National Council of Teachers of English suggested, in fact, that "such instruction made it difficult for most children to understand the joy and benefit of reading and writing—to make them lifetime readers and writers."

The current view is that learning to read and write is quite similar to learning to talk. Consider, for example, that when caregivers talk to their babies, they are not trying to *teach* them to use spoken language. They certainly do not produce isolated speech sounds in order to teach the phonology of the language. They do not speak single-word utterances in order to teach a vocabulary. They talk to their babies, sometimes in fun sentences and sometimes in babbled productions, in order to make *communicative* contact with them, even if it is a communication that is limited and simplistic. Caregivers tend to accept the child's most primitive productions as language-like behavior that should be appreciated and celebrated. Children learn to talk then, not by means of direct instruction from language experts, but through the process of hearing language, using language, and sharing language with the significant people in their lives. Current views about reading and writing suggest that children learn these processes in much the same way. That is, they observe the written word. They listen to people read. They read, and they write. In the process of observing and doing reading and writing, they learn to read and write.

Whereas oral language develops rapidly during the preschool years, the child's competence with written language develops much more slowly over a longer period of time. The foundations for reading and writing, however, are established during the child's earliest years. Research indicates that a number of variables contribute to the child's early literacy development, but the single most important factor, particularly in the development of reading, or the command of written language, is the child's home environment (Bernstein, 1989, p. 147). That is, the child who is exposed to the written word early will tend to develop competency in reading more easily than the child who is denied access to written language or print.

Even before babies can talk, they enjoy looking at books and having books or stories read to them. They are able to understand some of the content that is being read to them long before they can read, just as they are able to understand the meanings of some of the words they hear in speech months before they say their

Learning to enjoy books.

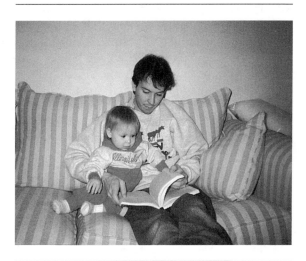

first words. Before children understand the content of stories, they enjoy the experience of having people read to them, being held closely, and hearing the soothing voices of loving adults (Fields & Spangler, 1989). The findings from the relevant research about children and their early experiences with the written word consistently lead us to the same conclusion: Reading to children is a successful way to teach them to read, and the influence of these early experiences is not limited to reading. Gordon Wells (1986), after a fifteen-year study of children in England, concluded that the academic success of these children was highly influenced by the frequency with which stories were read to them. Dolores Durkin's (1980) studies showed that the most common factor shared by children who read early is that they are read to frequently. The findings of other research indicate that children learn ways of constructing meaning for print as adults share and discuss stories with them (Altwerger, Diehl-Faxon, & Dockstader-Anderson, 1985; Fisher, 1991; Mason, 1989; Teale, 1988).

Parents and other caregivers can facilitate literacy development by reading stories to their children while encouraging them to follow the pictures, the sense of the story, and the words. As children listen to stories being read, and especially as they actively participate in the experience, they gain control over the language of books. In a very real and meaningful sense, they seem to be able to absorb this language (Doake, 1995). The adult reader can encourage the child to participate in the reading experience by using an invitational and conversational reading style. For example, if the reader pauses at certain highly predictable junctures in a story, the child will likely participate by filling in the gaps. The child might predict the word that is actually written, or he might use a word that closely approximates the target word, but accuracy is not the point. Participation is. Using whatever language the child has at this point in his communicative development, he gradually reproduces, with increasing accuracy, the meaning of the story for himself. At this point, adults often conclude that the child has memorized the words. While this is undoubtedly true, this is not a minor accomplishment because memorization is part of the process of constructing the meaning of the story. The emerging *reader* is demonstrating "reading-like" behavior, an important step in the process of reading development (Doake, 1995).

As children gain experience with their books and with the written language of their environments, they become increasingly aware that the print on the page actually carries the story. They also begin to connect what they are saying with what they are seeing. At this point, they are beginning to show a metalinguistic awareness of letter–sound relationships. They are independently discovering and demonstrating the role of phonics in a contextual, natural setting. Given the language competencies of preschool children, this can no longer be viewed as simply a preparatory period for the learning of reading and writing. What is happening at this time in development goes beyond mere preparation. In their wide-ranging studies of the literacy development of young children, Harste, Woodward, and Burke (1984a) found no evidence to suggest that "children's psycholinguistic and sociolinguistic strategies are qualitatively different from the kinds of decisions which more experienced language users make." They concluded that "the process children engage in is not a pseudo form of the 'real' process; it is that process" (p. 105).

As young children become increasingly engaged in the reading/language process, they begin to develop a genuine desire to read. While reading stories to children will help facilitate language development, the inherent value of reading goes beyond language development. In order to realize this value, children must want to read. Unless they want to read, they will not read enough to become proficient readers, and unless they become proficient readers, they will not derive the full value of the experience. As melodramatic as it may sound, when parents and other caregivers read stories to young children, they are introducing them to the magic of books. They are initiating the process that will, if all goes well, awaken in their children the desire to read. The sharing of high-quality literature with youngsters provides a glimpse of the excitement, the drama, and the beauty that is contained in books. When adults share enthusiasm with children for a good story, they provide a model for how to interact with text. Making the printed page come to life during an animated reading of a story demonstrates not just the *process* of reading, but the *power* of reading as well. As children reenact stories that have been read to them, and as they discuss these stories with adults, they gradually, and without pressure, construct understandings they need in order to become readers (Fields & Spangler, 1995).

The younger children are when they are introduced to the written word, the better their reading competencies will be. As adult literacy programs attest, it is never too late for a person to learn to read, but at a time when the written word is so pervasive and powerful in the world, the darkness of illiteracy is terribly restrictive and unnecessary. Children who have been immersed in the written word during their early years at home begin school with significant advantages over children who have had limited experiences with books. Some of these advantages might vanish when environmentally deprived children are given the encouragement and support to use their academic opportunities, but there is little doubt that early experiences with the written word are important for the development of both reading and writing.

From the most traditional perspective, parents send children to school to learn the three *R's, reading, writing,* and *arithmetic.* Hmm, methinks we should have placed a stronger emphasis on spelling. In any case, parents expect that their sons and daughters will learn how to read and write when they go to school. It is with some alarm then that we note the increasing number of children who are sent to resource rooms for help with reading, and the small percentage of students who are able to read critically by their senior year in high school (Applebee, Langer, & Mullis, 1988b). These trends, coupled with the staggering number of illiterate adults in our country, should cause American educators who are directly concerned with reading and writing to consider if teaching paradigms for these critical skills are consistent with the natural language/learning strategies used by children (Weaver, 1994).

Prior to the 1970s, most experts in the field of reading viewed reading as a visual-perceptual phenomenon. Reading instruction focused on words and on pronouncing words correctly. Children who were not successful with this exact word-bound model were often considered candidates for special help or for services outside the regular classroom. Children who needed more support with reading were enrolled in programs that focused on correct word pronunciation. In the 1970s and 1980s, reading experts began to explore the relationship between language and reading. Goodman (1986) asserted, for example, that "Children learn written language in the same way they learn oral language because it is language." This point of view led to an understanding that in order to help children who need special support in learning how to read, teachers must know more about language acquisition and about the functions of language in the early development of young children. According to this view, reading is a language-based activity. This view gave rise to assumptions underlying the two dominant reading instruction approaches currently used in American public schools.

Expressed most simply, one view suggests that reading is *taught.* The other view suggests that reading *develops* as part of the child's natural language development. Those who hold the first view teach reading skills in a direct and systematic manner. Teachers who believe that reading develops within the larger context of language development try to facilitate reading and writing in a manner that is as natural as possible. Some of the differences between these two points of view are reflected in their terminologies. Other differences are reflected in how terms they share in common are used. These differences will be noted in the two models of reading that support these divergent viewpoints: (1) the *transmission model* that supports the view that reading is taught, and (2) the *transactional model* that supports the view that literacy develops (Weaver, 1994).

Theoretical Models of Reading

In order to appreciate how each model explains how reading develops, one must first understand the more global view of each model as it relates to education in general. Underlying the *transmission model* of education are principles from behavioral psychology. Students are viewed as empty vessels into which knowledge is poured. Curriculum based on this model requires students to practice skills, memorize facts, and accumulate information, typically in a manner that isolates knowledge from the application of the skills learned and the information obtained. In this educational scheme, errors are to be avoided, and near perfection is expected. In principle, what is taught today will be practiced tomorrow, and will be tested for complete and accurate understanding the next day. The commission of errors is penalized in order to discourage the formation of inappropriate habits. When this model is applied, students often "fail" and are judged to be in need of remedial help (Weaver, 1994).

In the *transactional model,* students are viewed as people who bring significant language competence and a knowledge background to the process of education. The principles underlying this model are derived from what cognitive psychologists and psycholinguists have discovered about human learning, including the development of language. In applying this model, teachers encourage a constructivist view of learning by trying to create rich environmental contexts and situations in which students can learn. Students use their schemas to construct and advance their own knowledge. Taking risks, developing and refining hypotheses, and making errors are treated as essential components in the course of learning. Mastery of processes, such as speaking a language, reading, writing, and spelling, occurs over a period of years, and the learner will probably never reach a level of perfection in any of them (Weaver, 1994).

When applied specifically to reading, the *transmission model* suggests that reading must be taught in much the same way that arithmetic, geography, science, or any other subject is taught. A teacher who uses this model spends time preparing the child for reading, developing "reading readiness." The teacher invests considerable time teaching students to read and testing to determine if, in fact, students have learned to read. Students invest a great deal of time in practicing reading skills, completing worksheets and laboring in workbooks to hone their skills. There is a strong emphasis on producing words exactly as they are presented in print. Variations, even if they are semantically comparable to the target words, are not accepted and are discouraged. Reading is a separate subject in the curriculum and is even isolated from writing, its close academic cousin. The transmission model explains the development of reading in terms of stages through which all children move at presumably a comparable pace, and the term *development* is used in reference to the stage concept (Weaver, 1994).

The *transactional model* of literacy development presents a very different view of how children learn to read and how teachers can facilitate the development of reading. In this model, there is no dichotomy between readiness to read and learning to read. Literacy development, which includes reading and writing, is viewed as a uninterrupted process. Development is seamless, not divisible into discrete stages. The teacher and her students invest their time not in drill work, but in actual reading and writing. They talk about what they have read. Students read and write for pragmatic reasons, and they read and write for the sheer joy of doing so. The competency emphasis is not on exact pronunciations of the words in print but on understanding what words, phrases, sentences, paragraphs, and stories mean. The teacher explains various reading and writing strategies in meaningful context, and she encourages her students to discuss these strategies in this same context. The emphases are always on meaning, pragmatics, and on individual development. In the transactional model, the term *development* is used in reference to the concept that reading and writing literacy emerges in a continuous manner over a period of time (Weaver, 1994). Underlying the transactional model of reading is the belief that language development and the emergence of literacy cannot be separated. They are interactive partners in the development of communication. Language knowledge certainly prepares children for the development of literacy, and literacy provides children valuable tools in their attempts to understand the language they use, the process we have identified as metalinguistic awareness.

Children's Reading Development

Our discussion of literacy development, including both reading and writing, is based on the transactional model. Keep in mind that within the context of this model, development is not viewed in stages, but is viewed as a continuous, seamless process. We will identify categories of development, but these categories should not be understood as periods of mastery in which one category is completed before the next category begins. The reader will note instead that there is a great deal of overlapping as we move from category to category, and the emphasis is always on continuous development. Three broad categories will be identified and described in the following paragraphs: (1) *emergent,* (2) *developing,* and (3) *independent.*

Emergent readers are at the beginning of the reading adventure. They have learned that books contain stories, that they can visit these stories as often as they like, that the words will be the same each time they return, and that the pictures accompanying the stories help construct and more fully develop meaning. Emergent readers show progressively more interest in trying to read without assistance from others. They are able to discuss what is happening in a story, and they can predict what is likely to happen next. They are also beginning to recognize certain words in varying contexts.

It is important to choose books for emergent readers with their needs and competencies in mind. The books selected should provide opportunities for these children to enjoy literature even though they cannot yet read independently. The text and illustrations should be clear. The plots should be simple. The language should be repetitive, rhythmic, and natural. Ideally, the illustrations will precede the text that describes the illustrations in order to assist emergent readers in the process of predicting what the text might say and what is going to happen next in the story. Books suited for these children will possess an invitational tone that will encourage them to participate to the extent they can until they are able to read on their own. Within the context of the transactional model, it is most important that books for emergent readers be designed to guide children toward an understanding of what they are reading, rather than focusing on individual words. From the very beginning of literacy development, children should be made aware that the essence of reading, and indeed the essence of language in all its forms, is meaning (Department of Education, Wellington, 1985).

In the second category, we find **developing readers.** These are children who are becoming true readers. At this point in literacy development, children have established the habit of reading for meaning, at least in the sense that they understand that meaning is the reading bottom line. Developing readers are encouraged to use their own life experiences as context for what they read. As they process printed text, they are encouraged to take interpretative risks, to make approximations about what words are or what words mean. Developing readers use the text, illustrations, and their own knowledge of print conventions to sample, to predict, and to confirm printed words. These children also use letter–sound associations, within context, to help confirm their predictions about words. They are encouraged to move beyond unfamiliar words to find lexical content they do recognize, content that may help them figure out what the unfamiliar words are. They are also encouraged to re-read and self-correct when the process of interpreting meaning has been interrupted or when the printed words do not seem to make sense. You will recognize, of course, that these are strategies adult readers use when they have difficulty determining the meaning of printed words. What is important to understand is that these are strategies, according to the transactional model, that should be encouraged from the beginning of reading development.

In comparison to books chosen for emergent readers, books chosen for developing readers draw on a wider range of life experiences, and they expand readers' horizons to a significantly enlarged world, complete with more elaborate, mature understandings about how the world works. The vocabulary bases of these books match the rapidly growing vocabularies of the children reading them. They are designed, in fact, to increase readers' vocabularies and to introduce them to more complex and varied language structures. These books, in comparison to the books used by emergent readers, employ a wider variety of cues to help children sample, predict, and monitor what they are reading, and to construct and maintain meaning.

The third category includes **independent readers.** Independent readers read on their own, and they read when they are alone. These children are confident and competent readers who are integrating into the process of reading all the cueing systems available in language. They pay little conscious attention to the details of printed words because their focus is on constructing and maintaining meaning. For independent readers, the printed details are means, not ends. The ends are understanding, interpretation, and meaning. Independent readers are able to read increasingly longer and more structurally complex sentences with meaning. They are able to process a wide variety of prose and poetry. They are also learning to adjust reading rate to accommodate the purposes for which they are reading. One of the most obvious characteristics of independent readers is variety, not just in what they read, but in the data bases upon which they draw to make sense of what they read. To a much greater extent than developing readers, independent readers use knowledge gained from their personal experiences in their homes, schools, and communities, as well as knowledge gleaned from previously read books, movies, and television to understand what they are reading right now. As their reading choices expand, they encounter books that are increasingly challenging in terms of content, format, and style. They read stories about people and places far removed from their own lives in time and space. They read nonfiction as well as fiction. They read essays, poems, novels, plays, and, dare we acknowledge it, even textbooks. As their language becomes more complete, and their reading experiences become more varied, these children experience a knowledge explosion that cannot be fathomed by people who cannot read. The true miracle in this experience is that it all happens inside readers' minds, bounded only by the limits of their imaginations, and all this can take place in the family room or the classroom. The power of books in the hands of readers is truly amazing. As their reading experiences increase in frequency and variety, independent readers learn to enjoy reading. As they learn to enjoy reading, they risk becoming what are called *voracious* readers. You know these people. They are knowledgeable, interesting, creative, and productive people.

Throughout our discussion of language development, we have emphasized that children do not proceed through development at the same pace. We make the same emphasis here. While the general development of reading competencies will be the same for all children, they do not all achieve these competencies at the same ages. Rather than becoming unduly concerned about whether or not a child is on schedule in terms of literacy development, we should be concerned about doing whatever we can to facilitate development. What we can do is fairly simple. We can support and encourage children who are learning to read and write. We can trust that their natural language abilities, in combination with teaching/learning paradigms that foster natural, language-based reading instruction, will ultimately produce effective and efficient adult readers.

The Development of Writing

Even the casual observer will understand that reading and writing are closely related processes, sharing language as a common bond. Butler and Turbill (1987) note that reading and writing are also functional cousins in that each is an act of composing. More specifically, Butler and Turbill observe that "Readers, using their background of knowledge and experience, compose meaning from text; writers, using their background of knowledge and experience, compose meaning into text" (1987, p. 11).

In a very real sense then, reading and writing are different facets of a single process. In the development of reading and writing, the knowledge of each process is enhanced by the knowledge gained in the other. This means that the more a person reads, the more he will know about writing, and the more he writes, the more he will know about reading (Fields & Spangler, 1995). From the point of view of Butler and Turbill, the tie that binds reading and writing together is meaning. As the reader processes the printed symbols on the page, he constructs meaning, not by paying attention to every detail, but by sampling only those details he needs for meaning closure. You know from your own experience that if you are reading material with which you are not familiar, you process many more details of the printed symbols than if you are reading material you know well. The reader's knowledge and experience help him gauge how many details are enough in a given reading situation. Alas, sometimes the reader exhausts all the available details, and for want of more, never achieves meaning closure. We have all been there too.

Writing offers a different challenge. The writer begins with ideas, morsels of meaning, and must decide which symbols in which combination will best represent those ideas. If the writer understands the nuances of this kind of communication, he will also take into account the audience to whom he is directing his packaged morsels of meaning, and he will select the literary style he believes is most appropriate for conveying his message (Department of Education, Wellington, 1985). Consider the differences in symbols and literary styles that might be reflected in the following: writing a diary entry, writing a letter to a lover, writing a letter of inquiry about a job, and writing an essay for a philosophy professor on the relative dangers of optimism and pessimism in humankind's efforts to save the planet.

We should step back for a moment and consider what has been discussed about writing to this point. The opening paragraphs in this section have been devoted to what might be called *real writing,* in contrast to the act of copying letters or words a teacher has written on the chalkboard. It needs to be emphasized that *real writing* is not the same thing as *handwriting practice.* For many years, teachers assumed they were teaching writing when they taught their students how to print their letters and then produce them in cursive, the physical skills included in *penmanship.* Today, teachers recognize that while the physical skills involved in forming letters are important, the process of writing, real writing, is far more important. Teachers today value writing as a powerful communication tool. They believe their students have the potential to become authors, that they can actually compose meaning into text (Fields & Spangler, 1995). Writing is, as writing experts today remind us, about meaning, and it is about language. The developing child who processes meaning in the speech of others, and who learns how to create meaning in his own oral expressions, eventually extends these meaning-language skills into the processes of reading and writing. Just as he can express meaning in what he says, so can he express meaning in what he writes. Even though, as we have noted, there is a more powerful biological drive in human beings for the production of speech than for the production of language in written form, there can be little doubt that children have a natural inclination to write. They certainly show evidence of a strong desire to write even before they enter school. Preschoolers are infamous for marking up walls, sidewalks. and newspapers with crayons, chalk, pencils, and pens (Graves, 1983). If speech begins in cooing and babbling, writing certainly begins in the preschool child's scratches and scrawls.

The physical process of moving the fingers and hands to put letters on paper is closely related to drawing in that writing and drawing are both processes of symbolization (Dyson, 1983). Writing and drawing, however, are not the same thing. The child demonstrates that writing and drawing are differentiated processes when he is about three years old (Gibson & Levin, 1975). As soon as the child can hold and manipulate a pencil or crayon and is given an opportunity to experiment with these instruments of expression, he will begin to make marks on any surface that is available. These early marking and scribbling exercises form the foundations of writing. Especially if the young child has been exposed to printed language in books and magazines, he will try to make forms that resemble letters of the alphabet. These early attempts are crude approximations at best. At this point, the child does not know the names of the letters he is trying to form, nor does he understand that printed words represent spoken words, but he is beginning the journey that leads inexorably to written language (Sulzby, 1981).

The first word the typical child learns to write is his own name. Shortly thereafter, he will probably learn to write other words with which he is familiar, including "Mommy," "Daddy," and the names of his siblings. These personally familiar words provide the child with his first understanding that a connection exists between printed symbols and spoken sounds.

Very early in writing development, the child begins to make natural associations between the letters of the alphabet and the speech sounds they most commonly represent. These early sound-letter associations lead to what is called *graphophonemic awareness,* in which *graph* refers to printed symbols (letters) and *phonemic* refers to speech sounds. The child demonstrates graphophonemic awareness when, in a contextual setting, he makes a conscious effort to match letters to sounds (Read, 1981). It is at this juncture in the development of writing that the child begins to sense a need to spell, and it is at this juncture in our discussion that we need to be reminded that writing and spelling fit within the larger context of language. If it is true, as present-day language experts assert, that language acquisition occurs most efficiently when the child takes risks, when he experiments, develops hypotheses about rules, tests the rules, and revises them as necessary, the child must also risk, experiment, develop and refine rules in written language. Since written language includes spelling, common sense suggests that the child must be allowed, even encouraged, to risk and experiment with spelling. In fact, the typical child is likely to experiment with spelling even if he is not encouraged to do so. His earliest spelling risks and experiments result in some pretty interesting sequences of letters, often called *invented spellings*. The journey from invented to conventional spelling moves through the following four stages, each of which involves progressively more sophisticated spelling: (1) **prephonemic,** (2) **early phonemic,** (3) **letter-name,** and (4) **transitional** (Weaver, 1994).

In the **prephonemic** stage, the child is wantonly experimental and blithely uninhibited. When he tries to spell a word, he writes down letters in a manner that is clearly more capricious than calculated. He does seem to understand that longer words require more letters, and he knows that when letters are strung together, they "say" something, but he does not yet understand that there are specific, if not always consistent, relationships between the letters of the alphabet and the sounds of speech.

The changes in the **early phonemic** stage are not dramatic, but they are important because they reflect more sophisticated understanding about spelling and sounds. In this stage, the child often attends only to the first letter of a word. From the child's perspective, this single letter represents the entire word even if other letters are included. The other letters in the child's "written word" typically have no correspondence to the remaining segments of the target word. The child might know, for example, that the letter "D" makes the sound that begins "Daddy," but he writes "Daddy" as "DBMS." While the child is most likely to include the letter representing the first sound of a word, he may also include the letter that represents the last sound of the word. The middle of the word is a kind of mystery spelling package in the sense that no one, including the child, knows what letters might be included from one spelling attempt to the next on the same word. We do know that these attempts are not entirely random. For example, early phonemic spellings include consonants and exclude vowels. As the child gains more experience with letters and the sounds they represent, phonemic spellings begin to shade into spellings that more obviously reflect letter–sound relationships.

In the **letter-name** stage, the child is representing vowels as well as consonants. The child is attempting to spell more sounds, but he is most likely to use letters whose names sound like the speech sounds they purportedly represent. Nurtured in a risk-free environment, this understanding that there are relationships between printed symbols and speech sounds, or graphophonemic awareness, enables the child to move to the **transitional** stage of spelling.

In the **transitional** stage, the child will try a number of spelling strategies. He might use a particular spelling because he *remembers* seeing the word spelled that way in print. He might try to apply rules for spelling he has observed in his own reading. Perhaps he observed that when a word contains a double vowel (e.g., *teeth*), the vowel sound is long, or when a word ends with "e" (e.g., fin*e*), the preceding vowel is long. When asked to spell a word he does not know, such as *leaf,* he might assume, based on his knowledge of these rules, that the word should be spelled *leef,* or *lefe.* The child might continue to rely on letter-name spellings, so that when he is asked to spell *sugar,* he might write *shuger.* A writing sample of a child in the transitional stage of spelling might include productions based on several different spelling strategies, including the examples provided here and others. It would be a very rare child, at this stage of spelling development, who would rely on a single spelling strategy. The typical child is still experimenting. In fact, the development of spelling is facilitated by successful use of an expanding range of spelling strategies (Wilde, 1992). After all, a strategy that works well in one spelling challenge may be of absolutely no help in another. Given the inconsistencies between the way words are spelled and the way words are spoken, the child who aspires to be a competent speller must have a plethora of spelling strategy options at his disposal. Did I spell *plethora* correctly? The first vowel is not long, so it should not be a double *ee,* and the sound *uh* at the end is probably spelled with an *a,* and . . . The truth is, many of the strategies used in the transitional stage are used by adult spellers as well. The child learns much of what he will ever know about spelling patterns during the elementary school years, but most people continue to learn how to spell throughout their adult years, or at least until their brains are totally fried by television.

Obviously, much more is involved in writing than forming letters and spelling. Even as these foundational processes continue to develop, the child is learning to express himself through writing, and he is learning the rules of grammar, capitalization, and punctuation that make writing "correct." Whatever limitations others may see in the young child's writing abilities, he is typically unabashed about expressing himself on paper, and the products of these early attempts are often delightful. In the following essay written by a seven-year-old boy, you will notice spelling, punctuation, and capitalization errors, but you will also notice the simple elegance of the written message:

> spider live in hot dezerd.
> but not oll of them. sum live here.
> sum cude hurt you. they are deadles.
> I saw one before it was not deadles.
> It was a dade-long-legs he was on
> me. they are not fast
> they are not good jumpers at all
> THE END
> of the spiter story

By the time the child is in the third or fourth grade, he moves from writing designed mostly for his own amusement to writing for other people. He now examines his own written material and, using his knowledge of language, revises his copy so that it is more correct or complete (Bartlett, 1982; Graves,

1979). Although the child's oral language was dramatically superior to written language at the beginning of the school years, by the end of the elementary school years, his written language is more complex than his oral language (Gundloch, 1981). As the child moves into junior and senior high school, he becomes more proficient in the technical aspects of writing, but he also learns how to organize and develop his ideas and how to use written language to influence the thoughts, feelings, and attitudes of others (Nold, 1981).

And the Beat Goes On . . .

What a magnificent adventure this has been! The child, by virtue of his genetic background, was born to talk, but acquiring language and the abilities to express language through speech and writing is not as simple as acquiring freckles. Language acquisition depends on environmental opportunities and on the child's interactions with the important people in his life. It depends on motor, sensory, perceptual, and cognitive development. It is a complex process that begins before birth, accelerates through the child's first five or six years of life, and continues, only slightly abated, through the remainder of his school years. Even then the learning does not end. As adults, we learn new words. We understand syntactic rules more completely. We learn the multiple meanings of words, and we learn the differences between the denotations and connotations of words, which allow us to use words more effectively to convey the exact messages we intend. Language is indeed a wondrous and exciting phenomenon, and we continue to experience the wonder of language as long as we live and speak and listen and read and write.

This marks the end of our journey through the joys and travails of speech and language development, but three chapters remain. Throughout our discussion of language development, we have mentioned the sound system of speech but we have not specifically traced its development. In Chapter Seven, we take a closer look at phonology and the acquisition of speech sounds. In Chapter Eight, we examine language differences based on geography, culture, and gender. Finally, we review some of the common disorders of speech and language in Chapter Nine.

Review Questions

1. How does vocabulary growth parallel Jean Piaget's four stages of cognitive development? That is, what changes in intellectual development seem to account for the acquisition and use of vocabulary over the first fifteen years of the child's life?

2. What is the syntagmatic-paradigmatic shift and how is it related to vocabulary growth?

3. What is the difference between horizontal and vertical expansion in the development of word meanings?

4. Why do the child's definitions shift from personal to shared, and in what sense do his definitions become more "elaborate" as his language knowledge increases?

5. Define each of the following figurative language forms and provide several examples of each: metaphor, simile, idiom, and proverb.

6. What is the difference between reversible and nonreversible passive sentences? Provide several examples of each type.

7. What is the principle of minimal distance? Why does the child have more difficulty with words that inconsistently violate the principle than with words that consistently violate the principle?

8. Create several conjoined sentences using each of the following categories of conjunctions: conditional, causal, disjunctive, and temporal.

9. Why is "because" a troublesome conjunction for the developing child?

10. What morphological modifications does the child begin to master during the school years?

11. Describe each of the following advancements in conversational skills: shading, stacked repair sequences, and sophisticated versions of indirect request.

12. Describe the major changes that occur in the child's narratives as he moves through the school years.

13. Describe each of the following types of narrative discourse: *recount, eventcast, account,* and *fictionalized narrative.*

14. When do gender differences in communication begin to emerge? Why do you think these differences exist?

15. What new challenges does the child as communicator experience in the classroom?

16. What does metalinguistic awareness mean? What do we know about metalinguistic development in the following areas: phonology, semantics, syntax, and pragmatics?

17. What can parents do to facilitate literacy development in their children?

18. Compare and contrast the two dominant reading models underlying current reading instruction programs in American public schools: (1) *transmission* model and (2) *transactional* model.

19. Briefly describe the following categories of reading development: (1) *emergent,* (2) *developing,* and (3) *independent.*

20. What is the difference between *writing* and *penmanship,* and why is the difference important?

21. What is *graphophonemic awareness?*

22. Briefly describe the four stages of invented spelling: (1) *prephonemic,* (2) *phonemic,* (3) *letter-name,* and (4) *transitional.*

23. What is the moral of "the spiter story" for adults who teach reading and writing?

References and Suggested Readings

Abrahamsen, E., & Rigrodsky, S. (1984). Comprehension of complex sentences in children at three levels of cognitive development. *Journal of Psycholinguistic Research, 13*, 333–350.

Altwerger, B., Diehl-Faxon, J., & Dockstader-Anderson, K. (1985). Read-aloud events as meaning construction. *Language Arts, 62* (5), 476–484.

Ames, L. (1966). Children's stories. *Genetic Psychological Monographs, 73*, 307–311.

Applebee, A. N., Langer, J. A., & Mullis, I. V. S. (1988b). *Who reads best? Factors related to reading achievement in grades 3, 7, and 11.* Princeton, NJ: National Assessment of Educational Progress, Educational Testing Service.

Baldie, B. (1976). The acquisition of the passive voice. *Journal of Child Language, 3*, 331–348.

Bartlett, C. (1982). Learning to write: some cognitive and linguistic components. In R. Shuy (Ed.), *Linguistics and Literacy Series*, No. 2. Washington, DC: Center of Applied Linguistics.

Berko-Gleason, J., & Greif, E. (1983). Men's speech to young children. In B. Thorne, C. Kramerae, & N. Henley (Eds.), *Language, Gender, and Society.* Rowley, Massachusetts: Newbury House.

Bernstein, D. (1989). Language development: The school-age years. In D. Bernstein & E. Tiegerman, (Eds.), *Language and communication disorders in children* (2nd ed.). Columbus, OH: Merrill/Macmillan.

Biemiller, A. (1970). The development of the use of graphic and contextual information as children learn to read. *Reading Research Quarterly, 6*, 75–96.

Billow, R. (1975). A cognitive developmental study of metaphor comprehension. *Developmental Psychology, 11*, 415–423.

Brinton, B., Fujiki, M., Loeb, D., & Winkler, E. (1986). Development of conversational repair strategies in response to requests for clarification. *Journal of Speech and Hearing Research, 29*, 75–81.

Butler, A., & Turbill, J. (1987). *Towards a reading-writing classroom.* Portsmouth, NH: Heinemann.

Carey, S., & Bartlett, E. (1978). Acquiring a single new word. *Papers and Reports on Child Language Development, 15*, 17–29.

Carrell, P. (1981). Children's understanding of indirect requests: Comparing child and adult comprehension. *Journal of Child Language, 8*, 329–345.

Carrow, E. (1973). *Test of auditory comprehension of language.* Austin, TX: Urban Research Group.

Chall, J. (1983). *Stages of reading development.* New York: McGraw-Hill.

Cherry, L., & Lewis, M. (1976). Mothers and two-year-olds: A study of sex-differentiated aspects of verbal interaction. *Developmental Psychology, 12*, 278–282.

Cherry-Wilkinson, L., & Dollaghan, C. (1979). Peer communication in first grade reading groups. *Theory Into Practice, 18*, 267–274.

Chomsky, C. (1969). The acquisition of syntax in children from 5 to 10. Cambridge, MA: MIT Press.

Clark, H., & Chase, W. (1972). On the process of comparing sentences against pictures. *Cognitive Psychology, 3,* 472–517.

Committee on School Practices and Programs (1993). *Current research on language learning.* Urbana, IL: National Council of Teachers of English.

Corrigan, R. (1975). A scalogram analysis of the development of the use and comprehension of "because" in children. *Child Development, 46,* 195–201.

Corsaro, W. (1979). Young children's conception of status and role. *Sociology of Education, 52,* 46–50.

Craig, H., & Evans, J. (1991). Turn exchange behaviors of children with normally developing language: The influence of gender. *Journal of Speech and Hearing Research, 34,* 866–878.

Crais, E. (1990). World knowledge to word knowledge. *Topics in Language Disorders, 10,* 45–62.

Department of Education, Wellington, New Zealand (1985) *Reading in junior classes.* Katonah, NY: Richard C. Owen Publishers, Inc.

de Villiers, J., & de Villiers, P. (1978). *Language acquisition.* Cambridge, MA: Harvard University Press.

Doake, D. B. (1995). *Literacy learning: A revolution in progress.* Bothell, WA: The Wright Group.

Durkin, D. (1980). *Teaching young children to read.* Boston: Allyn & Bacon.

Dyson, A. (1983, April). *Early writing as drawing: The developmental gap between speaking and writing.* Paper presented at the American Educational Research Association convention, Montreal, Canada.

Edelsky, C. (1977). Acquisition of an aspect communicative competence: Learning what it means to talk like a baby. In S. Ervin & C. Mitchell-Kernan (Eds.), *Child discourse.* New York: Academic Press.

Ehrenreich, B. (1981). The politics of talking in couples. *Ms, 5,* 43–45, 86–89.

Emerson, H. (1979). Children's comprehension of "because" in reversible and nonreversible sentences. *Journal of Child Language, 6,* 279–300.

Emerson, H., & Gekoski, W. (1976). Interactive and categorical grouping strategies and the syntagmatic-paradigmatic shift. *Child Development, 47,* 1116–1125.

Ervin, S. (1961). Changes with age in the verbal determinants of word-association. *American Journal of Psychology, 74,* 361–372.

Ervin-Tripp, S. (1977). From conversation to syntax. *Papers and Reports in Child Language Development, 13,* 11–21.

Ervin-Tripp, S., & Gordon, D. (1986). The development of requests. In R. Schiefelbusch (Ed.), *Language competence: Assessment and intervention.* San Diego, CA: College-Hill Press.

Fields, M., & Spangler, K. (1995). *Let's begin reading right: Developmentally appropriate beginning literacy* (3rd ed.). Englewood Cliffs, NJ: Prentice-Hall, Inc.

Fisher, B. (1991). *Joyful learning.* Portsmouth, NH: Heinemann.

Frith, V. (1985). Beneath the surface of developmental dyslexia. In K. Patterson, J. Marshall, & M. Coltheart (Eds.), *Surface dyslexia: Neuropsychological and cognitive studies of phonological reading*. London: Erlbaum.

Gallagher, T (1977). Revision behaviors in the speech of normal children developing language. *Journal of Speech and Hearing Research, 20,* 303–318.

Gardner, H., & Winner, E. (1979). The child is father to the metaphor. *Psychology Today, 12,* 81–91.

Garvey, C. (1975). Requests and responses in children's speech. *Journal of Child Language, 2,* 41–63.

Gathercole, V. (1985). "Me has too much hard questions": The acquisition of the linguistic mass-count distinction in "much" and "many." *Journal of Child Language, 12,* 395–415.

Gelman, R., & Shatz, M. (1977). Appropriate speech adjustments: The operation of conversational constraints on talk to 2-year-olds. In M. Lewis & L. Rosenblum (Eds.), *Interaction, conversation, and the development of language.* New York: Academic Press.

Gerber, A. (1981). Problems in the processing and use of language in education. In A. Gerber & D. Bryen (Eds.), *Language and learning disabilities.* Baltimore, MD: University Park Press.

Gibson, E., & Levin, H. (1975). *The psychology of reading.* Cambridge, MA: MIT Press.

Goodman, K. (1976). Behind the eye: What happens in reading. In H. Singer & R. Ruddell (Eds.), *Theoretical models and processes of reading* (2nd ed.). Newark, DE: International Reading Association.

Goodman, K. S. (1986). *What's whole in whole language?* Richmond Hill, Ontario, Canada: Scholastic-TAB Publications.

Graves, D. (1979). What children show us about revision. *Journal of Language Arts, 56,* 312–319.

Graves, D. H. (1983). *Writing: Teachers & children at work.* Portsmouth, NH: Heinemann.

Greif, E., & Berko-Gleason, J. (1980). Hi, thanks, and goodbye: Some more routine information. *Language and Society, 9,* 159–166.

Grimm, H. (1975, September). *Analysis of short-term dialogues in 5–7 year olds: Encoding of intentions and modifications of speech acts as a function of negative feedback loops.* Paper presented at the Third International Child Language Symposium, London, England.

Gundloch, R. (1981). On the nature and development of children's writing. In C. Frederiksen & J. Dominic (Eds.), *Writing: The nature, development, and teaching of written communication* (Vol. 2). Hillsdale, NJ: Erlbaum.

Haas, A. (1979). The acquisition of genderlect. *Annals of the New York Academy of Sciences, 327,* 101–113.

Hakes, D. (1980). *The development of metalinguistic abilities in children.* Berlin: Springer-Verlag.

Hakes, D. (1982). The development of metalinguistic abilities: What develops? In S. Kuczaj (Ed.), *Language development: Vol. 2. Language, Thought and Culture.* Hillsdale, NJ: Erlbaum.

Harste, J. C, Woodward, V. A., & Burke, C. L. (1984). *Language stories and literacy lessons.* Portsmouth, NH: Heinemann.

Heath, S. (1982). Toward an ethnohistory of writing in American education. In M. Whiteman, (Ed.), *Writing: The nature, development and teaching of written composition* (Vol 1). Hillsdale, NJ: Erlbaum.

Hoffner, C., Cantor, J., & Badzinski, D. (1990). Children's understanding of adverbs denoting degree of likelihood. *Journal of Child Language, 17,* 217–231.

Hood, L., & Bloom, L. (1979). What, when, and how about why: A longitudinal study of early expressions of causality. *Monographs of the Society for Research in Child Development, 44.*

Horgan, D. (1978). The development of the full passive. *Journal of Child Language, 5,* 65–80.

Johnston, J. (1982). Narratives: A new look at communication problems in older language disordered children. *Language, Speech and Hearing Services in Schools, 13,* 144–155.

Kamhi, A., & Catts, H. (1986). Toward an understanding of developmental language and reading disorders. *Journal of Speech and Hearing Disorders, 51,* 337–347.

Kemper, S. (1984). The development of narrative skills: Explanations and entertainments. In S. Kuczaj (Ed.), *Discourse development: Progress in cognitive development research,* New York: Springer-Verlag.

Kemper, S., & Edwards, L. (1986). Children's expression of causality and their construction of narratives. *Topics in Language Disorders, 7,* 11–20.

Klecan-Acker, J., & Kelty, K. (1990). An investigation of the oral narratives of normal and language-learning disabled children. *Journal of Childhood Communication Disorders, 13,* 207–216.

Krauss, R., & Glucksberg, S. (1977). Social and nonsocial speech. *Scientific American, 236,* 100–105.

Leonard, L., Wilcox, J., Fulmer, K., & Davis, A. (1978). Understanding indirect requests: An investigation of children's comprehension of pragmatic meanings. *Journal of Speech and Hearing Research, 21,* 528–537.

Litowitz, B. (1977). Learning to make definitions. *Journal of Child Language, 4,* 289–304.

Lund, N., & Duchan, J. (1988). *Assessing children's language in naturalistic contexts.* Englewood Cliffs, NJ: Prentice-Hall.

Maratsos, M. (1974). When is a high thing the big one? *Developmental Psychology, 10,* 367–375.

Marsh, G., Friedman, M., Welch, V., & Desberg, P. (1981). A cognitive-developmental theory of reading acquisition. In G. McKinnon & T. Weller (Eds.), *Reading research: Advances in theory and practice,* New York: Academic Press.

Mason, J. (1989). *Reading & writing connections.* Needham Heights, MA: Allyn & Bacon Publishers.

Mattingly, J. G. (1972). Reading the linguistic process and linguistic awareness. In J. Kavanagh & J. Mattingly (Eds.), *Language by ear and by eye.* Cambridge, MA: MIT Press.

McNeil, D. (1970). *The acquisition of language: The study of developmental psycholinguistics.* New York: Harper & Row.

Menyuk, P. (1969). *Sentences children use.* Cambridge, MA: MIT Press.

Menyuk, P. (1971). *The acquisition and development of language.* Englewood Cliffs, NJ: Prentice-Hall.

Miller, L. (1990). The roles of language and learning in the development of literacy. *Topics in Language Disorders, 10,* 1–23.

Mitchell-Kernan, C., & Kernan, K. (1977). Pragmatics of directive choice among children. In C. Mitchell-Kernan & S. Ervin-Tripp (Eds.), *Child discourse.* New York: Academic Press.

Muma, J., & Zwycewicz-Emory, C. (1979). Contextual priority: Verbal shift at seven? *Journal of Child Language, 6,* 301–311.

Nelson, N. (1985). Teacher talk and children listening—Fostering a better match. In C. Simon (Ed.), *Communication skills and classroom success: Assessment of language-learning disabled children.* San Diego, CA: College-Hill Press.

Nelson, N. (1986). Individual processing in classroom settings. *Topics in Language Disorders, 6,* 13–27.

Nippold, M., & Martin, S. (1989). Idiom interpretation in isolation versus context: A developmental study with adolescents. *Journal of Speech and Hearing Research, 32,* 59–66.

Nippold, M., Martin, S., & Erskine, B. (1988). Proverb comprehension in context: A developmental study with children and adolescents. *Journal of Speech and Hearing Research, 31,* 19–28.

Nippold, M., & Sullivan, M. (1987). Verbal and perceptual analogical reasoning and proportional metaphor comprehension in young children. *Journal of Speech and Hearing Research, 30,* 367–376.

Nold, E. (1981). Revising. In C. Frederiksen & J. Dominic (Eds.), *Writing: The nature, development, and teaching of written communication* (Vol. 2). Hillsdale, NJ: Erlbaum.

Obler, L. (1989). Language through the life-span. In J. Berko-Gleason (Ed.), *The development of language* (2nd ed.) Columbus, OH: Merrill/ Macmillan.

Owens, R. (1996). *Language development: An introduction* (4th ed.). Needham Heights, MA: Allyn & Bacon.

Parlee, M. (1979). Conversational politics. *Psychology Today, 5,* 48–56.

Parsons, C. (1980). *The effect of speaker age and listener compliance and noncompliance on the politeness of children's request directives.* Unpublished doctoral dissertation, Southern Illinois University, Carbondale.

Perfetti, C., & Goodman, D. (1970). Semantic constraint on the decoding of ambiguous words. *Journal of Experimental Psychology, 86,* 420–427.

Peterson, C. (1990). The who, when, and where of early narratives. *Journal of Child Language, 17,* 433–455.

Peterson, C., & McCabe, A. (1983). *Developmental psycholinguistics: Three ways of looking at a child's narrative.* New York: Plenum.

Piaget, J. (1963). *The origins of intelligence in children.* New York: Norton.

Read, C. (1981). Writing is not the inverse of reading for young children. In C. Frederiksen & J. Dominic (Eds.), *Writing: The nature, development, and teaching of written communication.* Hillsdale, NJ: Erlbaum.

Richards, M. (1980). Adjective ordering in the language of young children: An experimental investigation. *Journal of Child Language, 6,* 253–277.

Rumelhart, D. (1977). Toward an interactive model of reading. In S. Dornic (Ed.), *Attention and performance* (Vol. 1). Hillsdale, NJ: Eribaum.

Sause, E. (1976). Computer content analysis of sex differences in the language of children. *Journal of Pycholinguistic Research, 5,* 311–324.

Saywitz, K., & Cherry-Wilkinson, L. (1982). *Age-related differences in metalinguisitc awareness.* In S. Kuczaj (Ed.), *Language development: Vol. 2. Language, thought and culture.* Hillsdale, NJ: Eribaum.

Shultz, T., & Horibe, F. (1974). The development of the appreciation of verbal jokes. *Developmental Psychology, 10,* 13–20.

Scollon, R., & Scollon, S. (1981). *Narrative, literacy and face in interethnic communication.* Norwood, NJ: Ablex.

Slobin, D. (1978). Cognitive prerequisites for the development of grammar. In L. Bloom & M. Lahey (Eds.), *Readings in language development.* New York: Wiley.

Snow, C. (1990). The development of definitional skill. *Journal of Child Language, 17,* 697–710.

Spector, C. (1990). Linguistic humor comprehension of normal and language-impaired adolescents. *Journal of Speech and Hearing Disorders, 55,* 533–541.

Stanovich, K. (1980). Toward an interactive-compensatory model of individual differences in the development of reading fluency. *Reading Research Quarterly, 16,* 32–71.

Stein, N. (1979). How children understand stories. In L. Katz (Ed.), *Current topics in early childhood education,* Vol. 2. Norwood, NJ: Ablex.

Stein, N. (1982). What's in a story: Interpreting the interpretations of story grammars. *Discourse Processes,* 319–335.

Stein, N., & Glenn, C. (1979). An analysis of story comprehension in elementary school children. In R. Freedle (Ed.), *New directions in discourse processing.* Norwood, NJ: Ablex.

Stein, N., & Policastro, M. (1984). The concept of story: A comparison between children's and teachers' viewpoints. In H. Mandl, N. Stein, & T. Trabasso (Eds.), *Learning and comprehension of text.* Hillsdale, NJ: Erlbaum.

Strong, C. & Shaver, J. (1991). Stability and cohesion in the speech narratives of language-impaired and normally developing children. *Journal of Speech and Hearing Research, 34,* 95–111.

Sulzby, E. (1981). *Kindergartners begin to read their own compositions.* Final report to the Research Foundation of the National Council of Teachers of English. Urbana, IL: The Research Foundation of the National Council of Teachers of English.

Sutter, J., & Johnson, C. (1990). School-age children's metalinguistic awareness of grammaticality in verb form. *Journal of Speech and Hearing Disorders, 33,* 84–95.

Sutton-Smith, B. (1986). The development of fictional narrative performances. *Topics in Language Disorders, 7,* 1–10.

Swacher, M. (1975). The sex of the speaker as a sociolinguistic variable. In B. Thorne & N. Henley (Eds.), *Language and sex: Difference and dominance.* Rowley, MA: Newbury House.

Teale, W. H. (1988). Developmentally appropriate assessment of reading and writing in the early childhood classroom. *The Elementary School Journal, 89* (2), 173–183.

Thorne, B., Kramerae, C., & Henley, N. (Eds.) (1983). *Language, gender, and society.* Rowley, MA: Newbury House.

Torrey, J. (1979). Reading that comes naturally: The early reader. In T. Waller & G. MacKinnon (Eds.), *Reading research: Advances in theory and practice.* New York: Academic Press.

Vanevery, H., & Rosenberg, S. (1970). Semantics, phrase structure and age as variables in sentence recall. *Child Development, 41,* 853–859.

Van Kleeck, A. (1990). Emergent literacy: Learning about print before learning to read. *Topics in Language Disorders, 10,* 25–45.

Vellutino, F. (1979) Alternative conceptualization of dyslexia: Evidence in support of a verbal-deficit hypothesis. *Harvard Educational Review, 47,* 334–354.

Vellutino, F. (1974). *Dyslexia: Theory and research.* Cambridge, MA: MIT Press.

Warren-Leubecker, A. (1982). *Sex differences in speech to children.* Unpublished master's thesis, Georgia Institute of Technology, Atlanta.

Weaver, C. (1994). *Reading process and practice: From sociopsycholinguistics to whole language.* Portsmouth, NH: Heinemann.

Wehren, A., DeLisi, R., & Arnold, M. (1981). The development of noun definition. *Journal of Child Language, 8,* 165–175.

Wells, G. (1986). *The meaning makers: Children learning language and using language to learn.* Portsmouth, NH: Heinemann.

Whorf, B. (1956). *Language, thought, and reality.* New York: Wiley.

Wilde, S. (1992). *You kan red this! Spelling and punctuation for whole language classrooms, K–6.* Portsmouth, NH: Heinemann.

Willis, F., & Williams, S. (1976). Simultaneous talking in conversation and the sex of speakers. *Perceptual and Motor Skills, 43,* 1067–1070.

Wing, C., & Schoinick, E. (1981). Children's comprehension of pragmatic concepts expressed in "because," "although," "if " and "unless." *Journal of Child Language, 8,* 347–365.

Wolf, M., & Dickenson, D. (1989). From oral to written language: Transitions in the school years. In J. Berko-Gleason, (Ed.), *The development of language* (2nd ed.). Columbus, OH: Merrill/Macmillan.

SEVEN

The Building Blocks of Speech

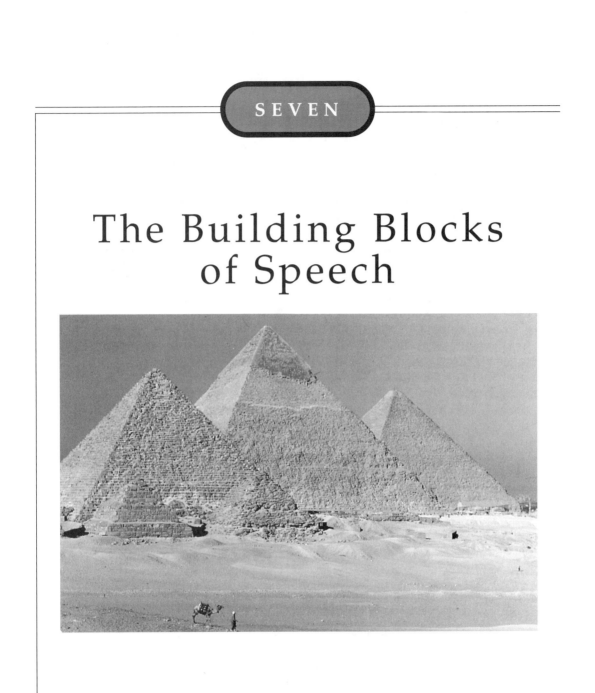

Chapter Objectives

The preceding chapters have focused primarily on language development, but we have made frequent references to speech, and we have made occasional references to speech sounds. We want to emphasize that for the normally hearing, normally developing child, the speech sound system does not exist apart from language, and we want to stress that the child is acquiring the sound system and learning its underlying rules at the same time that he is acquiring language. You must be reminded, however, as we noted in the opening chapter, that speech is not a synonym for language, and that speech can exist apart from language as it does when a mynah bird "talks," and language can surely exist apart from speech as it does when the deaf person communicates through sign language. Because speech is related to language, but in some ways separate from language, and because the speech sound system is mastered according to a different developmental schedule than language, we have chosen to devote a separate chapter to the speech component of the larger communication system. Specifically, this chapter is designed to facilitate understanding of the following topics:

- How speech sounds are described.
- The influence of co-articulation when sounds are sequenced into syllables, words, and phrases.
- An overview of phonological development.
- Theories of phonological development.

Whˢⁱᶻᵉen I was in high school, I lived in Egypt for two years. Although I had some extraordinary experiences during that time and saw many remnants of a remarkable ancient civilization, nothing impressed me as much as the great pyramids outside Cairo. From a distance, the surfaces of the pyramids appear relatively smooth, almost seamless. A closer view reveals structures of enormous size consisting of many huge blocks piled on top of one another in precise patterns. In the years since my visit to the pyramids, I have looked at modern buildings, especially brick buildings, with an eye not only to the total structure but to all the small pieces, the bricks, which together make the building complete.

We can think about human speech in much the same way. As senders and receivers of speech, we pay attention to the final product, the message, but even a simple sentence is actually a structure consisting of many small pieces. A sentence is a string of words, of course, but the words themselves are strings of speech sounds or **phonemes,** which are the building blocks, the bricks, of speech. And when someone speaks, there are no markers at the beginnings and endings of words. An utterance consists of a long, uninterrupted string of sounds. Only our knowledge of the language being spoken and our perceptual abilities allow us to know which segments of the string are words.

In a practical sense, there is little reason we should pay attention to the sounds of speech any more than we should pay attention to individual bricks in a building. Individual bricks become important only when they fall out or break, threatening the structural integrity of a wall. In much the same way, we usually pay attention to specific sounds of speech only when they are missing or misarticulated in ways that affect our ability to understand the words of which they are members.

One cannot fully appreciate human speech, however, unless one understands the sound system from which specific phonemes are drawn to make up spoken words. We call the study of speech sounds and the rules that determine how sounds can be sequenced into syllables and words, **phonology,** and that is the focus of this chapter. We take a look at how speech sounds are described and classified and how sounds interact with one another when they are joined to form syllables, words, and phrases, and we consider some of the major theories that attempt to explain how children acquire their sound systems as language is emerging.

Describing Speech Sounds

We begin by differentiating between sound differences that matter and sound differences that do not matter. A phoneme is often described as a distinctive speech sound. That is, a phoneme is a speech sound that is recognized as a specific sound and is distinctly different from all other speech sounds. Consider the words *seat* and *seed*. These two words, when spoken, are exactly the same except for one small, but important, difference. Each word consists of three sounds. The first sound in each word is *s*. The second sound in each word is the long vowel, *e*. Now notice the last sound in each word. Say each of these sounds aloud and feel what is happening in your speech mechanism during each production. Both the *t* and *d* are produced with the front portion of the tongue pressed against the alveolar ridge, and in both productions, the tongue is quickly released to complete the sound. The only difference between *t* and *d* and, in the example used, the only difference between *seat* and *seed* is that when the *d* is produced, the vocal folds vibrate and when the *t* is produced, the vocal folds do not vibrate. The difference between vocal fold vibration and no vibration, therefore, is a difference that makes a difference. It is a difference that can differentiate one phoneme from another.

Not all differences matter, however. In American English, for example, it does not matter if I produce the word *cat* with a release of air following the *t* or if I produce *cat* with no released air. The listener will hear both productions as *cat* and will perceive the final sound as *t*. The term **aspiration** describes a production in which there is a release of air following a sound like *t*. Although aspiration is a distinctive sound difference in some languages, it is a nondistinctive speech sound difference in English. That is, it is a difference that does not make a difference. A nondistinctive speech sound change is called an **allophone.** In the *cat* example, the aspirated *t* and the unaspirated *t* are allophones of the *t* phoneme. Think of the phoneme as a sound family. Allophones are members of the family. Each allophone is a little different from every other allophone, but allophones are so similar to one another in all important respects that they are recognized as members of the same family. After we examine the three approaches used to describe phonological productions, we will consider how allophones are created. All of this information is preliminary to a brief overview of phonological acquisition and a summary of major theoretical views about how the sound system of language emerges.

Traditional Phonetics

The most basic approach for describing consonant speech sounds is the threefold classification system used in traditional phonetics. Each consonant is identified according to place of articulation, manner of articulation, and voicing. **Place of articulation** identifies where in the oral cavity the essential articulatory contact or movement is being made. There are three major places of articulations: the *lips* for sounds such as "b," "p," "m," "w," "f," and "v"; the *teeth* and the *alveolar ridge* for sounds such as "th," "t,", "d," "s," "z," "n," and "l"; and the *hard* and *soft* regions of the *palate* for sounds such as "sh," "zh," "ch," "dg," "y," "r," "k," "g," and "ng." A fourth place of articulation, *glottal,* is included to accommodate the "h" which is the square peg of speech sounds searching for a round hole. *Glottal* refers to the *glottis,* which is the variable space between the vocal folds. When "h" is produced, the speaker simply forces a short burst of air through the glottis.

Manner of articulation describes how a consonant sound is produced. The term *plosive* or *stop* is used to describe a consonant produced by stopping the flow of air out of the mouth and then suddenly releasing it. It may be helpful to remember that a plosive sound is produced in a somewhat explosive manner. The plosive sounds in English are "p," "b," "t," "d," "k," and "g". A *fricative* sound is produced by forcing air through a narrow constriction, producing a friction-like sound. The following sounds are fricatives: "f," "v," "s," "z," "th," "sh," and "zh". The "h" is also considered a fricative in traditional phonetics even though one would be hard-pressed to identify where the constriction is. This is another dimension of the "h" as a square peg still in search of its round hole. An *affricate* is a unique sound that combines plosive and fricative qualities. There are two affricates in English, "ch" and "dg." The "ch" sound is actually a "t" and a "sh" pushed together into a single sound that retains qualities of both original sounds. In the same way, "dg" combines "d" and "zh." A *nasal* consonant is produced with nasal resonance. The only consonants in English that should be produced with nasal resonance are "m," "n," and "ng." All others should be produced with oral resonance only. A consonant is considered *lateral* if its production involves directing the flow of air out of the mouth along the sides of the tongue. There is only one lateral consonant in English, and it is easy to remember because it is the first and last sound in *lateral,* the "l" sound. *Glides* are also called *semivowels,* and both names are helpful in understanding how they are produced. They are called *glides* because their productions involve movement. They are called *semivowels* because they are somewhat vowel-like in the sense that they involve a relatively free and continuous flow of air through the oral cavity, unlike other consonants, which involve varying degrees of constriction or closure. Once again, the "h" is a classification problem. As is true of the glides, the "h" does not have the constriction or closure of other consonants, but neither does it have the continuous flow of air characteristic of glides. The "h" just cannot decide what it wants to be!

Voicing is simple. A consonant either involves vocal fold vibration or it does not. The majority of consonants are *voiced.* Those consonants that are *voiceless* are partners with voiced consonants. We call these voiced and voiceless partners *cognate pairs.* A cognate pair consists of two consonants produced in the same place and in the same manner but differing in voicing. For example, "p" and "b" are both produced with the two lips and both are produced in a plosive manner, but "p" is voiceless and "b" is voiced. They are a cognate pair. Cognate pairs account for 16 of the 24 consonants we use in English. The 8 consonants that are not members of cognate pairs are all voiced . . . except for that incorrigible "h," which is voiceless.

Classifying vowels in traditional phonetics is more difficult than classifying consonants, primarily because vowels are so variable in their production. Consider the vowel "e" as in the word *bee.* The "e" is classified as a high, front vowel. That is, the tongue is positioned at the front of the mouth in a relatively high position, but with very little effort, you will discover that you can produce the "e" with the tongue in almost any position. In fact, with a little dexterity, you can produce an "e" with your tongue protruding from your mouth. How and where vowels are produced depends on the sounds that precede and follow them, and vowels can adapt to virtually any phonetic environment. The traditional phonetics classification for vowels, therefore, is a general guide based on the production of these sounds in isolation.

A threefold classification is also used to classify vowels: height of tongue (i.e., high and low), location of primary resonance (i.e., front, central, and back), and tension of the tongue (i.e., tense or lax). **High vowels** have narrow resonating spaces. **Low vowels** have wider resonating spaces. Examples of high vowels include the "e" in *bee* and the "u" in *shoe.* Low vowels include "a" in *cat,* and "a" in *father.* The "e" in *bee* and the "a" in *cat* are **front vowels.** The "u" in *shoe* and the "a" in *father* are **back vowels.** The vowel "u" in *cut* is a **central vowel. Tense vowels** include the "e" in *bee* and the "u" in *shoe.* **Lax vowels** include the "i" in *bit* and the "u" in *cut.*

Throughout this discussion of the description of speech sounds using traditional phonetics, you may have noticed that the classification of speech sounds is based on certain basic contrasts. For example, in cognate pairs we contrast voiced and voiceless sounds. We contrast nasal sounds with all other consonants that are oral. Plosives are contrasted with fricatives on the basis of how they are produced, plosives by stopping the airstream completely before release and fricatives by forcing air through a narrow constriction. With the vowels, we contrast high and low, front and back, tense and lax. The idea of classifying speech sounds by contrast eventually led to a more elaborate system of describing speech sounds known as the *distinctive feature approach.*

Distinctive Features

Many of the distinctive features are replications of contrasts we have already identified in traditional phonetics: *voicing, nasality, lateral* for consonants, and *high, low, back,* and *tense* for vowels. The remaining features make smaller distinctions among speech sounds, especially the consonants, than are made in traditional phonetic analysis. The two most basic features, *consonantal* and *vocalic,* are designed to make the most basic contrast among speech sounds. A sound is *consonantal* if it is produced with constriction or closure somewhere in the oral cavity. A sound is *vocalic* if it is produced without constriction or closure, and if air flows relatively unimpeded through the oral cavity. These two features effectively contrast consonants and vowels, but they also help us to understand that some sounds, such as "l" and "r," have characteristics of both features, and other sounds, such as "w," "y," and "h," do not clearly possess the characteristics of either feature. The feature, *continuant,* makes an important differentiation among sounds that involve constriction or closure. That is, some of these sounds involve more constriction or closure than others. Sounds such as "p," "b," "t," and "ch", for example, involve a great deal of closure and are not marked for the continuant feature. Sounds such as "f," "th," "s," and "sh" are marked for this feature because, while they involve constriction, they involve less constriction than other consonants. The feature, *coronal,* referring to the front portion of the tongue, separates sounds that depend on the front part of the tongue from sounds that either use the middle or back portion of the tongue, or do not use the tongue at all. Sounds such as "s," "t," "l," and "n" are marked for the coronal feature. Sounds such as "m," "p," and "b" are not coronal because they do not involve the tongue at all, and sounds such as "k," "g," and "ng," are not coronal because they use the back portion of the tongue. The feature, *anterior,* makes a place of articulation distinction. Any sound produced on the alveolar ridge or forward is considered an anterior sound. Sounds such as "t," "d," "n," and "l" are considered anterior because they are produced with the tongue on the alveolar ridge. Sounds such as "p," "b," "m," and "f," are also marked for the anterior feature because they are produced in front of the alveolar ridge, but "ng," "k," and "g" are not marked for this feature because they are produced behind the alveolar ridge. The last of the consonant features, *strident,* separates some fricatives from others. A fricative is strident if the vibrating air produced by the primary constriction point hits a second constriction point, usually the upper lip or upper teeth, to produce even more turbulence. The sounds "s," "z," "sh," and "zh" are strident. The affricates, "ch" and "dg" are also strident because they include "sh" and "zh" qualities in their productions. The other fricatives, including "f," "v," and "th" are not strident because they are produced so far forward that there are no structures to create the additional turbulence characteristic of stridency.

As already noted, the distinctive features used to describe vowels are the same contrasts used to describe vowels in traditional phonetics with one possible exception, *rounding.* A vowel is considered round if it is produced with natural lip rounding. The round vowels include the "u" in *blue,* the "oo" in *look,* the "o" in *goat,* and the "aw" in *law.*

Phonological Processes

The distinctive features approach to phonology built upon and extended traditional phonetics by making finer distinctions among consonant phonemes than were possible with the threefold classification of place, manner, and voicing. The phonological processes approach, which dominates present theoretical and intervention discussions of phonology, represents a further extension. In addition to the concepts and terms already introduced by phonetics and distinctive features, the phonological approach gives attention to the effects of syllabic structure, to the sequencing of sounds, and to the effects sounds have on one another in the production of words and phrases. It should also be noted that while traditional phonetics and distinctive features are used to describe standard speech sounds so that we can better understand phonological errors, the phonological approach is designed specifically to describe productions that vary from standard targets.

The concept of phonological processes was introduced by Stampe in 1969 and became the subject of his doctoral dissertation completed in 1973. Phonological processes have been described in a variety of ways, but if we cut through most of the discussion and debate, we come down to this: *Phonological processes are rules children use to make productions that fit into their phonological understandings and abilities.* In most cases, these rules appear to *simplify* adult forms, although those who take a phonological processes approach are careful to point out that these rules *describe* rather than *explain* children's productions. It is tempting to conclude, for example, that faced with the task of producing an adult form consisting of four or five syllables, two or three sequences of consonants, and several sounds he cannot yet articulate accurately, the child makes decisions to reduce the word to one or two syllables, reduce the sequences to single sounds or eliminate them entirely, and omit or substitute for the sounds he cannot articulate. It is tempting to conclude, as Stampe first suggested, that the child uses a *mental operation* to transform the adult target into something he can produce, but the truth is we cannot know what cognitive manipulations, at what levels of consciousness, determine what the child produces. However processes are ultimately explained, it is clear that the child's phonological productions are not random or capricious. He does apply rules, called *processes,* in a fairly consistent and logical manner. For example, he might reduce all multisyllabic words by deleting the unstressed syllable or syllables. He might reduce all consonant sequences to single phonemes. He might always delete a single consonant in the final position if the consonant is a member of a cognate pair.

It is not within the scope of this book to include a detailed description of all common phonological processes, but the inclusion of a few examples may help the reader grasp what these rules contribute to our understanding of children's phonological productions. Actually, a few have already been mentioned. If a child reduces multisyllabic words by deleting unstressed syllables, the rule he is applying is called **syllable reduction** or **weak syllable deletion.** Reducing the number of segments in a sequence or cluster of consonants is called **consonant sequence reduction.** The child might use this process on the word *street* to make it *teet.* If he deletes the final consonants of words like *dog, cat,* and *house* to produce *do___ , ca___ ,* and *hou___ ,* he is using a process called **postvocalic singleton consonant deletion.** Some processes are considerably more complicated. For example, the child might produce *foon* for *spoon,* using a process called **coalescence.** He replaces two adjacent phonemes, "s" and "p" with a single phoneme, "f," that retains the fricative quality of "s" and the labial quality of "p." Rather than reducing the number of sounds in a word, the child might actually add sounds, using a process called **epenthesis.** The word *blue,* for example, might become *balue,* or *fork* might become *fwork.* The child might take voicing out of consonants at the ends of words, producing *dok* instead of *dog* or *bat* instead of *bad.* This process is known as **postvocalic devoicing.** If the child adds voicing to sounds at the beginning of words, it is called **prevocalic voicing.** Sometimes the child will include all the sounds in a word but will transpose a couple of the sounds. This process, called **metathesis,** is applied when the child says *aminal* for *animal* or *ephelant* for *elephant.*

The processes I have included here are only examples. Hodson and Paden (1991) describe nearly 40 processes, not including idiosyncratic rules, which are processes unique to individual children. We will probably never have a complete list of processes precisely because children are very inventive in their phonological strategies. Just when we think we have heard them all, we will find a child who uses a rule we have never heard before.

With all three phonological descriptions in mind, consider how each would be used to describe what a child does when he makes "errors" on speech sounds. Using the traditional phonetics point of view, if the child says *bu___* for *bus,* we simply say that he has an "s" problem. A distinctive features specialist might speculate that the "s" is deleted because the child has not yet mastered the strident feature. The phonological processes specialist, taking into account other productions in which final consonants are deleted, might conclude that the problem has nothing to do with "s" specifically, or even with the strident feature. The child says *bu___* for *bus* because he applies the process, postvocalic singleton consonant deletion, to all words that end with consonants.

Each of these approaches to describing phonological productions leads to a somewhat different interpretation about how phonology develops. The traditional phonetic view suggests that phonemes develop as whole entities. The distinctive features view suggests that the child masters features. When he has all the features for which the "s" sound is marked, for example, he will produce "s." The phonological processes view suggests that the child masters the adult phonological system by gradually suppressing his rules or processes in favor of adult rules. The two-year-old, for example, applies the rule, postvocalic singleton consonant deletion, to all words ending in consonants, but by the time he is four or five years old, he has suppressed that rule in favor of the adult rule that says that some words do, in fact, end in consonants.

Before we consider specific theories of phonological development, we need to further set the stage by addressing two additional topics. The first, *co-articulation*, is concerned with how speech sounds interact with one another in connected speech. The second, *landmarks of phonological development*, is a description of the real time acquisition of the speech sound system, independent of the debate about why what happens when it happens. The *why-what-when* questions are the prickly issues incorporated into theories of phonological development.

Co-articulation: The Mix of Sounds in the Making of Speech

If you had never experienced speech, you might assume that a child learns individual speech sounds before he combines them, in much the same way as children learn the alphabet as the foundation for learning to spell, read, and write. If you listen to children who are just beginning to acquire speech, however, you will not hear them practicing sounds in isolation. Even their earliest utterances involve combinations of sounds. These combinations, even in simple syllables or words, involve complicated interactive adjustments of the speech mechanism.

In the opening of this chapter, speech sounds were compared to bricks in a wall. As is true of most analogies, the brick comparison has limitations. It is true that any given word consists of a finite number of sounds just as a wall, no matter how large, consists of a finite number of bricks. In the case of a brick wall, however, each brick retains its individual identity. It looks and feels the same whether it is in the wall or separate from the wall. When speech sounds are joined into words, they lose some of their individual characteristics. They blend together and influence one another so that the final product is something other than the sum of the sounds. We call the influence sounds have on one another in context, **co-articulation.**

Many years ago, Hockett (1955) wrote an interesting description of co-articulation that is helpful in understanding the process, but like the brick analogy, it has limitations. He explained it this way:

Imagine a row of Easter eggs carried along a moving belt; the eggs are of various sizes, and variously colored, but not boiled. At a certain point, the belt carries the row of eggs between the two rollers of a wringer, which quite effectively smash them and rub them more or less into each other. The flow of eggs before the wringer represents the series of impulses from the phoneme source. The mess that emerges from the wringer represents the output of the speech transmitter. (p. 210)

Hockett's analogy, captures the idea that sounds are merged together in a manner that blurs their separate identities, but it also gives the impression that this process is random and not governed by rules. Although there is still much we do not understand about co-articulation, we do know that it is an orderly and lawful process, and therefore, predictable.

We know, for example, that co-articulation works in a forward and a backward manner. That is, an early appearing sound sometimes affects how a following sound will be produced, and sometimes a later appearing sound will affect how an earlier sound is produced. When an early sound affects a later sound, it is called **retentive co-articulation.** In producing the word *new*, I cannot avoid producing the "ew" with nasality because of the influence of "u." That is, nasality is retained on the "ew." If I put the nasal sound after a vowel, the same influence will occur in the other direction. When I produce the word *aim*, the vowel is nasalized because I am anticipating the nasal sound, "m." This is called **anticipatory co-articulation.**

Feel what happens to your lips on the production of the two "s's" as you say the word *seesaw*. Now say the sound "s" in isolation a few times. Repeat *seesaw* a few more times and sense the lip adjustment again. What is happening here? The sounds influencing the "s" productions are the vowels "ee" and "aw." The "ee" is a front vowel produced with the lips slightly spread, so the "s" in the first syllable is produced with the lips in a slightly spread position. The "aw" is a back vowel produced with lip rounding, so the "s" in the second syllable is produced with the lips rounded. These are examples of anticipatory co-articulation. What is truly amazing is that you have no idea you are making these adjustments, and if I asked you how you knew to make them, you could not provide an answer.

Consider what happens when you put two or more consonants together in a cluster or blend as in the words *cluster* and *blend.* In both words, you actually begin to produce the "l" before you release the first sound. Try to produce the beginning of each word in slow motion. In *cluster*, you are using the back of the tongue for "k" at the same time you are moving the front of the tongue to the alveolar ridge for "l." In saying *blend*, you contact the alveolar ridge for the "l" before you release the bilabial closure for "b."

We may not be able to explain *how* we co-articulate, but we should be able to understand *why.* Co-articulation allows us to speak in the most efficient manner possible within the limits of our speech mechanisms. I retain nasality as I move from the "n" to the "ew" in *new*, for example, because I cannot close the velopharyngeal mechanism quickly enough to eliminate nasal resonance on the vowel. I produce the "ai" in *aim* with nasal resonance because I cannot wait for the "m" to begin before I open the velopharyngeal port. Just as a drawbridge begins to open long before a ship arrives because it takes time to accomplish the opening, so the velopharyngeal port begins to open before the nasal sound arrives because it is a slow adjustment.

Articulation follows the path of least resistance, which means that the speaker is constantly adjusting according to the challenges presented by the sounds combined in a word or phrase. The adjustments sometimes result in compromises. In saying the word *little*, for example, the "t" is usually produced as a "d" because every other sound in the word is voiced, and it's too much trouble to turn off the larynx for one sound, and the "d" is produced with lateral emission rather than frontal emission because it is surrounded by "l's," which are laterals. When I say *windmill,* I leave out the "d" entirely because the adjustment from nasal alveolar "n" to non-nasal alveolar "d" to another nasal, "m," is just too difficult. I compromise in this case by just saying "winmill," a much easier production than "windmill." Because we all co-articulate according to the same rules, these adjustments and compromises have no effect on the ability of people to understand one another. In fact, if we concisely articulated every sound in every word, we would sound a little strange. Speech that sounds too perfect is not normal!

The Landmarks of Phonological Development

Since we have been down the developmental road with cognition and language already, a few simple reminders about ages and stages should suffice here. Children do not progress through the stages of phonological development on a predetermined schedule. In fact, there is considerable age variation at each stage, but the order of development will be the same for all children. No one knows exactly how many stages there are in phonological development any more than we can say with certainty how many stages there are in cognitive development or in language development. We describe development in stages as an academic convenience, recognizing that there will be overlapping of behaviors at every juncture. With these reminders in mind, which is where reminders belong, we will consider the development of phonology in four general stages.

Phonology Before Language: Laying the Foundation for a Speech Sound System

Even the most uninformed person knows that human babies are not mute at birth. In fact, the visual and auditory impression most of us have about the newborn is that he or she enters the world screaming. This is not always true, of course, but if the neonate does not cry with his first breath, he does not wait long before he tests his noise-making equipment.

During his first year, the infant produces a wide range of vocalizations. The first of these vocalizations are reflexive, or unlearned. They include cries, coughs, gurgles, and hiccups. It is generally understood that the child's first cries and certainly the other reflexive noises he produces are automatic responses reflecting the child's general physical condition. When he is hungry, uncomfortable, or in pain, he will cry. If something is threatening to invade his larynx, he will cough. If he swallows too much air with mother's milk, he will burp. If he is perfectly content with the state of his world, he will be silent.

By the time the infant is two or three months old, we begin to hear vocalizations we call *cooing*. These are vowel-like productions the child produces when he is contented. Some children quickly add consonant-like sounds to their vocalizations to produce a behavior commonly called *babbling*. At this point, the child might produce vowel-like productions at times and productions that sound like consonant–vowel syllables at others. The "vowels" resemble adult back vowels as in *shoe* or *look*, and the "consonants" resemble adult back consonants such as "k" or "g." It must be emphasized, however, that these are not true speech sounds because they are not purposive and they are not used, either alone or in combination, to convey specific meanings.

By the time child approaches his fifth or sixth month, he is engaging in what is commonly referred to as *vocal play*. He has not abandoned vowel-like productions, and he continues to produce what appear to be consonant–vowel syllables, but he has added a number of other vocalizations that certainly impress adult listeners as playful. These include squeals, grunts, screams, growls, and the always popular "raspberries." Some children seem to fixate on one particular kind of noise for a few days before moving on to another noise and then sometimes returning to an old favorite for a time.

The child's earliest syllable-like forms are not produced with adult-like prosody. They are produced at a slower rate, and whatever intonational patterns are superimposed are irregular in nature. By the time the child is about eight or nine months old, the prosody superimposed on these syllable-like forms sounds more adult-like. That is, the overall rate has increased, and adults believe they hear stresses and meaningful intonational patterns. The fact that the child is superimposing all of this on reduplicated consonant–vowel forms resulting in productions such as "mamama" or "dadada" leads many adults to erroneously conclude that the child is producing meaningful words at this stage. Although it is not impossible for a child to produce meaningful words at nine months, it is highly unlikely. The test for *meaningful* is that productions be purposive, consistent, and used to convey specific meanings. At this stage in phonological and language development, productions, while not random, tend to be more playful than communicatively purposive, and they are not aimed at particular semantic targets. The sounds the child is producing do not have the consistency of adult phonemes, but they most closely resemble the plosive, nasal, and glide consonants, and lax vowels of adult phonology. As the child enters the last quarter of his first year, he tends to produce the velar sounds ("k" and "g") less frequently and alveolar sounds ("t," "d," "n") more frequently. Although we hear more labial sounds such as "p," "b," "m," and "w" at this point, the alveolar sounds are still more common.

During the last two months of the first year, the child produces *variegated babbling*. Most productions are still consonant–vowel forms, but as the term suggests, we hear fewer reduplicated forms, and we hear a wider variety of consonants and vowels in more complicated productions such as "gubadee," or for those with musical connections to the 1960s, "doowadidee!" Even though the child is expanding his consonant-like inventory, the sounds we most often hear continue to most closely resemble the plosives, nasals, and glides of adult phonology. The child will occasionally produce sounds that resemble fricatives, affricates, and even liquids, but he does not venture down these phoneme avenues very often.

Although there is considerable disagreement about how phonology develops in a general sense, as we will see when we sample common theories of phonological development, experts generally agree that what happens during the first year of phonological development is largely the result of physical maturation in combination with the human instinct to talk. The best evidence of this is that children from widely varying language and cultural backgrounds sound remarkably similar during this first stage of phonological development.

Before we leave this first stage of phonological development, we should briefly address a central controversy regarding the relationship between *babbling* and *true speech*. The controversy was sparked by two very different interpretations of this relationship. The first view, *babbling drift*, is probably most closely associated with Mowrer (1952). According to this view, the vocalizations the child produces that most closely resemble the speech productions of his caregivers are selectively reinforced by his caregivers so that the child's emerging phonological system is gradually shaped to fit the phonological system of his caregivers' language. That is, the child's babblings *drift* into adult speech. Opposing this view is the *discontinuity theory* most closely associated with Jakobson (1968). According to Jakobson, babbling and true speech are two entirely separate stages of development. Whatever relationship they might have to one another is almost coincidental. During babbling, the child produces a wide variety of sounds common to many of the world's languages. When the child begins to produce meaningful speech, he stops babbling. He might even experience a period of silence before he begins to acquire the true sounds of his native language. The acquisition of true speech sounds, according to this view, is a slow and deliberate process.

There are problems with both of these views. If the babbling drift theory were correct, we would expect that children from varying language backgrounds would sound different from one another by the end of the first year because their babblings would be differentially reinforced. That is, a Japanese child's Japanese-like sounds would be reinforced. A Russian child's Russian-like sounds would be reinforced. An American child's English-like sounds would be reinforced, and because of the phonological differences among these languages, these three children would sound different. But they do not. If the discontinuity theory were true, we would expect that there would be dramatic differences between the sounds we hear in babbling and the sounds we hear in early speech productions, and we would expect that babbling would have a definite ending and true speech a clearly defined beginning. Neither of these expectations is supported by research. Most children continue to babble for several months after they produce their first true words, and the sounds we hear in true words are remarkably similar to the sounds we hear in babbling.

If neither view is correct, what do we conclude? We conclude that even if we do not fully understand the purposes served by babbling relative to the emergence of speech, the facts of development speak for themselves. That is, the child does not stop babbling one day and begin to produce true words the next. For several months covering the end of the first year and the beginning of the second, babbling and true speech co-occur. To make matters even more interesting, as noted in an earlier chapter of this book, the child will produce what are called *proto-words* or *vocables* during the transition period between babbling and true speech. A proto-word is a word in the sense that it is used consistently with clear communicative intent. It does have phonemic and semantic consistency, but it is not an adult word, and it may not even be an attempt at an adult word. The child might call his high chair a *baki*, for example. If he uses this production consistently in reference to the same object, it is a proto-word, and it is just as meaningful as *high chair*. The transition then from babbling to true speech is just that, a transition. It is not the end of Act I and the beginning of Act II. Perhaps the most important conclusion we can reach about babbling itself is that, based on the evidence we have gathered and examined so far, phonological development begins during babbling, before the child begins to produce his first true words (Lowe, 1994, p. 37).

Phonology in the Child's First Meaningful Words

While the child continues to babble and while he is producing proto-words, he is also trying to produce words based on the models provided by his caregivers. His first attempts are far from perfect, of course, but given his limited neurophysiological abilities and his limited language competence at the beginning of his second year of life, he does pretty well. His first words are typically single-syllable productions or reduplicated forms. He might say, "hi," "bye," "mama," or "wawa." Consonant–vowel–consonant forms, such as "hot," do occur, but infrequently.

The most common manners reflected in the phonology of first words are plosive, nasal, and glide. Not surprisingly, these are the same manners we observed during the latter half of the first year, the manners we hear most often in babbling. The most common places of articulation reflected in the early phonology of meaningful speech are labial and alveolar, although the child will also produce some palatals and velars. Again, these are the same places of articulation we observe in babbled sounds.

When we examined first words from a language point of view, we suggested that the child often chooses his first words based on the personal importance of their referents, as well as their semantic properties and grammatical functions. To this list of selective factors we can also add phonological characteristics. That is, if the language and personal factors are equal, the child will select words that contain phonological segments that are included in his speech sound system, and he will avoid words that contain phonological information he does not yet possess. This means that given a choice between the targets, *dog,* and *miniature Schnauzer,* the young child will attempt to say *dog* because its phonological makeup is more consistent with his developing sound system than the phonological makeup of *miniature Schnauzer.*

Once the child acquires his first few words, vocabulary development occurs quickly. By the time he is 18 months old, the typical child will have about 50 words in his productive vocabulary, but do not forget the caution about age. It would not be unusual for a child to be using 50 words as early as 13 or 14 months, and it would not be at all unusual for a child to be producing his first 50 words as late as his second birthday.

Putting the Phonological Pieces Together

Most of phonological development occurs in the period between 18 months and 4 years, during which there are significant advances in language development. The inventory of consonant sounds that has been limited primarily to plosives, nasals, and glides now expands to accommodate all phoneme classes, although this does not mean that all phonemes are correctly produced all the time. Syllable structures become more complex as the child sequences consonants both within syllables and across syllables, and he produces more true multisyllabic words, not just reduplicated forms.

To this point, the child has demonstrated little understanding of phonemes as individual sound segments, and he has not shown much evidence that he uses the same phonological rules used by adults. Early in development, he seems to contrast words, not phonemes. The rules he uses are processes, rules that often simplify adult forms, based on his current knowledge and his present abilities. As the child's phonological knowledge expands, and as his articulatory abilities improve, he uses a phonological system that increasingly resembles the adult system. He contrasts phonemes, not just whole words, and he knows how to generalize phonological rules from one phonetic context to another related phonetic context.

By the time the child is four years old, he has either suppressed, or is well on the way to suppressing, the phonological processes he has been using. He is producing the majority of consonants correctly, and is using the remainder correctly at least on occasion, and he is demonstrating an understanding of all phonemic contrasts. Phonological development is not complete by the time the child is four years old, but most of the acquisition is complete, and he is ready to begin tying up the loose ends of his speech sound system.

The Finishing Touches: Completing Phonological Development

Between the ages of four and eight years, the child finishes phonological development. Those phonemes he has been producing correctly but inconsistently now become increasingly correct. If there are any sounds he has not been producing at all, perhaps the liquids, they now begin to emerge, and by the end of this final stage, these sounds are mastered. When the child learns to read and write, his metalinguistic awareness increases. As he associates sounds with the letters of the alphabet, his understanding of speech sounds as individual segments solidifies. Because of the inconsistencies in our language between written symbols and the speech sounds they represent, the child may always struggle with some pronunciations and some spellings, but by the time he reaches the end of his elementary school years, he will grasp the obvious written and spoken connections well enough that he will be able to encounter new words in either oral or printed form and make a pretty good guess about how printed words should be pronounced or how spoken words should be spelled.

Theories of Phonological Development

Since the speech sound systems of languages can be described in different ways, it is not surprising that there are varying theories about how phonological systems develop in children. In this section, we will look at a sample of the views that experts have expressed over the last fifty years.

The Phoneme-by-Phoneme View of Development

The first systematic studies of phonemic acquisition were conducted by Wellman, Case, Mengert, and Bradbury (1931), Poole (1934), and Templin (1957). These studies were designed to establish norms for phonemic acquisition by assessing the phonemic abilities of large numbers of children within a broad age range. Although the specific methodologies of these studies varied, there was a fairly consistent general design. That is, attempts were made to include a reasonable distribution of subjects by socioeconomic level, although Templin weighted her sample toward the lower end of the socioeconomic continuum and included only children from urban areas. In each study, children with hearing problems and language delay were excluded. Responses were typically elicited by asking the subjects to name pictures or objects. In the Wellman and Templin studies, if a subject did not produce a word spontaneously, a model was presented and an imitated response was accepted. Poole accepted only spontaneous productions. In all three studies, sounds were elicited in the word-initial, word-medial, and word-final positions, depending upon the positions in which a particular sound is produced. For example, "ng" was elicited in only the word-medial and word-final positions because it does not occur in the word-initial position in English. Each of these large, cross-sectional studies established a criterion for age of mastery. In the Wellman and Templin studies, a

Phonemes	Age of Mastery		
	Wellman et. al. (1931) 75% criterion for mastery	**Poole (1934)** 100% criterion for mastery	**Templin (1957)** 75% criterion for mastery
p	4	3.5	3
b	3	3.5	4
t	5	4.5	6
d	5	4.5	4
k	4	4.5	4
g	4	4.5	4
f	3	5.5	3
v	5	6.5	6
voiceless th	–	7.5	6
voiced th	–	6.5	7
s	5	7.5	4.5
z	5	7.5	7
sh	–	6.5	4.5
zh	–	6.5	7
h	3	3.5	3
voiceless w	–	7.5	–
ch	5	–	4.5
dg	6	–	7
m	3	3.5	3
n	3	4.5	3
ng	–	4.5	3
w	3	3.5	3
y	4	4.5	3.5
l	4	6.5	6
r	5	7.5	4

FIGURE 7-1 Summary of Phonemic Development Studies

sound was considered mastered if it was correctly produced in all appropriate word positions by 75 percent of the subjects at a given age level. In Poole's study, a sound was considered mastered if it was correctly produced in all appropriate word positions by 100 percent of the subjects at a given age level. In spite of methodological differences and different mastery criteria, the results of these studies were remarkably consistent, as indicated in Figure 7-1. The (–) indicates that this sound either was not tested or was not mastered by the requisite number of subjects.

Templin (1957) compared her results with the findings of the two preceding studies. She noted that among the seventeen sounds included in all three studies, there was a spread in age of mastery of one year or less on eleven sounds, and a spread of two or more years on only six sounds. Considering the differences in subject populations, the element of chance that always enters this kind of research, and the differences in experimental designs, this is significant agreement.

There were few surprises in these data. The sounds we would expect to emerge early because they appear in children's initial words are apparently mastered early. Among children's first words are productions such as "mama," "papa," "wawa," and "no," and the consonants in these productions are mastered, according to Templin's data, by three years. Sounds we would consider difficult are late to emerge, including "r," "l," "s," "z," voiced and voiceless "th," "sh," "zh," "ch," "dg." It is also interesting that the greatest differences in age of acquisition among the three studies occur on many of these sounds. Additional examination of the findings reveals that plosives are acquired fairly early and continuing sounds are acquired later and that the voiced sounds in cognate pairs tend to be mastered later than their voiceless partners.

Even though these data seem to provide general normative guidelines concerning the mastery of phonemes, they should be viewed with caution. Sander (1972), after reviewing and reanalyzing the data from the Wellman et al. (1931) and Templin (1957) studies, suggests that the ages of mastery derived from these findings should be not understood as representing average ages of mastery. Sander argued that because of the stringent criterion levels used in these early cross-sectional studies, the ages of mastery represent the upper limits for phonemic acquisition. According to Sander (1972), we should distinguish between the age of customary production and mastery. **Customary production** is correct production of a phoneme in two of three word positions by 50 percent of the subjects at a given age level. **Mastery** is correct production of a phoneme in all appropriate word positions by 90 percent of the subjects at a specified age level. This distinction results in very different interpretations of phonetic acquisition by age levels. Using Sander's reanalyzed data, for example, "g" is produced correctly in at least two word positions by 50 percent of two-year-old children, but it is not produced correctly in all three positions by 90 percent of children until the age of four years. The phoneme "b" is customarily produced by children younger than two years but is not mastered until four years. The distinction between customary production and mastery is useful because it acknowledges that there are individual variations among children while still allowing a sense of what we can expect in phonemic acquisition by age levels.

Consider what we can conclude about phonemic acquisition based on the findings of large, cross-sectional studies, and specifically the studies mentioned here. We can conclude that there is a tendency for some sounds to emerge before others, but we must be careful not to assume that there is a specific order of mastery. As we have already noted, there are wide individual differences among children, which are reflected, to some extent, even in the data provided by these researchers. For example, most of Templin's subjects were producing "r" by four years, but some of Poole's subjects did not produce "r" correctly until 7.5 years. All of Poole's subjects were producing "t" correctly by 4.5 years, while most of Templin's subjects were six before they mastered the "t." This latter difference is an excellent example, however, of how even a small methodological variation can affect results. As Sander (1972) noted, Templin (1957) found a late age of mastery for "t" because her younger subjects did not produce a voiceless "t" in the word-medial position. She did not take into account the fact that in American English, when "t" occurs in the word-medial position and follows a stressed vowel, it is typically produced with voicing. This means that any speaker is likely to say a word such as "*dating*" as though it were "*dading*." An unrealistic expectation, therefore, undoubtedly resulted in a spuriously high age of mastery. It is also prudent to note that longitudinal, or diary, data on phonemic acquisition in individual children and the results of studies of small groups of children attest that the individual variability in phonemic acquisition is so great that establishing reliable norms is difficult at best. We should use ages of customary production and mastery, therefore, only as general guidelines for understanding phonemic acquisition and for making determinations about how an individual child is progressing in his own phonemic development.

Finally, we must consider the perspective maintained by those who conducted the early cross-sectional studies of phonemic development. They took the view that children acquire phonemes as whole units. Acquisition, therefore, is an all or nothing proposition. This means that if a child is producing voiceless "th" for "s," he is given no credit for what he obviously knows about the target sound. He knows that "s" is a fricative, that it is voiceless, and that it is produced in the anterior portion of the mouth. His production is just slightly off target in terms of place of production. Instead of having the tongue tip against the alveolar ridge, he has moved it forward between the teeth. There is the assumption in the phoneme-by-phoneme view of acquisition that unless the target sound is produced in a completely correct manner, the phoneme does not exist in the child's sound system. Considering that the voiceless "th" for "s" substitution reflects more knowledge of the target sound than ignorance, this seems a harsh assumption. As you will see, more recent theories give the child credit for understanding the pieces of the phonemic jigsaw puzzle, not just the complete puzzle.

The Behaviorist Theory

One of the most popular theories of phonological acquisition during the 1950s and 1960s was the Behaviorist Theory. It was originally formulated by Mowrer (1952) but was later adapted by other influential phonologists (Olmsted, 1966; Winitz, 1969). This theory emphasizes selective reinforcement and the role of the child's caregiver in the acquisition process.

Mowrer suggests that there are fairly discrete steps through which the child's vocalizations are gradually shaped as they become more and more similar to the speech patterns of his adult models. In the beginning, the child identifies with the primary caregiver, usually the mother, and attends to her speech patterns during pleasurable activities like feeding, bathing, and fondling. As the child associates the mother's speech patterns with the pleasures of these nurturing activities, the mother's speech patterns themselves become secondary reinforcers. Because the infant's speech-like productions resemble the mother's speech patterns in certain basic respects, they also develop secondary reinforcing traits. The mother, other adults, and the child himself will selectively reinforce those utterances produced by the child that are the most adultlike until the child's phonological system includes just those sounds that are germane to his language.

Even though this theory is appealing because it emphasizes the role of the mother, and most of us would like to believe that mothers, or other caregivers, play a major role in all aspects of child development, it is not a widely accepted theory today. Critics point out that we do not have evidence supporting the dominant role of reinforcement in the acquisition process, and we do not have evidence that mothers, or other caregivers, selectively reinforce the adultlike productions in their children's speech. Most importantly, the Behaviorist Theory suggests that children learn phonology in much the same way animals are conditioned to learn tricks, a view not consistent with the present belief that children are not passive and manipulated creatures but are very active in phonological acquisition. That is, they explore, discover, create, apply, retain, and throw away until all the pieces are finally in place.

Structuralist Theory

This theory was formulated by Jakobson in 1941 and was translated into English in 1968. While this theory and the Behaviorist Theory both focus on the relationship between babbling and the emergence of meaningful speech, they are contrasts in at least one important respect. The Behaviorist Theory suggests that babbling is continuous with meaningful speech in the sense that babbling drifts into meaningful speech. The Structuralist Theory is based on the discontinuity view that suggests that babbling and meaningful speech are two clearly separate periods of speech production. During babbling, the child's productions are random, transitory, and extremely diverse, reflecting sounds heard in many of the world's languages. Furthermore, the sounds in babbling do not emerge in any particular or meaningful order. When meaningful speech begins, the child loses his ability to produce an unlimited variety of sounds. His sound inventory is dramatically reduced, and true speech sounds emerge slowly, in a predictable order, until the phonological system of the child's native language is complete.

Phonological development in meaningful speech follows a predictable, universal, and innately determined order, based in large part, on fundamental contrasts among speech sounds. In the beginning, the child's productions reflect mastery of major contrasts, such as vowel versus consonant and oral versus nasal. As development proceeds, the child makes narrower contrasts, filling the gaps between the larger contrasts. When he has mastered all the contrasts inherent in the phonological system of his language, he will produce all the sounds included in that system.

Longitudinal studies of phonological acquisition and the large-scale studies completed by Wellman et al. (1931), Poole (1934), Templin (1957), and Sander (1972) suggest an order of acquisition of phonemes that is consistent with Jakobson's assertions about an order of contrasts. For example, these studies confirm, as suggested by Jakobson's claims, that children acquire plosives and nasals before they acquire fricatives, affricates, and liquids, and that front consonants emerge before back consonants. Critics point out, however, that we have no evidence supporting Jakobson's assertion that this order is universal. More importantly and contrary to the basic premise of the Structuralist Theory, we know that the emergence of sounds in babbling is not irregular or random. We know that babbling and true speech are not two distinct and unrelated periods of vocalization, that children babble for several months after they begin to produce meaningful words.

Natural Phonology Theory

According to the Natural Phonology Theory (Stampe, 1969, 1973; Donegan & Stampe, 1979), the child does not actually *acquire* a phonological system. Rather, he suppresses processes that do not occur in the phonological system of his language. Stampe, like Jakobson, asserts that phonological development is universal. Jakobson saw universality in the contrasts the child must master in order to acquire his sound system. Stampe argues that all children are born with the same set of phonological processes, rules by which "phonological oppositions" are modified to reflect the natural "restrictions of the human speech capacity." The child's challenge, as he puts his phonological system together, is to discover the processes that must be suppressed in his language. The English-speaking child, for example, must suppress **consonant sequence reduction, postvocalic consonant devoicing,** and **liquid gliding** because in English phonology, consonant sequences must be complete, postvocalic consonants are sometimes voiced, and there is a phonemic difference between a liquid and a glide.

Some of the criticisms leveled at the Natural Phonology Theory focus on Stampe's most basic theoretical tenet that phonological processes are "mental operations." Since we cannot identify the cognitive functions associated with the use of phonological processes or with their suppression, it is difficult to determine how one can prove or disprove Stampe's assertion. A more common criticism of this theory concerns Stampe's assumption that children perceive words and their segmental components the same way adults do, and that whatever differences there are between the speech forms of children and the speech forms of adults reflect production constraints, not perceptual limitations, on the part of children. Data to support this assumption about the perceptual abilities of children during the phonological acquisition period are not available, and yet the assumption is key to the theory's viability.

Prosodic Theory

In at least one important respect, the Prosodic Theory (Waterson, 1971, 1981) stands in stark contrast to the Natural Phonology Theory. While Stampe assumes that children's perceptual abilities are complete and accurate at the beginning of true speech production, Waterson believes that the child's perceptual abilities, like his production abilities, are incomplete and emerging when language development is beginning. Furthermore, she believes that words, rather than speech sounds, should be viewed as the most basic phonological structures. Accordingly, she describes words in terms of their suprasegmental features as well as their segmental features. According to this view, the child attends to and perceives the salient characteristics of words. These salient characteristics might include segmental features such as nasality, voicing, and manner class, but they also include prosodic or suprasegmental features such as intonational patterns and stress. In the early stages of phonological development, the child struggles to match adult models in terms of segmental and surprasegmental features. The child's phonological system matures as a consequence of mastering information in both parts of the system, that part concerned with phonemes and that part concerned with the prosodic characteristics superimposed on sounds sequenced into syllables, words, and phrases. Because the Prosodic Theory takes a wider view of phonological development than other theories, it provides a reasonable explanation for the great variability of phonological productions by context. That is, if a child's productions are influenced not only by his attention to phonemic characteristics, but also by his attention to elements of prosody, we would expect wide variations in production because the combination of segmental and suprasegmental features will vary widely from one linguistic context to another. Unfortunately, this theory deals only with the earliest stages of phonological development, and while it accounts for intrapersonal variability, it does not account for the common patterns of phonological development we observe in children as a group.

Cognitive Theory

As is true of the Prosodic Theory, the Cognitive Theory, or the similar Interactionist-Discovery or Problem-Solving Theory, focuses on the early stages of word acquisition (Ferguson, 1978, 1986; Macken & Ferguson, 1983; Menn, 1976, 1983). Both the Prosodic Theory and the Cognitive Theory suggest that during the early stages of production, the child addresses words rather than the sound segments of words, and both theories emphasize individual variations in phonological development. The Cognitive Theory is, in part at least, a reaction to the assertion in other theories that phonological development occurs in a universal, highly predictable, linear manner, and to the failure of other theories to account for individual variability in phonological development.

The Cognitive Theory suggests that while all children face the same challenges in mastering the phonological system of their language, and while they all devise strategies for meeting these challenges, they do not all develop the same strategies. While proponents of this theory concede that there are some universal or nearly universal patterns in phonological development, they believe these tendencies are the products of the uniform development of children's auditory and speech systems. The primary focus of the Cognitive Theory is on what happens as each child confronts the challenges he perceives in the words he hears. Each child notices phonological patterns in his developing vocabulary. These patterns may reflect understandings of what adults know as distinctive features or syllabic shapes. The child then formulates phonological rules he applies to new words that contain the sound features he knows or the syllabic shapes with which he is familiar. Different children will recognize different patterns and develop different rules, but they will choose words to add to their vocabularies that are characterized by the patterns they recognize, and they tend to reject words characterized by patterns they do not recognize. As development proceeds, the child continues to develop new hypotheses about how the phonological system works. If these hypotheses seem viable within his communicative experiences, he retains them. If a given hypothesis is not viable, he will revise it and test it again. This process presumably continues until the child's hypotheses are consistent with those that underlie the rules of the adult phonological system. Along the way, he will generalize when generalizations are not appropriate according to adult usage, he will reduce long words by deleting syllables, and he may even appear to regress because he will replace words he acquired as whole units with words designed according to his rules. He might, for example, produce a word such as "blue" with both sounds of the prevocalic cluster intact, only to reduce the word to "bue" a few months later. While this might seem to be a clear regression, it may be that the child is applying a newly formulated phonological rule regarding prevocalic clusters, which is that two-segment clusters should be reduced to one segment, and if one of the two segments is a liquid, that is the segment that will be deleted.

While the Cognitive Theory appeals to those who believe the child is an active agent in phonological development, it may go too far in its emphasis on individual exploration and hypothesis building and testing. Critics suggest that this theory does not adequately account for limits on learning imposed by the physical and psychological maturation of the child. It does not address later phonological development, and it gives too little attention to the universal patterns of phonological acquisition noted in large-scale studies.

Biological Theory

As the name implies, the Biological Theory (Locke, 1980, 1983, 1990; Locke & Pearson, 1992) suggests that phonological development, especially its early stages, can be explained on the basis of biological forces. All children, regardless of the language environments in which they are reared, are born with the same basic perceptual abilities and tendencies. All children are innately predisposed to produce the same articulatory motor acts. Vocalizations during babbling, for example, are the products of these innate abilities and tendencies, and for this reason, the babblings of children from widely varying language environments sound the same. Because the sounds heard in late babbling and the phonological patterns in early words are remarkably similar, Locke argues that the phonological patterns observed in early words are also universal. When the child begins to produce true words, the influence of his language on his phonological system begins, but this influence is minimal until the child's vocabulary begins to expand dramatically at about eighteen months. At this point, in what Locke sees as the third of three major stages of phonological development, the biological forces that have been primarily responsible for development begin to interact with cognitive factors, eventually driving the child to complete the phonological system of his native language.

Most theorists are reasonably comfortable with the notion that biological forces influence the earliest stages of speech development, and most would probably accept the idea that there are some universal phonological patterns during these early stages. Critics of the Biological Theory suggest, however, that Locke places too much emphasis on the innateness of the acquisition process and gives too little attention to the variability of development that has been well-documented in the research literature, including evidence that a child's native language might influence productions during the first year (de Boysson-Bardies & Vihman, 1991).

What Do We Make of All This?

The differences that exist among current theories of phonological development bring us back to the old nature versus nurture debate. Is phonological development a universal experience and primarily the product of biological forces as suggested by the Structuralist Theory and the Biological Theory, or is it primarily the product of environment as suggested by the Behaviorist Theory? What is the role of the child in phonological acquisition? Is he a fairly passive experiencer as suggested by the Behaviorist Theory and the Natural Phonology Theory, or is he an active and creative participant in the process as suggested by the Cognitive Theory or its close cousin, the Interactionist-Discovery Theory? We find that some theories successfully account for individual differences that exist among children who are acquiring their sound systems but fail to account for universal tendencies, and other theories focus on general or universal patterns without giving adequate attention to individual variations in phonological acquisition.

As is almost always true in this kind of debate, we will eventually find that the answer lies somewhere in the middle of the argument's extremes. The Self-Organizing Theory (Lindblom, 1992) seems to represent a step in that direction. This theory takes both biological factors and language environment into account. It begins with the assumption that the phonological systems of all languages have been gradually shaped to accommodate the perceptual needs of listeners and the productive needs of speakers. That is, speakers need phonological features that make production manageable, and listeners need phonological features that make sounds and words easy to discriminate. When the needs of both speaker and listener are met, we are given phonological systems that contain segments common to most languages and segments that are unique to languages that have exceptionally large phonemic repertoires. Part of phonological development, from this point of view, involves the discovery of universal patterns, but the development of a particular language's phonological system will not be complete until the child also discovers the patterns unique to that language.

Whatever we might conclude about the value of any of the theories briefly described in this section, we can certainly agree that the process of phonological acquisition is far more complex than envisioned by Wellman, Poole, and Templin. We can also agree that we are still searching for a theory that addresses all relevant aspects of development. Such a theory will address the cognitive and perceptual aspects of oral communication as well as the productive aspects. It will account for how developing cognitive and perceptual abilities are related to the neuromuscular requirements for speech. It will certainly attempt to reconcile universal patterns of phonological development with individual variations in acquisition tied to language environment and to the child's active role in the process of discovering phonological patterns, formulating hypotheses about how these patterns work and should be applied to newly acquired words, testing his hypotheses in real-life communication challenges, and using his communicative experiences to help build the phonological system of his language.

Someone once observed that the more you know, the more you know what you don't know, and that is certainly true in our attempts to understand speech and language, even in an area like phonology, which at one time seemed so simple. A half century ago, researchers like Wellman, Poole, and Templin thought all we needed to do was count the bricks, the sounds of speech, but the more we have learned about phonology, the more complex we have discovered it to be. It is impossible to separate what the child produces from what he hears. It is impossible to separate what the child performs from what he understands, and it is impossible to separate what he knows and understands from the physical processes that generate speech sounds. Although we are learning more about these intricately interconnected relationships every day, we must accept that a complete understanding of the development of phonology lies somewhere in the future.

Review Questions

1. Define the following terms: *phonology, phoneme,* and *allophone.*
2. What are the three means by which consonants are classified in traditional phonetics?
3. How are vowels classified in traditional phonetics?
4. What is a cognate pair? Identify three cognate pairs among English consonants.

5. What does it mean to say that the distinctive features approach to phonology *extends* traditional phonetics and that the phonological processes approach to phonology *extends* the distinctive features approach?

6. What is a phonological process?

7. What is co-articulation? What is the difference between anticipatory and retentive co-articulation?

8. What accounts for changes in the child's vocalizations over the course of his first year?

9. Differentiate the following terms: *cooing, babbling,* and *variegated babbling.*

10. Briefly explain the babbling drift theory and the discontinuity theory. Why has each, as a sole explanation of the relationship between babbling and true speech, been dismissed?

11. What are proto-words? What does the existence of proto-words suggest about the relationship between babbling and true speech?

12. What are the most common manners and the most common places of articulation of the sounds used by the child in his first true words?

13. How does the metalinguistic awareness facilitated by learning to read and write help the child better understand his phonological system?

14. Briefly describe each of the following views of phonological development: Phoneme-by-Phoneme, Behaviorist Theory, Structuralist Theory, Natural Phonology Theory, Prosodic Theory, Cognitive Theory, and Biological Theory.

15. How does the nature-versus-nurture argument fit into the varying theories of phonological development?

16. In what sense is the Self-Organizing Theory a compromise between the nature and nurture extremes?

17. Identify the essential issues that should be addressed by a viable and comprehensive theory of phonological development.

References and Suggested Readings

Bernthal, J., & Bankson, N. (1988). *Articulation and phonological disorders* (2nd ed.). Englewood Cliffs, NJ: Prentice-Hall.

Blache, S. (1978). *The acquisition of distinctive features.* Baltimore: University Park Press.

Blache, S. (1982). Minimal word-pairs and distinctive feature training. In M. Crary (Ed.), *Phonological intervention, concepts and procedures* (pp. 66–96). San Diego, CA: College-Hill Press.

de Boysson-Bardies, B., & Vihmann, M. M. (1991). Adaptation to language. *Language, 61,* 297–319.

Chomsky, N., & Halle, M. (1968). *The sound patterns of English.* New York: Harper and Row.

Donegan, P, & Stampe, D. (1979). The study of natural phonology. In D. A. Dinnsen (Ed.), *Current approaches to phonological theory* (pp. 126–173). Bloomington, IN: Indiana University Press.

Eisenson, J. (1985). *Voice and diction: A program for improvement* (5th ed.). New York: Macmillan Publishing Company.

Ferguson, C. A. (1978). Learning to pronounce: The earliest stages of phonological development in the child. In F. D. Minifie & L. L. Lloyd (Eds.), *Communicative Competence and Cognitive Abilities.* Baltimore, MD: University Park Press.

Ferguson, C. A. (1986). Discovering sound units and constructing sound systems: It's child's play. In J. S. Perkell & D. H. Klatt (Eds.), *Invariance and Variability of Speech Processes.* Hillsdale, NJ: Lawrence Erlbaum.

Hockett, C. (1955). A manual of phonology. In *International Journal of American Linguistics (Memoir II).* Baltimore: Waverly Press.

Hodson, B., & Paden, E. (1983). *Targeting intelligible speech.* San Diego, CA: College-Hill Press.

Hodson, B., & Paden, E. (1991). *Targeting intelligible speech* (2nd ed.). Austin, TX: Pro-Ed.

Hoffman, P. (1990). Spelling, phonology, and the speech-language pathologist: A whole language perspective. *Language, Speech, Hearing Services in Schools, 21,* 238–243.

Ingram, D., Christensen, D., Veach, S., & Webster, B. (1980). The acquisition of word-initial fricatives and affricates in English by children between 2 and 6 years. In G. Yeni-Komshian, J. Kavanaugh, & C. Ferguson (Eds.), *Child phonology, Vol. 2. Production.* New York: Academic Press.

Jakobson, R. (1968). *Child Language, Aphasia, and Phonological Universals* (A. R. Keiler, trans.). The Hague: Mouton.

Katz, W., Kripke, C., & Tallal, R (1991). Anticipatory coarticulation in the speech of adults and young children: Acoustic, perceptual and video data. *Journal of Speech and Hearing Research, 34,* 1222–1249.

Lindblom, B. (1992). Phonological units as adaptive emergents of lexical development. In C. A. Ferguson, L. Menn, & C. Stoel-Gammon (Eds.), *Phonological Development: Models, Research, Implications.* Parkton, MD: York Press.

Lleo, C. (1990). Homonymy and reduplication: On the extended availability of two strategies in phonological acquisition. *Journal of Child Language, 17,* 267–278.

Locke, J. L. (1980). The prediction of child speech errors: Implications for a theory of acquisition. In G. Yeni-Komshian, J. F. Kavanaugh, & C. A. Ferguson (Eds.), *Child Phonology, Volume 1.* New York: Academic Press.

Locke, J. L. (1983). *Phonological Acquisition and Change.* New York: Academic Press.

Locke, J. L., & Pearson, D. (1992). Vocal learning and emergence of phonological capacity: A neurobiological approach. In C. A. Ferguson, L. Menn, & C. Stoel-Gammon (Eds.), *Phonological Development: Models, Research, Implications.* Parkton, MD: York Press.

Lowe, R. (1994). *Phonology, Assessment and Intervention Applications in Speech Pathology.* Baltimore, MD: Williams and Wilkens.

Macken, M., & Ferguson, C. (1983). Cognitive aspects of phonological development: Model, evidence and issues. In K. E. Nelson (Ed.), *Children's language, Vol, 4* (pp. 256–282). Hillsdale, NJ: Erlbaum.

Menn, L. (1976). Evidence for an interactionist-discovery theory of child phonology. *Papers and Reports on Child Language Development, 12,* 169–177.

Menn, L. (1983). Development of articulatory, phonetic, and phonological capabilities. In B. Butterworth (Ed.), *Language Production, Volume 2*. London: Academic Press.

Mowrer, O. (1952). Speech development in the young child: The autism theory of speech development and some clinical applications. *Journal of Speech and Hearing Disorders, 17*, 263–268.

Ohde, R., & Sharf, D. (1992). *Phonetic analysis of normal and abnormal speech*. Columbus, OH: Merrill/Macmillan.

Olmsted, D. (1966). A theory of the child's learning of phonology. *Language, 42*, 531–535.

Paul, R., & Jennings, P. (1992). Phonological behavior in toddlers with slow expressive language development. *Journal of Speech and Hearing Research, 35*, 99–107.

Poole, I. (1934). Genetic development of articulation of consonant sounds in English. *Elementary English Review, 11*, 159–161.

Prather, E., Hedrick, D., & Kern, C. (1975). Articulation development in children aged two to four years. *Journal of Speech and Hearing Disorders, 40*, 179–191.

Sander, E. (1972). When are speech sounds learned? *Journal of Speech and Hearing Disorders, 37*, 55–63.

Spencer, A. (1996). *Phonology, Theory and Description*. Cambridge, MA: Blackwell Publishers.

Stampe, D. (1969). The acquisition of phonetic representation, in *Papers from the fifth regional meeting of the Chicago Linguistic Society* (pp. 433–444). Chicago: Chicago Linguistic Society.

Stampe, D. (1973). A dissertation on natural phonology. Unpublished doctoral dissertation, University of Chicago.

Stoel-Gammon, C., & Dunn, C. (1985). *Normal and disordered phonology in children*. Baltimore: University Park Press.

Templin, M. (1957). Certain language skills in children: Their development and interrelationships. *Institute of Child Welfare Monographs, Vol. 26*. Minneapolis: University of Minnesota Press.

Vihman, M. (1996). *Phonological Development, The Origins of Language in the Child*. Cambridge, MA: Blackwell Publishers.

Waterson, N. (1971). Child phonology: A prosodic view. *Journal of Linguistics, 7*, 179–211.

Waterson, N. (1981). A tentative developmental model of phonological representation. In T. Myers, J. Laver, & J. Anderson (Eds.), *The Cognitive Representation of Speech*. Amsterdam: North-Holland.

Wellman, B., Case, I., Mengert, E., & Bradbury, D. (1931). *Speech sounds of young children* (University of Iowa Studies in Child Welfare). Iowa City: University of Iowa Press.

Winitz, H. (1969). *Articulatory acquisition and behavior*. Englewood Cliffs, NJ: Prentice-Hall.

EIGHT

Language Diversity: Regional, Social/Cultural, and Gender Differences

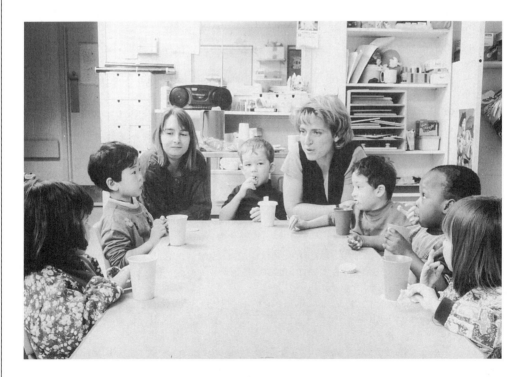

Chapter Objectives

Throughout this book, we have stressed that language is a universal human phenomenon. People are all born with the same genetic predispositions for language use, and although people have different experiences with their speech and language models, most are exposed to adequate samples of speech and language and have normal interactive relationships with their models. We do not have to travel very far outside of our homes or neighborhoods, however, to discover that there are some significant differences in language. In some cases, of course, people speak different languages, but even within a single language, there are differences. In this chapter, we consider differences within a national language, differences called dialects. We examine some of the characteristics of major dialects and consider how they have evolved. We also consider differences in language that are the products of gender. Specifically, this chapter is designed to facilitate understanding of the following topics:

- Variables that influence the acquisition of language and language behaviors.
- Meanings of key terms such as dialect, accent, standard dialect, and nonstandard dialect.
- Lexical characteristics of several easily recognizable regional dialects.
- Language and phonological characteristics of two social/cultural dialects of American English: Black English and Hispanic English.
- Educational implications of social/cultural dialects in America.
- Gender differences in language.

Although the child is born to talk, he is not born to speak a particular language or to speak a particular variation of a language. If a child is born in Paris to French-speaking parents, he will speak French. If a child is born to Korean parents but adopted shortly after his birth by English-speaking parents who live in Peoria, Illinois, he will speak English, and he will speak the same kind of English modelled for him by his adoptive parents. A black child reared by white parents will speak the dialect of his parents, not Black English, and a white child growing up in a predominantly black community will speak the dialect to which he has been exposed. I have purposely belabored the message here in the hope that it will be clearly understood and not soon forgotten. That is, the language one speaks and the variation of the language one speaks are not products of biology. They are products of environment.

According to Taylor (1990, p. 132), seven major variables influence the acquisition of language and language behaviors: (1) race and ethnicity; (2) social class, education, and occupation; (3) region; (4) gender; (5) situation or context; (6) peer group association or identification; and (7) first language community or culture. It should be obvious that these factors operate in an interactive manner to determine the language one speaks, and it should be equally obvious that the language one uses in one situation with one group of people may differ from the language one uses in another situation with a different group of people. This might mean, for example, that the Vietnamese child who emigrated to the United States with his family speaks Vietnamese to his parents but speaks English to his American friends. It might also mean that a black child uses Black Standard English when conversing with his family but uses General American English at school, and it might mean that a white child attending a predominantly black school uses Black English Vernacular when talking with his black friends even though he speaks General American English at home.

What Is a Dialect?

It should be apparent that the issue of language variation is fraught with sensitivities. We must take care to approach this topic with thoughtful and considerate respect, beginning with an understanding of dialect. The term **dialect** is used often, and it is often used with incomplete understanding. Wolfram and Christian (1989) suggest that dialect should be understood in a "technical" sense as well as the "popular" sense. Wolfram and Christian (1989, p. 1) define dialect as "any given variety of a language shared by a group of speakers." Taylor (1990, p. 131) offers a more elaborate version of the same definition: "A dialect is a variety of language that has developed through a complex interplay of historical, social, political, educational, and linguistic forces." All students of dialectology and sociolinguistics would agree that dialect should be understood and treated as a neutral term. A dialect typically corresponds with other differences among groups of people who happen to be united by culture, social class, or region. That is, people who live in the same region and who share cultural, ethnic, educational, and social values tend to speak the same variety of their national language. The dialect spoken by any given group of people is neither superior nor inferior to the dialect spoken by any other group of people. It must also be understood that every speaker of a given language speaks a dialect of that language. There is no Absolute Standard English, for example, against which variations are evaluated. There are dialects of English spoken by many people, and dialects spoken by fewer people, but number of speakers does not indicate superiority or correctness. Every dialect of English is linguistically correct within the rules that govern it, and every dialect of English is as valid as any other.

There are at least two problems with the popular or common lay understanding of dialect. First, some people use the term *dialect* as a synonym for *language*, especially when they are not adequately informed about the languages in a particular region of the world. Most people would not refer to the languages spoken by people living in Europe as dialects because they are familiar with some of the common languages of Europe, including French, Spanish, German, Russian, etc., but they might refer to the languages spoken by people living in Africa as dialects because they do not know the languages of Africa. At the same time, these people might not realize that there are many distinct dialects of Chinese, and that there are dialects of French, Spanish, German, and all major languages of the world.

A second and more troubling problem associated with the popular understanding of dialect centers on evaluating language differences as good/bad or standard/nonstandard. Such judgments are social rather than linguistic because, as we have already noted, every dialect is linguistically legitimate. A person from a northern state might judge the dialects of people from the southern states to be nonstandard or inferior, but a person from a southern state might make the same negative judgments about the speech of Yankees. In reference to English, it is best to understand that there are a number of standard dialects. A standard dialect is a variety of a language spoken by people of relatively high status who have economic, political, social, and educational power. Those who speak a standard dialect often maintain condescending attitudes toward other dialects and the people who speak them, but one must always keep in mind that standard is relative. The standard dialect of the rich and powerful in Texas is not the same as the standard dialect of the rich and powerful in New York, so that what is standard in one place may be nonstandard in another place.

If we accept that there are standard dialects of English, we must accept that there are nonstandard dialects as well. This is not a problem, as long as we remember that nonstandard does not mean inferior. Another term sometimes used for nonstandard dialect is **vernacular dialect.** This may be a better term because it does not connote value. Vernacular emphasizes what Wolfram and Christian (1989, p. 3) refer to as the "indigenous community dimension of these language varieties."

Whether dialects are standard or vernacular, the differences that separate them occur in grammar, phonology, semantics, vocabulary, pragmatics, and all other dimensions of language. In our discussion of dialects, we consider some of these differences in several major categories of language differences: (1) regional, (2) social/cultural, and (3) gender.

What Is an Accent?

Before we continue with our discussion of dialect, we should differentiate between dialect and accent. These terms are sometimes treated as synonyms by lay persons. Is there a difference, for example, between a southern dialect and a southern accent? The two terms can be separated if one understands **accent** to indicate characteristics of speech or variations in pronunciation, and **dialect** to indicate language differences as well as speech differences (Abercrombie, 1967, p. 19). Understood in this way, dialect is the broader term and subsumes accent. If a listener perceives only pronunciation differences in the speech of someone else and no language differences, he is perceiving an accent. If he hears pronunciation and language differences, he is hearing a dialect which differs from his own.

Regional Dialects

For the sake of convenience, we assume greater homogeneity within each identified regional dialect than actually exists. In fact, it is difficult to clearly separate social dialect and regional dialect. Technically, a **regional dialect** refers to a variety of language used by people living in a restricted geographic area, but within that area there may be several social dialects spoken by people who are grouped by factors other than geography, including social class, ethnicity, educational level, occupations, and religion. The social dialect is influenced by the regional dialect, however, so that a group of people linked by factors such as those identified here have a different dialect in Texas than in Boston. In other words, regional and social dialects interact, producing variations within dialects of language.

As you might imagine, not all experts agree about the number of regional dialects because they do not all draw lines on dialectal maps in exactly the same places, and regional dialects are defined according to geographic boundaries. Taylor suggests that there are at least ten regional dialects in the United States (1990, p. 133). According to Craig Carver (1987), a specialist in regional American dialects, there are six major regions, which can be divided into many layers and subregions. There are five places along the eastern and southern coasts of the United States from which most American regional dialects have evolved: Boston, Philadelphia, tidewater Virginia, Charleston, and New Orleans (Carver, 1987, p. 7). These centers are called **cultural hearths.** In some cases, as in Boston, the original dialectal influences remain strong. In others, the original dialect has been largely lost. In all cases, American dialects constantly evolve as a result of changes in population centers. Because we tend to be increasingly mobile and increasingly connected to one another through a variety of mass media, dialects will continue to evolve, eroding many of the speech and language differences that now exist.

Our discussion of regional dialects includes samples of language differences that have been noted and explained by Craig Carver (1987). This analysis is certainly not complete in breadth or depth but provides you with a sense of the dialectal differences that exist in the United States. Regional dialects are characterized by differences in all components of language, including phonology, grammar, and semantics, but the dimension most affected is vocabulary. Certain words that are common to the vocabularies of people living in New England may be unknown to people living in the Midwest. Some words are used and defined differently from region to region. Our discussion focuses on selected examples of these vocabulary differences in just three of the six regions identified by Carver (1987).

The New England and Northeast Region

When many of us think about the speech of people who live in New England, especially in the Boston area, we think about what these people do with the *r*. That is, they drop the *r* when it should be present in a word, and they sometimes add it where it does not belong. The Bostonian might say *ca* for *car,* for example, but he might say *tuber* for *tuba.* As with all regional dialects, however, the most notable features of the dialects in this region are in word usage.

The past and present of New England have been powerfully influenced by the sea, and this influence is observed in the language of the people in this area. They use words such as *nor'easter* and *nor'wester* to describe the movements of winds and storms. When the wind calms, they say it is *lulling down,* and when the wind increases, they say it is *breezing up.* Some words that were originally nautical terms have developed broader usage. For example, a *bulkhead* refers to a partition between compartments of a ship. The term is now used in New England to refer to the sloping doors of a cellar.

Those who came to this part of the country from England sometimes found new phenomena for which they had no vocabulary, so they adapted words to describe these things. The weather in England, for example, is fairly constant, but the weather in New England changes rapidly and often. Nautical folks in the eighteenth century referred to a sunny day as an *open* day, so that over time the expression *open-and-shut day* came to mean a day when the clouds come and go. Settlers from England were also unfamiliar with mountain passes, so using a word known to them, they called this kind of opening between mountains a *notch.*

Many terms in the dialects of this region reflect, not influences of the sea, but experiences of rural living. *Creepers,* for example, are metal cleats fastened to boots for the purpose of providing sure footing on ice. A bobsled is called a *double runner, double ripper,* or *traverse sled.* When one hauls something, he *carts* or *teams* it. If a horse

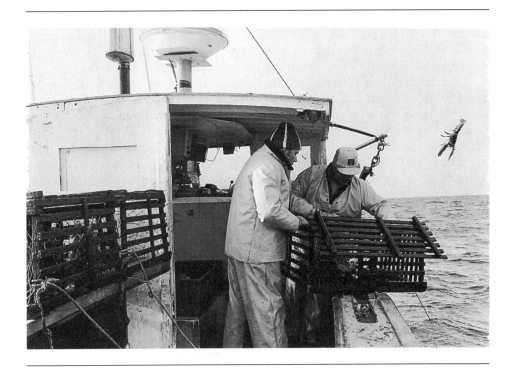

The influence of the sea is apparent in New England dialects.

or cow is uncooperative or mean, it is described as *ugly,* but an *ugly top cow* is a bull, and not necessarily an ill-tempered bull. Cow or horse manure is called *top dressing* or *meadow dressing.* A *wheel harrow* is a farm implement used to break up clumps of plowed dirt, and a *bush scythe* is used to clear brush or weeds. When the farmer spreads his hay so that it can dry, he *tedders* it. After he tedders the hay, he *tumbles* it, which means that he stacks it for curing, and then he *mows it away,* which means that he stores it in a barn.

This region has produced many unique terms for food items. Some of these terms, such as *Boston brown bread* or simply *brown bread,* refer to recipes unique to the region, but most are terms used to name food items found throughout the country. For example, a submarine sandwich is called a *grinder,* and a soft drink is called a *tonic.* Hamburger and frankfurter are often shortened to *hamburg* and *frankfurt.* A poached egg is called a *dropped egg,* a term unique to New England dialects.

Many other terms peculiar to this region do not fit the categories already identified. For example, older residents of the region may refer to a funnel as a *tunnel,* and if liquid poured through the funnel comes out slowly, it is coming out in *dribs and drabs.* An apartment building is called a *tenement,* and a veranda or open porch is called a *piazza.* Someone who is especially rigid or fastidious is called a *fusspot* or *fussbudget.* Taking a shortcut is *cutting cross-lots.*

The Northeast region beyond New England includes New York, most of New Jersey, and Pennsylvania (Carver, 1987, p. 44), but the influences of the dialects in this region extend to the north and west. Since this portion of the region was settled by New Englanders migrating westward, many of the terms used in New England are used by other speakers in the region. Some words, however, are associated with specific areas of this region beyond New England. Although the term *cruller,* referring to a doughnut, is widely used in many areas of the country today, it was originally a word unique to speakers from the Hudson Valley. Speakers from New York refer to a freeway or expressway as a *throughway,* to curdled or sour milk as *lobbered milk,* and to a whisk broom as a *brush broom.* Speakers from the greater New York metropolitan area, including northern New Jersey, refer to a particularly large and aggressive mosquito as a *Jersey mosquito* or *Jersey bomber.* Other words are common to speakers throughout the region, including *nightwalker* for nightcrawler or large earthworm, *soda* for soft drink, *scallion* for small onion, and *grass* for asparagus. There are also slang words or phrases characteristic of the dialects in this region, including *can* in reference to buttocks, *nanna* in reference to one's grandmother, and *get a wiggle on* to mean *hurry up!*

The Northern and Midwest Region

The boundaries of this area are difficult to define with great precision, but it may be useful to think of this region as spreading from coast to coast with the Ohio River as a rough dividing line between North and South. Even though this region covers a wide geographic area, the dialects have been primarily influenced by only two cultural and linguistic hearths: New England and southeastern Pennsylvania. As these cultures moved westward across the United States, they mixed and influenced one another, eventually producing a shared dialect. There are variations within this broad dialect, of course, but our focus is primarily on the common features.

Although some dialects, including the New England dialect, still show influences of older English and include words borrowed from other European languages and American Indian languages, the dialects of this region are remarkably free of these influences. A few words such as the German word *fest,* meaning festival or holiday, are retained in the dialects of the northern/midwest region, but *fest* is most often included within the words *gabfest* or *talkfest* to refer to an informal conversation or gossip session. Other self-explanatory words have been coined from the morpheme *fest,* including *beerfest, slugfest,* and *funfest.* Another word borrowed from German and used in this region is *gesundheit,* an expression used in response to a sneeze. Some speakers who use this expression may believe it means *God bless you,* but it is actually just a way of saying, *I wish you good health.*

There are a number of slang and colloquial expressions that are used throughout the country, but are most common in this region. For example, when one works hard, he sweats *like a butcher*. A cigar is called a *rope* and a cigarette is called a *coffin nail*. A common euphemism for regurgitate is *toss one's cookies*.

Speakers in this region refer to large earthworms as *nightcrawlers* and to fuzzy caterpillars as *woolly bears*. A snapping turtle is called a *snapper,* and bullfrogs are called *croakers*. Tree sap is called *pitch,* and the sugar maple tree is called a *hard maple*.

Speakers in the upper portion of the north region use *squealer* in reference to an informer, *milquetoast* in reference to someone who is shy and timid, *crusty* in reference to someone who is aggressive and nervy and *souse* to mean a drunk. There are also phrases common to this area, as shown here. The meanings of these phrases should be clear in the following:

I wouldn't run a marathon for *all the tea in China*.

He's always trying *to get the best of* his friends.

Jim's brother is *meaner than dirt*.

Why, I haven't seen that movie *in a dog's age*.

Our television has been *on the fritz* since the storm.

Sally is so boy-crazy. She's always *on the make*.

It's been great talking to you. *See you in church!*

Other words that are especially common in the most northern section of this region include *pollywog* for tadpole, *bloodsucker* for leech, *sticker* for a prickly weed, *sliver* for splinter, *mammoth* for large, *shuck* for removing the covering of something, and *heave* for throw.

The Southern Region

We tend to think of the speech of people who live in the southern states as representing a single dialect. In actuality, there are a variety of dialects in the south, but we treat the south as one region and provide dialectal examples from throughout the region. The dividing line between north and south extends westward from central Delaware, along the traditional Mason-Dixon Line and the Ohio River to an area west of the Mississippi River, including some or all of Texas, depending upon whose version of the region one accepts.

The dialects of this region are characterized by uniquely American words and phrases, including *snake doctor* for dragonfly, *calling the hogs* for snoring, *egg turner* for spatula, and *cooling board* for the slab upon which a corpse is laid. Other words are adaptations of common English words, including *puny* to mean not only small and weak but also sickly, *harp* for harmonica, *rogue* for a thief or scoundrel, *spew* for gush, *slouch* for a bungler or clod, and *piddles around* for wasting time.

Because the south is primarily a rural area, there is a definite rural flavor to the dialects of the region. Words relating to the farm experience include *hand* for farm worker, *overseer* for supervisor, *dusky dark* for twilight, *critters* for animals, *juicing* for milking cows, and *cowlot* for pasture. If a farmer works too hard, he may feel *wore out,* and if he continues to work too hard, he may *take sick,* and he might lose weight or *fall off* a bit.

Other common words and phrases heard in the dialects of the south include *fussing* for fighting, *draw up* for shrink or squeeze, *slosh* for spill or splash, *johnny* or *commode* for toilet, *booger* for child, *sowbelly* for pork, *calaboose* for jail, *ruther* for preference, *earbob* for earring, *dead cat on the line,* meaning that something is suspicious, and *jumped the broom stick,* for getting married.

One of the more distinct subregions in the south includes Louisiana and especially the area around New Orleans. The French were among the first to settle this area, and even though settlers came from other parts of the world, including Germany, Spain, and what is now known as Nova Scotia, the French influence has remained strong through the years. It is, in fact, this French influence that gives New Orleans its unique character. The dialect of this region retains a distinct French flavor. Carver refers to this dialect as Louisiana French (1987, p. 141). It contains words borrowed directly from French and incorporates other words borrowed from British English, Spanish, and Indian languages. Words common to Louisiana French include *armoire* for a dresser or bureau, *gallery* for porch, *lagniappe* for modest gift or bonus, *bayou* for a marshy stream or creek, *pirogue* for canoe, *marais* for swamp, and *coulee* for dry creek bed,

Many people associate New Orleans with excellent French food. Louisiana French includes culinary terms such as *praline* (candy made with pecans and brown sugar), *gumbo* (stew containing meat or seafood and vegetables), *jambalaya* (rice with tomatoes and herbs along with chicken, ham, oysters, or shrimp), *brioche* (coffee cake), *bisque* (cream soup), and *pigeonnier* (roast pigeon).

Social/Cultural Dialects

In introducing the concept of a social/cultural dialect, it is important to reiterate that dialects are not products of biology. In this section, we consider the characteristics of two social/cultural dialects: Black English and Hispanic English. One must not assume, however, that all African-American speakers use the same dialect. In fact, some African-Americans do not speak Black English as their primary dialect and may not use Black English at all. On the other hand, many whites living in areas where the dominant dialect is Black English use the patterns of that dialect. In the same way, not all Hispanic speakers sound the same. In fact, one should not assume that speakers from a Mexican Spanish background will produce a dialect of English that is exactly the same as the dialect derived from Puerto Rican Spanish. All possible variations of English that fit within the broad Black and Hispanic English categories are the products of social, cultural, ethnic, educational, and occupational influences. These dialects are then influenced by regional dialects so that Black English in Atlanta, Georgia, differs from Black English in Philadelphia, Pennsylvania, and Hispanic English in New York differs from Hispanic English in Miami.

Black English

Without question, the most studied and most controversial dialect in American English is Black English, which is also called Black Dialect, Black English Vernacular, African American English, and Ebonics (Taylor, 1990, p. 140; Smitherman, 1994, p. 1). The controversy surrounding Black English is the result of misunderstanding, ignorance, and the continuing racial prejudices that tend to divide all black/white issues into "good" and "bad." Based on what has been presented in this chapter, you should understand that good and bad have no relevance in any discussion about dialects, because no dialect is inherently superior to any other. Furthermore, it is absolutely unreasonable for any educated person to believe that all African-Americans speak Black English. Although there is risk even in the following generalization, it may be relatively safe to say that Black English is the dialect spoken by most working-class African-Americans living in working-class African-American communities.

Each dialect of a language has its own social and cultural history. Black English has a long, diverse, complex history. According to the **creolist theory,** Black English is a complicated hybrid derived from several African languages and from Portuguese, Dutch, French, and English (Taylor, 1990, p. 141). Most of the Africans brought to the United States as slaves came from the west coast of Africa. On the east coast, Swahili was the dominant language, but natives of Africa's west coast spoke hundreds of languages which, although similar in terms of phonology and syntax, had different vocabularies (Taylor, 1972). When speakers of these various languages interacted, they developed common languages so they could communicate with one another. A common language, called a **pidgin,** develops as speakers of a nondominant language accept a few key words, usually related to business or trade, from the dominant language. A pidgin begins as an informal language consisting mostly of nouns and many gestures. As it develops, the pidgin becomes more formal. The vocabulary of the dominant language is absorbed into the nondominant language, which retains revised versions of its original phonological and grammatical systems. When the pidgin becomes the primary language of a group of people, it is called a **creole** language. At this point, the original nondominant language ceases to exist. As the language evolution continues, the creole language becomes increasingly similar to the language of the dominant culture, a process called **decreolization** (Taylor, 1972, pp. 6–7; Taylor, 1990, pp. 141–142). Part of the development of Black English then can be traced to the creolization of the west coast African languages. Elements of these creoles came with the people who were brought to America as slaves.

The influences of European languages on Black English can be traced to the trade initiatives of European countries in Africa. In the early 1500s, Portugal sent ships to West Africa for commercial purposes. Since the Portuguese traders could not learn all the African languages in this area, the Africans learned Portuguese. As one would expect, however, the Portuguese language that became the trading lan-

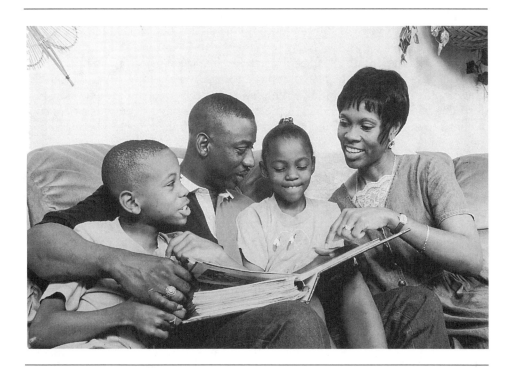

Black English is a valid and valued dialect.

guage of West Africa evolved into a creole, the product of Portuguese merged with various African languages. Black Portuguese came to America with the slaves who were brought to Portuguese and Spanish colonies. The Dutch took over Portuguese trading bases in the early 1600s, adding mostly Dutch vocabulary to Black Portuguese. At about this same time, England and France were becoming trading powers in Africa, and their languages were thrown into the mix. The French especially were active in the slave trade, but unlike the Dutch, they did not adopt Black Portuguese as their trade language. Their involvement in the slave markets of Africa, therefore, produced another creole, Black French. The original Black English also came to America by way of the slave trade. Unlike Black Portuguese and Black French, however, Black English became widely and firmly established in the United States because of the constant and intensive contacts between slaves and their English-speaking owners (Taylor, 1972, pp. 6–9).

Although Black English has changed considerably over the years, mostly as a result of social and educational pressures, it remains a distinct dialect with its own identifiable characteristics and rules. All variations between Black English and Standard English must be understood, not as errors, but as characteristics of a viable and valid dialect. According to Williams and Wolfram (1977), there are at least twenty-nine linguistic rules of Black English that vary from Standard English rules. As should be expected, many of these twenty-nine rules overlap the rules of other dialects of American English, especially the standard and nonstandard dialects of the south. Since African-Americans have strong historical connections to the southern states, this overlapping of dialects should be viewed as inevitable.

A complete analysis of Black English would require an entire book. Our purposes will be met by including a summary of selected characteristics of Black English. The selections include some features most of you will readily recognize and features that may be less familiar. Unlike regional dialects that are characterized primarily by vocabulary or lexical differences, Black English differs from Standard English in a variety of ways. There are phonological and syntactic differences as well as lexical differences.

Although the phonological system of Black English contains the same number of sounds as in Standard English, the rules for using and combining sounds are not the same. For example, in Black English the second of two sounds in a final consonant cluster is often deleted so that *rust* is produced as *rus* and *bend* becomes *ben*. Among the most recognizable features of Black English are the substitutions for voiced and voiceless "th". That is, "f" is commonly substituted for voiceless "th" in the word final position, as in *toof* for *tooth*, "d" is substituted for voiced "th" in the word initial position, as in *dat* for *that*, and "v" is substituted for voiced "th" when it occurs between vowels, as in *breaving* or *breavin* for *breathing*. In Black English, voiced plosives are typically devoiced in the postvocalic position so that *lid* becomes *lit* and *flag* becomes *flak*. In the word final position, "ng" is often produced as "n" as in *bringin* for *bringing* and *goin* for *going*, although this is a common feature in the speech of many people who do not use Black English. The "r" is often deleted when it occurs between two vowels so that *carrot* sounds like *cat*, and it is typically deleted when it occurs in the word final position or when it precedes another consonant, so that *car* becomes *ca* and *bark* becomes *bak*. In Black English, the "l" is often deleted in the postvocalic position and when it precedes "t," "d," "p," resulting in *te* for *tell*, *bet* for *belt*, *tod* for *told*, and *hep* for *help* (Taylor, 1990; Naremore, 1980, Bernthal and Bankson, 1993, p. 149).

Some of the grammatical differences between Black English and Standard English center on whether a rule is obligatory or not. In Standard English, for example, there are obligatory rules for marking plurality and possession. *Dog* is made plural by adding *s* to produce *dogs*. *Dog* is made possessive by adding *'s* to produce *dog's*. In Black English, plurality may be indicated by adding *s*, but it may also be indicated by using words that identify quantity either specifically or generally. This rule results in productions such as *I have two dog* or *I have many dog*. The rule for possession in Black English is similar. That is, possession is understood as long as the possessor is identified, resulting in sentences such as *That's Jim car* or *Mary is John mother.* In Standard English, a marker for past tense is obligatory, but in Black English a past tense marker is not required, resulting in sentences such as *She talk to me yesterday,* or *We walk to the park last night.* In Standard English, the copula and auxiliary forms of the verb *to be* are obligatory. In Black English, they may be deleted. For example, *He **is** a handsome man* might be produced as *He a handsome man.* The auxiliary verb in *They **were** running fast* might be deleted, resulting in *They running fast.*

Some irregular rules in Standard English are made regular in Black English. In Standard English, for example, the third person singular form of a verb differs from the first and second person forms, resulting in *I hit* (first person), *You hit* (second person), and *She hits* (third person singular). In Black English, the irregularity for third person singular forms is eliminated, resulting in *I hit, You hit, She hit.* The past tense copula and auxiliary forms in Standard English change according to person and number, resulting in productions such as *I **was** running, You **were** running, He **was** running,* and *They **were** running.* The rule in Black English is regularized so that *was* is used in all cases, resulting in sentences such as *I was running, You was running, He was running,* and *They was running.* Likewise, the present tense forms that change according to person and number in Standard English are regularized to *is* in Black English, resulting in sentences such as *I is running, You is running,* and *They is running.* In Standard English, the article (*a* or *an*) used depends on whether the word modified begins with a vowel or consonant, resulting in ***a** car* and ***an** automobile.* In Black English, the rule is made regular by using *a* in all cases to produce *a car* and *a automobile.* In Standard English, *those* is used in the subject position of a sentence, and *them* is used in the object position, resulting in sentences such as ***Those** cars are new,* and *We washed **them** yesterday.* The rule in Black English is regularized so that *them* is used in both the subject and object positions, resulting in sentences such as *Them dogs are ours.*

There are at least two differences between Standard English and Black English in the production of negation. *Ain't* is a common feature in many dialects of American English as a substitution for *am not, isn't,* and *aren't.* In Black English, *ain't* is substituted for these forms, but it is also used for *haven't, hasn't,* and *didn't* (Taylor, 1990, p. 143). For example, the sentence *She didn't go to school,* becomes *She ain't go to school.* We all learned about double negatives in school, and we were all probably taught that two negatives cancel out into a positive, so that *She don't got no money* means that she does, in fact, have money. Despite the warnings, all children and many adults of all dialects use double negatives occasionally. In Black English, the rule is that the more negative terms there are, the more negative the sentence, so that *Joe ain't going to no doctor at no time no how!* conveys a fairly powerful message about what Joe intends *not* to do.

One of the most interesting characteristics of Black English is a syntactic device called "aspect" (Warren-Leubecker & Bohannon, 1989). Most readers will recognize this feature, since it is often included in imitations of Black English. When the speaker wants to convey that an action or state of being is continuing or occurs intermittently, he uses the verb *be*. For example, if the speaker is referring to someone who talks constantly and is now talking, he would say *He be talking*. If the speaker is referring to someone who seldom talks but is now talking, he would say *He talking*. In Standard English, both observations would be expressed in the same sentence, *He is talking*. In Black English, *been* is used to describe an action or state of being that occurred a long time ago but no longer exists. To say *Joe been sad* means that Joe was sad a while ago, but he is feeling better now. The Standard English equivalent of this sentence is *Joe had been sad*. In Black English, the sentence *I been had this cough* means that this is not a recently developed cough but a cough I have had for a long time. What is most interesting about this feature is that there is no directly comparable version of it in Standard English. Labov (1966) has identified aspect as a feature of several West African languages. It would be reasonable to speculate that this feature of Black English is a remnant of the creole used by the West Africans who were brought to America as part of the slave trade.

As one would expect, there are also vocabulary or lexical differences between Black English and Standard English. The following are examples of words that are part of the Black English vocabulary and their Standard English equivalents (Smitherman, 1994)

Black English	Standard English
ace cool	best friend
airish	cool and breezy
bad	good, excellent, fine
banger	member of a gang
bank	large sum of money
bees	that's how it is
blue	police
curb	ugly, undesirable
dead Presidents	money
hawking	staring at someone
oil	liquor
Q	barbecued ribs
righteous	excellent
salty	angry, mad
seeds	one's children
sprung	hopelessly in love
woman	a man's wife or girlfriend
yo-yo	a weak, stupid person

You will notice, of course, that many of these terms have worked their way into other dialects of English. As we have already noted, language is never static. It con-

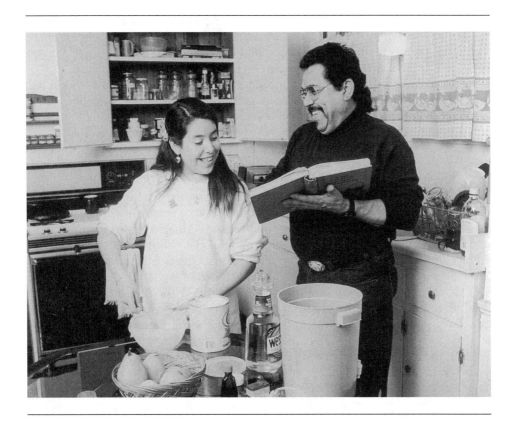

Hispanic English is a widely used dialect in the United States.

stantly changes, and each dialect of a language changes as speakers of a variety of dialects interact. As time passes, it is often difficult, perhaps impossible, to trace the origins of rules and words that become integrated into the many dialects of a national language.

Hispanic English

American English is spoken by people from so many national backgrounds that it would be impossible to identify and describe all the varieties of English that have derived from these influences. It should be understood, however, that every language will influence the speaking of English in different ways because although there are common characteristics shared by all languages, every language has its own unique features as well. The influence that one language has upon another depends upon their similarities and their differences and upon how divergent their differences are. In this section, we focus on Hispanic English because there are more speakers in the United States today who must deal with the interferences between English and Spanish than between English and any other language.

In describing the influences of one language upon another, linguists talk about **interference points.** An interference point is an area where the two languages differ in terms of how a form is represented. Perhaps the most obvious differences between English and Spanish are in their vocabularies, but there are also differences in the phonological and syntactic systems of the two languages. Because there is not a single variety of Spanish spoken in America, and because various Spanish-speaking Americans are confronted with a wide variety of English dialects, it is impossible to compile a list of interference points that would adequately describe the problems faced by every Spanish-speaking person learning English as a second language. Furthermore, some of these individuals are learning English as adults. Some children are learning English and Spanish simultaneously. Some children begin school as competent bilingual speakers. Others enter school with excellent language skills in Spanish but little or no experience with English. Still others come to school with strong English skills and limited abilities in Spanish. Some children come from families that emphasize the importance of retaining their cultural background, including their native language. Others are children of parents who want to be fully and immediately integrated into American culture and who put little or no priority on retaining Spanish as a first or second language. All these factors, and many others, make only the most general discussion of interference points meaningful and appropriate.

A number of phonological differences between English and Spanish result in productions that most of you will readily associate with Hispanic English. For example, Spanish does not include the vowel in *bit,* but it does include the vowel in *bee,* two vowels that are included in English phonology and are similar in classification. The Hispanic English speaker, therefore, often substitutes what is commonly called a long "e" for a short "e" in producing *beeg* for *big.* Spanish phonology does not include the vowel in *cat* or the vowel in *cut.* The vowel in *yet* is substituted to produce *cet* for *cat,* and the vowel in *father* is substituted to produce *cot* for *cut.* There are also several interference points involving consonants. The Hispanic English speaker typically substitutes "ch" for "sh" in the prevocalic and postvocalic positions, resulting in *choe* for *shoe* and *butch* for *bush.* Spanish has "s" but not "z," so "s" is substituted for "z" as in *soo* for *zoo* and *sipper* for *zipper.* Neither the voiced nor the voiceless "th" occur in Spanish, so the Hispanic English speaker substitutes either "t" or "s" for the voiceless "th" as in *tumb* or *sumb* for *thumb,* and he substitutes "d" for voiced "th" as in *dough* for *though.* In Spanish, there is no distinction between "b" and "v" so that *van* is produced as *ban.* The liquids, "l" and "r," occur in Spanish but are produced differently than in English, and the Hispanic English speaker often substitutes the Spanish versions for their English equivalents. In the final position of words, "n" is often substituted for "ng," resulting in productions such as *rin* for *ring* and *sin* for *sing,* although we note again that the substitution of "n" for "ng" at the ends of words is very common in many dialects of American English. Because prevocalic voiceless plosives are not aspirated in Spanish, obscuring the voiced/voiceless contrast, *kick* may sound like *gick.* On the other hand, all postvocalic plosives are voiceless so that *log* sounds like *lok* (Naremore and Hopper, 1990, p. 159; Taylor, 1990, p. 145; Bernthal & Bankson, 1993, pp. 152–155).

Syntactic interference points affect the use of verbs, adverbs, adjectives, pronouns, and articles, as well as the application of rules for creating questions, negation, plurality, and possession. Forms of the verb *to be,* for example, may be missing in some constructions. The Hispanic speaker typically produces the English sentence *He is going home* as *He going home.* In other cases, the Hispanic speaker substitutes *has* or *have* for *to be* as in *He **has** sadness* instead of *He **is** sad.* The third person singular form of regular verbs is produced without the *-s,* so that *He walks fast* becomes *He walk fast.* Past tense endings may be omitted, resulting in productions such as *He work yesterday.* The Standard English sentence *He is going to work tomorrow* is produced as *He go to work tomorrow.* Consistent with the Spanish rule, the Hispanic speaker places locative adverbs as close to the verb as possible, resulting in sentences such as *I saw her putting down the dog,* instead of the Standard English version *I saw her putting the dog down.* In Spanish, the comparative and superlative forms of adjectives are created by adding words rather than adding the suffixes, *-er* and *-est.* Rather than saying *His house is bigger,* therefore, the Hispanic speaker says *His house is more big.* Although the Hispanic speaker uses pronouns, he often deletes a pronoun as the subject of a sentence when the antecedent is obvious from the immediate context. Applying this rule, the Standard English production *Jack bought a new car. I think he will really like it* becomes *Jack bought a new car. I think will really like it.* Because articles are used differently in Spanish than in English, the Hispanic speaker often omits them in English, resulting in productions such as *He is handsome boy* instead of *He is a handsome boy.* In creating questions, the modal *do* is often omitted, resulting in constructions such as *You want to go to the park?* instead of *Do you want to go to the park?* When creating questions that require a word order change in Standard English, the Hispanic speaker may use the declarative sentence order so that *Can Joe go with us?* becomes *Joe can go with us?* The Hispanic speaker might use *no* to indicate negation in situations that call for negative contractions in Standard English. The sentence *Don't leave this room* might be produced as *No leave this room.* When Standard English calls for marking plurality or possession by adding *-s,* the Hispanic speaker may omit the marker, resulting in sentences such as *There are four dog* and *That's John car* (Naremore & Hopper, 1990, p. 159; Taylor, 1990, p. 146).

As has been stressed throughout this section, it is important that the features of Hispanic English and Black English not be viewed as errors or as simplifications of more sophisticated forms. Both of these varieties of American English are legitimate, rule-governed language systems. What appears to be an error is the product of a different form, the substitution of one form for another, or a compromise necessitated by the incompatibility of two widely divergent forms. Some of the forms and rules in Hispanic English and in Black English differ from the forms and rules in Standard English, but different is neither better nor worse. Different is simply different.

The Educational Implications of Social/Cultural Dialects

The controversies surrounding the legitimacies of social/cultural dialects have created problems for speakers of these dialects in all aspects of their lives, but the arenas of the most troubling and important battles have been the public schools. We have focused on the two primary social/cultural dialects in the United States, but there are many others. All of these languages and their dialects from Asia, Latin America, and Africa have mixed with all the dialects of American English to create a language confusion in many public schools that makes communication difficult at best. If the ability to communicate is diminished or lost in the educational process, all of our children suffer, but especially those who come into the schools without the advantage of speaking the same language as their teachers. In the long term, the nation suffers whenever the education of its children is compromised, and the education of those children who speak any language other than a Standard Dialect of American English is surely being compromised in many American schools today. This is not a problem that is disappearing. On the contrary, it worsens as the number of children who do not speak Standard American English continues to grow. Within the next twenty years, these children will constitute the majority of our public school population (Bowman, 1989).

One solution to this problem is to insist that all children who attend public schools speak the same dialect of the same language, a solution that is as offensive as it is impractical. The United States is not now, nor has it ever been, a culturally and socially homogeneous nation. One of the great strengths of our country is its almost unlimited diversity. We are one nation of many cultures, many political points of view, many religions. We are a people of widely varying beliefs and values. The various languages of the people who come to the United States and the many dialects of those who have lived here for generations are parts of our cultural diversity. These language differences are inherent characteristics of our cultural heritages. To the extent possible in an era that absolutely requires communicative integrity, we want to preserve our language differences, and according to the principles of the American way of life, we have a right to preserve these differences.

It may be difficult for many Americans who speak versions of Standard American English to understand what all the commotion is about. After all, why should anyone object to sounding like the good people of Hometown, USA? We should all consider this issue from an empathic point of view. If you speak Standard American English, for example, how would you feel if you or your children were required to speak Black English or Hispanic English, or how would you feel if all

Americans were required to speak the dialect of a region other than your own? How would you feel if basic words in your vocabulary were considered slang and not worthy of inclusion in anything other than informal conversations among people like you? How would you react if the rules of your dialect were considered errors or simplifications of standard or correct rules? The problem with a single dialect, of course, is that someone must decide what is correct and proper in terms of vocabulary and all the rules that govern the way people speak. Can you think of any group of people to whom you would be willing to give this responsibility?

Perhaps you can accept the idea that dialects of a national language are inevitable. You may even accept that dialects are valuable characteristics of our cultural diversity, but what about the issue of all people speaking one language? If people choose to live in the United States, should they not speak English since English is our national language? There is no question that a single language would simplify communication, and there is no question that if all children in our public schools spoke English with the same high degree of proficiency, the educational process would be easier and more efficient. Unfortunately, this wishful thinking just does not match the reality of our nation as it exists today. The United States cannot welcome immigrants and the cultural diversity they bring with them while insisting that they leave their heritages, including their languages, at the shore, and let us be clear about the importance of one's native language. A person's language is as much a part of his cultural heritage as his religion and his feelings of nationalism. People who come here from Asia or Latin America do not come because they want to forsake their countries or their cultures. They typically come here to find a better life in a country that offers freedom of religion, freedom of political thought, and freedom from tyranny.

The problem in all this is obvious—not simple, not easily solved, not without need for accommodation, but obvious. Even though we are a multicultural, multipolitical, multireligious nation, we do have a single national language. Those people who wish to take advantage of the opportunities afforded them in the United States find that understanding and speaking English are essential. Even those people who speak a dialect of American English other than what is considered a standard dialect find that many doors of social and vocational opportunity are narrowed or closed if one does not speak the language of the decision makers. There seems little question then that our children must be given the opportunity and encouraged to learn the national language. They must also be given the opportunity to learn those varieties of the national language that will give them the best chance of succeeding as students and as adults. We must recognize, however, that children can learn American English without surrendering the languages, cultures, and values of their native countries. Children can learn other dialects without abdicating their natural dialects and their associated cultural values. It is not only possible to accommodate multiple languages and multiple dialects within the American educational system, it is the right thing to do. The problem then needs to be addressed, not by trying to make all children fit the same social/cultural mold, not even by compromise, which suggests surrender from both ends, but by accommodation. To accommodate means to adapt or reconcile. It implies that variances are allowed in a manner that promotes harmony.

Barbara Bowman (1989) offers six suggestions, paraphrased below, that will help teachers more effectively reach their educational objectives while preserving the multicultural interests and rights of all students:

1. Teachers must recognize that although children from a variety of backgrounds learn many of the same things before they enter school, they do not all develop their knowledge and skills in the same way. All children, for example, learn to recognize, categorize, and understand the things, people, and events in their environments, but not all children encounter the same things, people, and events, and they certainly do not all categorize and understand according to a universal set of rules. All children learn a primary language, but not all children learn the same language or the same dialect of a given language. Furthermore, even though the order of language development is the same for all children, not all children meet developmental milestones at the same ages. All children come to school with skills in interpersonal communication, but because of environmental, cultural, and individual differences, there are wide variations in interpersonal communication styles and competencies. The point is, teachers must expect diversity in the knowledge and skills children bring to school.

2. Since not all children develop their basic skills and knowledge in the same way according to the same schedule, it is important that teachers do not value some developmental strategies more highly than others. Behaviors, including language behaviors, that differ from the behaviors of the majority may be erroneously and insensitively viewed as deficient or substandard. Teachers must keep in mind that the child who perceives that his language is not understood and appreciated will be reluctant to communicate. Communicative disengagement may be the first step toward educational disengagement.

3. Instruction, particularly in the introductory phase, is facilitated by the use of content with which children are familiar and by use of an interactive communicative style which directly and immediately involves children as participants. This may mean that early instruction is given in the child's native language or in the child's natural dialect. It may mean that the teacher will use management techniques with which children are comfortable. It may mean that the topics around which lessons are taught will depend on the social and cultural experiences of the students. Whatever is done relative to curriculum and teaching style, the teacher must first establish communicative relationships with students, and this inevitably means that accommodation is necessary.

4. What the child learns and achieves in school will have little long-term significance unless academic achievements are valued in the home. This does

not necessarily mean that parents must teach at home exactly what is being taught at school, but it does mean that the educational process will founder unless family members and community leaders reinforce the importance and worth of academic effort, accomplishment, and excellence. The teacher, along with all other members of the educational system, must help parents and community leaders understand and appreciate academic goals and procedures so that learning will be valued by all people who influence children as they grow up.

5. There will be times when what is taught in school will conflict with what is being taught or experienced at home or in the streets. The lessons of the real world are often brutal, and they often violate the principles of justice and fairness we teach our children in school. Sometimes the differences between school and home or the community are simply cultural and social. Whatever the conflicts, the teacher must be prepared to deal with differences directly and must take care to facilitate understanding without being unnecessarily judgmental. The teacher can develop lessons that take into account the cultural and social differences among students, but it is most important that the teacher be interested, compassionate, and responsive. The teacher who is able to relate to students culturally, socially, and personally will be far more effective in helping children put conflict, confusion, and misunderstanding in perspective than the teacher who remains aloof and disinterested.

6. The teacher must recognize that children from different social and cultural backgrounds will react to a given communicative attempt in different ways. As we have already noted, dialects differ in the way words are used and defined. In fact, some words used in a given dialect may be unknown to speakers of other dialects. The same kinds of differences we observe in language can be observed in the nonverbal aspects of communication. There is then a great potential for miscommunication when classrooms are filled with children from differing cultural and social backgrounds and when the teacher may or may not share the cultural/social background of any of the students. It may be impossible to always avoid communicative confusion, but the teacher should certainly keep this potential in mind when developing and using teaching or assessment materials and techniques.

In closing this section, it must be emphasized that there will be greater cultural diversity in the classrooms of tomorrow than today. The proportion of children who are bilingual and bidialectal will continue to increase. An educational system that fails to adjust to the increasing social and cultural diversity of students is a system that will fail to educate. The consequences for failing to adequately educate all of our children will go far beyond the walls of our school buildings to permeate in destructive ways every aspect of American life as we hope and expect it to be.

Gender Differences in Language

In Chapter Six, we briefly discussed the emergence of gender differences in language. We noted that many of the language differences between men and women begin to show up in the communicative efforts of children as young as four and five years, and children recognize gender differences in the messages of others at a very young age. As we consider gender differences in language, we must always keep in mind that some differences between the sexes may be explained on the basis of biology, but very often they reflect variations in the way males and females are socialized. It is highly likely that many of the gender differences we observe in language are socialized differences and are not biologically based. We should take care, therefore, to understand these as differences without drawing unwarranted conclusions about how they have developed or what they mean.

Assuming Gender Roles

Consider the following riddle that has made its rounds for several generations. A young man was in a serious automobile accident and suffered injuries that required immediate surgery. He was rushed to the emergency room of the nearest hospital. It was obvious that the young man needed surgery, but the surgeon on duty, although not the patient's father, declined to perform the operation, saying, "I can't operate on this patient because he's my son." Why did the surgeon refuse to operate? Some people speculate that the surgeon was the patient's stepfather. Others assume that the surgeon was confused because the patient resembled his son. Some people, who are not myopic about gender roles, correctly conclude that the surgeon could not operate because she was the patient's mother.

When my youngest daughter was about eight years old, she came home from school one day in an especially excited mood. She could not wait to tell me that she had decided what she wanted to be when she grew up. She proudly announced that she wanted to be a nurse. When I asked why she did not want to be a doctor, she laughed. She told me that I was being silly because boys are doctors and girls are nurses. This was certainly not a perception consciously or deliberately taught at home, and when I asked her where she got the idea that girls could not be doctors, she could not tell me. Gender roles are so powerfully socialized, even though sometimes in subtle ways, that we may grow up and accept our roles without ever giving any thought to their origins or their validity.

Even though linguists argue about how much language affects the way we perceive things, most would agree that language does shape the way we think just as surely as the way we think shapes our language. Are perceptions of gender roles shaped by language? Are perceptions of gender roles reflected in the language we use? Both questions must be answered in the affirmative. Men refer to their boats

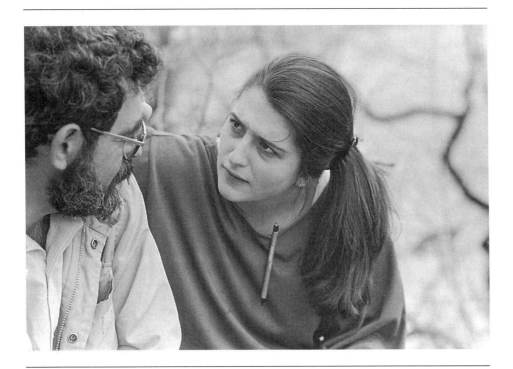

The gender gap in communication.

and cars as *she.* Draw your own conclusions about what these references suggest. When men refer to women as *babes* and *chicks,* what do we learn about their perceptions of women? When boys and girls grow up hearing the sexist labels we attach to both men and women, why are we surprised that they accept the stereotypical perceptions reflected in the labels?

Some gender differences in language are almost imperceptible but just as meaningful as the slang terms we use to identify men and women. Richmond and Gorham (1988) studied the use of gender referents in the written language of children in grades 3 through 12. The task was to write a story about a hypothetical classmate of unspecified gender. After reading a brief description of this student, the subjects were instructed to write a story about "how the hypothetical classmate would do in school." The investigators found that the male subjects of all ages used significantly more masculine referents (e.g. *he, his, him, the boy*) and fewer neutral referents (e.g. *they, their, the student*) than did the female subjects. Their female subjects, especially those in the lowest and highest grades, used nearly as many masculine referents as neutral referents. The males at all grade levels used almost no feminine referents (e.g. *she, her, the girl*). Among the female subjects, the number of feminine referents declined dramatically as age increased. Richmond and Gorham concluded that the trends in their research tend to support an earlier assertion (Nilsen, 1977) that young boys tend to perceive a neutral person as being male, and young girls tend to perceive a neutral person as being female, but the female perception does not endure. As females learn the language rule that when gender is not identified, assume male, they are less likely to perceive neutral persons as female. Boys, on the other hand, continue to perceive neutral persons as male, a perception reinforced by common language usage. In such subtle but powerful ways are language differences between the sexes created.

He Said . . . She Said

We have already identified some gender differences in Chapter Six. Let's review the highlights. Even though men and women include the same words in their vocabularies, they tend to select different words when they talk (Thorne, Kramerae, & Henley, 1983). Men tend to use profane and crude words more often than women, and women are more likely than men to use polite words such as *please, thank you,* and *you're welcome* (Greif & Berko-Gleason, 1980). Women also use words such as *darling, lovely,* and *adorable* more often than men and are more likely to name shades of colors. Men talk more than women (Swacher, 1975). Men are more likely to interrupt during conversations than women, and are more likely to interrupt women than men (Parlee, 1979). Only about one-third of the new topics introduced into conversation by women are retained, but almost all of the new topics introduced into conversation by men are retained (Ehrenreich, 1981). Mothers talk to their preschool daughters more than they talk to their preschool sons (Cherry & Lewis, 1976), and fathers use more endearing nicknames for their daughters than for their sons (Berko-Gleason & Greif, 1983).

Even though some writers caution that there is little solid empirical evidence of gender differences in American English (Warren-Luebecker & Bohannon, 1989), many writers and readers find the possibilities of sex-related language differences interesting and potentially enlightening. Are some differences clearly biological? Do language differences by gender tell us anything about what it means to be a man or woman? Is sexism reinforced by the way men and women use language, especially in reference to one another? Can we change the way people think about gender roles by changing the way they use language? We cannot satisfactorily answer all of these questions, but we can add some additional grist for your thoughts about these matters.

There is at least one aspect of oral communication that is, to some extent at least, biologically determined. The voice of the average man is lower in pitch than the voice of the average woman because adult males tend to have longer, thicker vocal folds than women. What is interesting, however, is that some of the vocal differences between men and women may be environmentally or socially determined. For example, women adjust their voices so that they sound like women, and men adjust their voices to sound like men (Sachs, Lieberman, & Erickson, 1973, p. 78). This means that a man may force his habitual pitch lower than it naturally should be, and a woman may force her habitual pitch higher than it should be to match some unspecified social standards for male and female voices. Another aspect of speech that may be socially determined is vocal variation. Women tend to use a wide range of pitches in all speaking situations, and they use their voices more expressively than men. Men tend to use their voices in a somewhat subdued and monotonous manner when they talk to adults, but use much greater vocal variation when they talk to young children (Warren-Leubecker & Bohannon, 1984). In other words, although both genders have the capability of vocal variation, men are much more selective about when and with whom they vary their voices.

What We Have Here Is a Failure to Communicate

Gender differences in communication are no more apparent than when men and women try to talk to one another. Sometimes even the most innocent topics create tension, frustration, and anger because men and women seem to be on different pages of the communication manual. Why do we have so much trouble talking to one another? When and why did the trouble begin? Deborah Tannen, a linguist and author of the best-selling *You Just Don't Understand: Women and Men in Conversation,* believes she has some answers to these questions.

According to Tannen (1990), the failure of men and women to communicate can be traced to the way boys and girls grow up. Although brothers and sisters may grow up in the same house with the same parents, they grow up in different worlds. Boys tend to play in large groups, and their play is activity-oriented. Their games have winners and losers, and there are elaborate rules about which the participants frequently argue. Boys brag about their own skills and argue about who is best. Speech is used in the context of play to achieve status and establish a hierarchy of superiority. They tell stories and jokes, and they interrupt and challenge one another to determine who is the quickest or wittiest. Boys with high status give orders to those with lower status. Speech is used as a tool of aggression, not only to establish one's status, but to defend one's position when verbally attacked.

Girls, according to Tannen (1990), play and communicate in very different ways. They tend to play in small groups or in pairs. Many of their activities, such as jump rope or playing house, do not have winners and losers. In fact, taking turns and sharing in the experience are emphasized, not winning. They do not boast about their skills, but are often self-deprecating because they want to be accepted and not be offensive. Rather than giving orders, girls are more inclined to try to manipulate the behaviors of others by offering suggestions or indicating their preferences. They do not maneuver for status because they are concerned that such maneuvering will cause others not to like them. Speech is used as a means for interacting with other people and for sharing feelings and thoughts.

Given their early life experiences, it is not surprising that adult men and women communicate differently, and that these differences often make communication between the sexes difficult. Tannen (1990) argues that while all people need intimacy and independence, women are more concerned with intimacy and men are more concerned with independence. The relative importance each gender gives to these needs is clearly reflected in the ways they talk to members of their own sex and to members of the opposite sex. Men use talking to convey information, to solve problems, to establish their positions within hierarchies of status. They often perceive the words of others as threats to their independence or challenges to their status. Many men who feel a strong need to be self-reliant are comfortable in giving information or advice to others but are not at all comfortable about accepting advice or information. Women, on the other hand, use talking to connect and interact with other people. They are very comfortable in using language to express their feelings. They talk to share, to demonstrate that they understand how the other person feels, and to be supportive. Many women are just as comfortable receiving information and advice as they are in giving it. It must be emphasized, of course, that all of these observations are generalizations. There are women who, in some circumstances if not all, communicate as men do and with the same apparent motivations. Likewise, there are men who have many of the communicative traits identified here with women. Furthermore, it is probably safe to assume that all speakers, regardless of gender, share some of the communicative needs and characteristics of the opposite sex some of the time. Nevertheless, the generalized differences are interesting.

Have you ever wondered, for example, why someone who is talkative in one situation may be silent in others? There are many reasons, of course, but Tannen (1990) suggests that there are gender reasons in many cases. Men tend to engage in what she calls "report talking." That is, they use talking to inform, impress, or persuade. This is the kind of talking one does in public settings such as at work, in meetings, or at parties. A man who is very talkative in these settings may be relatively silent at home because at home he does not have to prove himself. At home he is free to be quiet. Women, on the other hand, engage in what Tannen calls "rapport talking." They talk to establish, maintain, and cultivate relationships. They engage in very personal forms of communication. A woman who is talkative at home, a setting that allows for personal communication, may be relatively quiet in public settings because she is less comfortable in the role of information conveyor and more fearful of the negative and personal reactions her words might prompt. This gender difference creates a real and common problem. A wife cannot understand why her husband does not want to talk at home even though he cannot shut up at parties, and a husband cannot understand why his wife insists on talking at home when she says little or nothing in public meetings. The wife interprets her husband's silence at home to mean that he does not care about what she thinks or feels. The husband interprets his wife's insistence on conversation at home about what he perceives as trivial matters as nagging. What we have here is a classic case of a failure to communicate about communicative needs and expectations.

In her latest book, *Talking from 9 to 5, Women and Men in the Workplace: Language, Sex and Power,* Tannen (1994) suggests that the gender differences in communication can be observed in the way men and women try to get things done at work, they way they interact with their bosses and those they supervise, the way they develop relationships with their co-workers, and the way they try to position themselves to move up the corporate ladder. Even though some of these differences may cause you to smile or giggle knowingly, few of them will surprise you.

Tannen (1994, pp. 27–28) notes, for example, that while men at work are very willing to give information, they are reluctant to seek information. It may be that they are concerned about what others will think about them if they admit they do not know everything, and they may believe that asking for information puts the person who asks in a one-down relationship with the person from whom information is being solicited. Women, on the other hand, are quite willing to seek information. They apparently place far more importance on getting information they need than on how others will perceive them if they ask.

The communicative aggressiveness we observe in young boys continues to be part of the male style at work (Tannen, 1994, pp. 29–30). When men negotiate for the division of duties, for example, they will often try to grab what they want as early in the negotiating process as possible. A woman is more likely to open negotiations by asking the other person what he or she would like to do. If the other person is a man, he will likely interpret the question to be an invitation to seize what he wants, but the woman is probably extending an invitation to discuss the division of responsibilities before any decisions are made. The woman, just as she did as a child, attempts to be conciliatory in negotiations. She tries to create a win-win situation in that each party has a chance to identify what he or she would like to do and to explain why. After the discussion, the responsibilities will be divided according to ability and interest to the satisfaction of everyone. It does not always work out this way, of course, but that's the plan.

In reference to boys and girls, Tannen (1990) noted that boys play and interact in a manner that places a premium on being right, being the best, and being confident. Girls often react negatively to other girls who are too sure of themselves, too sure they are always right, or who are too confident for any reason. These same tendencies show up in adults at work (Tannen, 1994, pp. 35–36). Men are "more likely to downplay their doubts," whereas women are "more likely to downplay their certainty." It is interesting and revealing that adults of both sexes react to girls the same way that girls react to overly confident girls. While boys are often praised for being aggressive, girls are expected to keep their confidence and their aggressiveness in check. It does not require much of a stretch to see how these perceptions and expectations spill over into the adult world of work. A man who is assertive and confident is viewed positively. A woman with the same traits is often viewed negatively, by both men and women.

Conversation, including casual conversation, is a necessary part of the work experience. The fact that men and women talk differently can lead directly to communication breakdowns. A common communicative habit on the part of women is saying, "I'm sorry," when an apology is not called for and when an apology is not intended (Tannen, 1994, pp. 43–46). For example, a woman might give instructions to a subordinate. The subordinate, because of inattention or incompetence, fails to carry out the instructions. When the woman and the subordinate discuss what happened, the woman might begin by saying, "I'm sorry . . ." She is not apologizing in this case. She is trying to restore communicative balance. It's her way of saying, "We obviously had a breakdown in communication. Let's try again." Unfortunately, a man listening to or taking part in this exchange, might perceive that the woman is putting herself down. Men, you see, are far less likely than women to apologize, even when apologies are appropriate.

Tannen notes that the communicative rituals of apologizing, softening criticism, and thanking are more common in women than in men (1994, p. 56). All of these rituals depend on mutuality or balance. If a woman apologizes, for example, in a situation that clearly does not call for an apology and the other person accepts the apology, balance has been lost and the woman may be frustrated. If the other person dismisses the apology by saying something like, "There's no need to apologize. I'm the one who forgot what time we were supposed to meet," mutuality or balance has been maintained.

There are also communicative rituals involved in confrontational situations, and men and women tend to react differently to confrontation. Tannen (1994, p. 61) implies that men enjoy confrontation and women do not. Whereas men seem to thrive in situations where there are winners and losers, women would rather work things out so that all parties save face and remain friends.

The gender differences related to conversational topics follow through from childhood to adulthood. When men talk to men at work, their conversations are laced with comments about sports and politics. When women talk to women at work, they include comments about their personal lives, and women who are reluctant to share in these personal exchanges are viewed as cold or aloof. The topic differences are important because when people share a workplace, they establish personal and professional relationships by talking to one another, and the line between personal and professional is always a little fuzzy. It should be easy to understand why a man working in an office staffed by mostly women, if closed out of the personal conversations, would feel somewhat ostracized at a professional level. It is also easy to understand that a woman who does not feel welcome to join men when they talk about the NFL, the assets and liabilities of the 3-4 defense, and who will go high in next year's draft, will also feel left out as a co-worker.

Can the Gender Gap Be Bridged?

Is it possible for men and women to change the ways they talk and listen to one another? It is possible, of course, but as Tannen (1990, 1994) notes, most people expect the other person to change. We tend to view the way we communicate as not being in need of repair and probably as being superior to the way the other person communicates. A more reasonable expectation for both men and women is that we learn to understand and appreciate the communication needs, expectations, and strategies of both sexes. Two personal examples may illustrate common problems and reasonable solutions.

For many years, my wife and I have repeated the following scenario more times than I care to admit. She comes home from work after a troubling day during which she has felt overwhelmed by the volume of her work and frustrated by confrontations with one or more people with whom she must interact in the course of fulfilling her duties. I have always listened, but not always patiently, and certainly not with understanding, because as I listen, I am identifying the problems and conflicts that I believe are contributing to her vocational unhappiness. My responses to her are suggestions about how to solve her problems. She reacts with irritation to my suggestions. I am hurt because I believe I am trying to be helpful. In the context of Tannen's (1990) explanations of gender differences in communication, I now understand that my wife's recounting of the events of the day has nothing to do with identifying problems that beg for solutions. She wants to share with me, to be intimate about her feelings of frustration and anger. She does not want my advice. She just wants me to listen and express support and understanding. Knowing her needs, I am trying to become a better listener, and if necessary, I will bite my lip until I draw blood to prevent myself from offering advice when advice is not requested.

The second example is really the flip side of the first. When I have a particularly trying day, I want to retreat into the silence my home offers. For at least a few hours, I do not want to talk to anyone. Over the years, my wife has often interpreted this silence to mean that I am not happy to be home or that I am angry or upset about something. Because she is a rapport talker, she wants to connect with me. As my silence continues, she presses me for reasons, and if I say that nothing is wrong and I just do not want to talk, she perceives rejection. Now that she recognizes and understands the gender differences that account for my silence, she is more tolerant of my reticence. She leaves me alone for a time to revel in my quiet retreat. I, in turn, recognize that she has a powerful need to connect during our first few hours at home, so I compromise my silence after what seems an appropriate interval and give her an opportunity for the rapport talking she needs.

The conversational style differences between the sexes become problems only to the extent that we allow them to be problems. Understanding and compromise will not eliminate the differences, but they will do much to eliminate the gender friction that can be caused by the differences.

In closing this section, it must be emphasized that just as there is no language or dialect that is superior to any other language or dialect, there is no right or wrong about the way men and women talk. There is validity and value in the conversational style of each gender. Some of the disagreements that occur between men and women are exacerbated by differences in conversational style. When men and women argue, for example, men often use logical and reasonable arguments and accuse women of being too emotional. If we understand that because men use language to convey information and to impress and persuade, they tend to argue in a manner that emphasizes logic and reason, and that because women use language to connect and establish rapport, they tend to argue in a manner that emphasizes feelings and attitudes, the argument can focus on the issue of the conflict and not on the manner in which the argument is being waged. In the final analysis, we should consider that we may communicate best as we develop an integrated style of communication which includes elements of the male and female styles. Perhaps that is the most important lesson to be learned from gender differences in language and communication.

Review Questions

1. Identify language differences you associate with each of the seven variables that influence the acquisition of language and language behaviors according to Taylor (1990).

2. Differentiate the following terms: language, dialect, and accent.

3. What are the issues surrounding the use and understanding of labels such as standard dialect and nonstandard dialect?

4. What are some of the factors that account for the development of regional dialects in the United States?

5. Identify some of the lexical features of the dialects spoken in each of the following regions and offer an explanation for how these dialectal features have developed: New England Region, Northern and Midwest Region, and the Southern Region.

6. Trace the origins of Black English, incorporating explanations of the terms pidgin, creole, and decreolization.

7. How does the production of negation in Black English compare to the production of negation in Standard English?

8. What is the syntactic device, aspect? Provide examples of aspect expressed in Black English.

9. What are interference points, and what impact do they have on the development of social/cultural dialects?

10. Identify several phonological and several syntactic features of Hispanic English and explain why they occur.

11. What problems are created in American classrooms by a mix of dialects? How can we address these problems without violating the social and cultural rights of students from widely divergent backgrounds?

12. What do gender differences in communication seem to suggest about differences between women and men, girls and boys?

13. How do gender differences interfere with communication between women and men?

14. How might gender communication differences impact how work is conducted when a woman is the boss and many of her subordinates are men? When a man is the boss and many of his subordinates are women?

15. How might a woman's communicative strategies affect her ability to negotiate for a raise or for a promotion?

16. Can the gender gap be bridged? If so, how? If not, why not?

References and Suggested Readings

Abercrombie, D. (1967). *Elements of general phonetics.* Edinburgh: University Press.

Allen, H., & Linn, M. (Eds.) (1986). *Dialect and language variation.* Orlando, FL: Academic Press.

Bailey, G., & Maynor, N. (1989). The divergence controversy. *American Speech, 64,* 12–13.

Battles, D. (1983). Social dialects. *ASHA, 25,* 23–24.

Bebout, L., & Arthur, B. (1992). Cross-cultural attitudes toward speech disorders. *Journal of Speech and Hearing Research, 35,* 45–52.

Berko-Gleason, J., and Greif, E. (1983). Men's speech to young children. In B. Thorne, C. Kramerae, & N. Henley (Eds.), *Language, gender, and society.* Rowley, MA: Newbury House.

Bernthal, J., and Bankson, N. (1993). *Articulation and Phonological Disorders.* Englewood Cliffs, NJ: Prentice Hall.

Bowman, B. (1989). Educating language-minority children: Challenges and opportunities. *Phi Delta Kappan, 71,* 118–120.

Bryen, D. (1978). *Variant English: An introduction to language variation.* Columbus, OH: Merrill.

Campbell, L. (1993). Maintaining the integrity of home linguistic varieties: Black English vernacular. *American Journal of Speech-Language Pathology, 2,* 11–12.

Campbell, L. (1994). Discourse diversity and Black English vernacular. In D. Ripich & N. Creaghead (Eds.), *School Discourse Problems* (2nd ed.). San Diego, CA: Singular Group Publishing.

Carver, C. (1987). *American regional dialects: A word geography.* Ann Arbor, MI: University of Michigan Press.

Cherry, L., & Lewis, M. (1976). Mothers and two-year-olds: A study of sex differentiated aspects of verbal interaction. *Developmental Psychology, 12,* 278–282.

Cole, P., & Taylor, O. (1990). Performance of working class African-American children on three tests of articulation. *Language, Speech, Hearing Services in Schools, 21,* 171–176.

Cummins, J. (1989). A theoretical framework for bilingual special education. *Exceptional Children, 56,* 111–119.

Dillard, J. (1973). *Black English: Its history and usage in the United States.* New York: Vintage Books.

Edwards, W., and Winford, D. (1991). *Verb Phrase Patterns in Black English and Creole.* Detroit, MI: Wayne State University Press.

Ehrenreich, B. (1981). The politics of talking in couples. *Ms, 5,* 43–45, 86–89.

Fasold, R. (1984). *The sociolinguistics of society.* London: Basil Blackwell.

Figueroa, R. (1989). Psychological testing of linguistic-minority students: Knowledge gaps and regulations. *Exceptional Children, 56,* 145–152.

Francis, W. (1987). *Dialectology: An introduction.* New York: Longman, Inc.

Greif, E., & Berko-Gleason, J. (1980). Hi, thanks, and goodbye: More routine information. *Language in Society, 9,* 159–166.

Hakuta, K., & Garcia, E. (1989). Bilingualism and education. *The American Psychologist, 44,* 374–379.

Harbaugh, M. (1990). Celebrating diversity. *Instructor, 100,* 45–48.

Haskins, J., & Butts, H. (1973). *The psychology of black language.* New York: Harper & Row Publishers.

Labov, W. (1966). *The social stratification of English in New York City.* Washington, DC: Center for Applied Linguistics.

Naremore, R. (1980). Language variation in a multicultural society. In T. Hixon, L. Shriberg, & J. Saxman, (Eds.), *Introduction to communication disorders.* Englewood Cliffs, NJ: Prentice-Hall.

Naremore, R., & Hopper, R. (1990). *Children learning language* (3rd ed.). New York: Harper & Row Publishers.

Nilsen, A. (1977). Sexism in children's books and elementary teaching materials. In A. Nilsen et al. (Eds.), *Sexism and language.* Urbana, IL: National Council of Teachers of English.

Parlee, M. (1979). Conversational politics. *Psychology Today, 5,* 48–56.

Richmond, V., & Gorham, J. (1988). Language patterns and gender role orientation among students in grades 3–12. *Communication Education, 37,* 142–149.

Ripich, D., and Creaghead, N. (Eds.) (1994). *School Discourse Problems* (2nd ed.). San Diego, CA: Singular Publishing Group.

Robbins, J. (1988). Employers' language expectations and nonstandard dialect speakers. *English Journal, 77,* 22–24.

Sachs, J., Lieberman, P., & Erickson, D. (1973). Anatomical and cultural determinants of male and female speech. In R. Schuy & R. Fasold (Eds.), *Language attitudes: Current trends and prospects.* Washington, DC: Georgetown University Press.

Schneider, E. (1989). *American Earlier Black English.* Tuscaloosa, AL: The University of Alabama Press.

Smitherman, G. (1994). *Black Talk, Words and Phrases from the Hood to the Amen Corner.* New York: Houghton Mifflin Company.

Suhor, C. (1988). "English only" movement emerging as a major controversy. *Educational Leadership, 46,* 80–81.

Swacher, M. (1975). The sex of the speaker as a sociolinguistic variable. In B. Thorne & N. Henley (Eds.), *Language and sex: Difference and dominance.* Rowley, MA: Newbury House.

Taylor, O. (1972). An introduction to the historical development of Black English: Some implications for American education. *Language, Speech, and Hearing Services in the Schools, 3,* 5–15.

Taylor, O. (Ed.) (1986). *Nature of communication disorders in culturally and linguistically diverse populations.* San Diego, CA: College-Hill Press.

Taylor, O. (1990). Language and language differences. In G. Shames & E. Wiig (Eds.), *Human communication disorders* (3rd ed.). Columbus, OH: Merrill/Macmillan.

Tannen, D. (1990). *You just don't understand: Women and men in conversation.* New York: William E. Morrow & Company.

Tannen, D. (1994). Talking from 9 to 5, women and men in the workplace: Language, sex and power. New York, Avon Books.

Terrell, S. (1983). Effects of speaking Black English upon employment opportunities. *ASHA, 25,* 27–29.

Thorne, B., Kramerae, C., & Henley, N. (Eds.) (1983). *Language, gender, and society.* Rowley, MA: Newbury House.

Warren-Leubecker, A., & Bohannon, J. (1984). Intonation patterns in child-directed speech: Mother-father differences. *Child Development, 55,* 1379–1385.

Warren-Leubecker, A., & Bohannon, J. (1989). Pragmatics: Language in social contexts. In J. Berko-Gleason (Ed.), *The development of language* (2nd ed.). Columbus, OH: Merrill/Macmillan.

West, C., & Garcia, A. (1988). Conversational shift work: A study of topical transitions between women and men. *Social Problems, 35,* 551–571.

Wiener, F., Lewnau, L., & Erway, E. (1983). Measuring language competency in speakers of Black American English. *Journal of Speech and Hearing Disorders, 48,* 76–84.

Williams, R., & Wolfram, W. (1977). *Social dialects: Difference versus disorder.* Rockville, MD: American Speech-Language-Hearing Association.

Winsboro, B., & Solomon, I. (1990). Standard English vs. the American dream. *Educational Digest, 56,* 51–52.

Wolfram, W., & Christian, D. (1989). *Dialects and education: Issues and answers.* Englewood Cliffs, NJ: Prentice-Hall.

NINE

Speech and Language Disorders

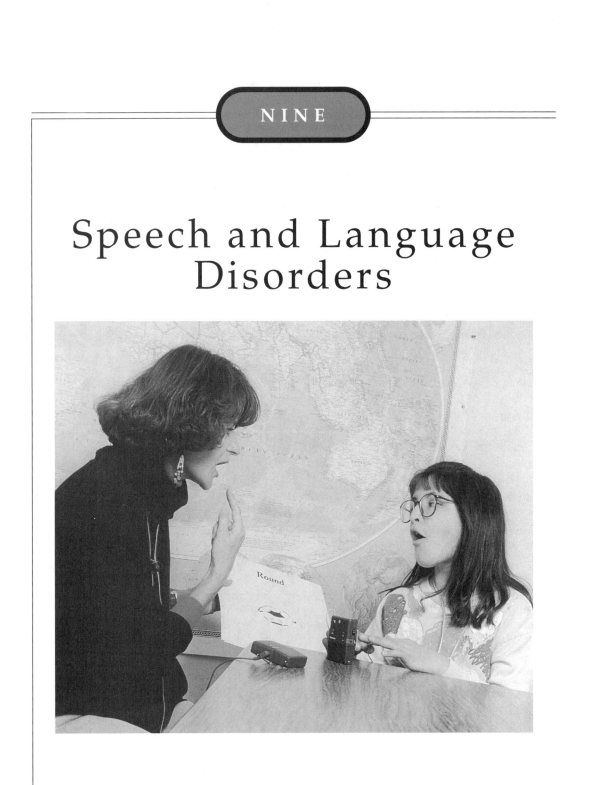

Chapter Objectives

The overwhelming majority of humans acquire speech and language without difficulty, but occasionally there are problems, either during the acquisition period, or later in life after speech and language have been normal for a time. Communication disorders develop for many reasons, including environmental deprivation, faulty learning, emotional conflicts, disease, and physical trauma. In this chapter, we consider some common speech and language disorders, with special attention to those disorders most likely to affect children. Specifically, this chapter is designed to facilitate understanding of the following topics:

- Differentiating between normal and abnormal speech and language.
- The classification of communication disorders.
- The use of the terms *organic* and *functional* when categorizing disorders according to etiology.
- Phonological disorders.
- Language impairments.
- Voice disorders.
- Fluency disorders, with an emphasis on stuttering.

The acquisition of speech and language is so natural that we may not truly appreciate the complexities and power of human oral communication unless or until something goes wrong. About 10 percent of Americans have speech, language, or hearing problems (Larkins, 1985; Leske, 1981a and 1981b), and this number is likely to increase as people live longer. Some may be surprised that this many people have communication disorders. When I consider how much language knowledge the child must acquire, how quickly he acquires it, and the incredible neuromuscular mechanisms that must be coordinated to make speech work, I am amazed more people do not have communication problems. In fact, I often wonder how any of us master the mysterious and magical processes of speech and language.

Falling Short of Normal Communication

Before we proceed, it is important to note that the 10 percent prevalence figure we have cited tells only part of the story about how many people have communication problems. If we exclude hearing disorders, for example, the prevalence figure drops considerably. Fein (1983) suggests that the prevalence of speech and language disorders in the United States is about 4 percent. Shewan (1988), using numbers from several sources, suggests it may be about 6 percent. More importantly, Shewan and Malm (1990) emphasize that a single prevalence figure for speech and language disorders is misleading because communication disorders are not evenly distributed throughout the population. Prevalence figures vary depending upon age, gender, racial/ethnic background, and even geographic region.

Defining Communication Defects

In this chapter, we will examine the major communication disorders affecting children. We must begin by addressing the issue of **abnormality.** What constitutes a communication defect? This may seem a simple question, but it is, in fact, such a difficult question that experts in speech-language pathology have failed to come to any uniform definition. The problem in defining communication defects becomes immediately obvious when we try to define **normal** speech and language.

How many words are included in a normal vocabulary? How fast is normal speech? What is a normal voice? How hesitant or nonfluent must speech be before we call it stuttering? How precisely must one produce speech sounds to be considered normal? I trust you are beginning to see a trend here. The range of normal along every dimension of speech is tremendous. We have no exact standards for how much language a normal speaker has or even for how well he uses the language he has. We have vague ideas about acceptable male and female voices, but most of us have a tolerance for voices that go beyond even our own standards. We may notice that well-known television journalists like Tom Brokaw and Barbara

Walters have some problems with "r" and "l," but few of us would consider these individuals speech-defective. There are people we would all agree are normal speakers who are more nonfluent than other people we would all agree are stutterers. So how do we determine what is a communication defect?

One of the most widely used definitions of defective speech is offered by Van Riper and Erickson (1996, p. 110): "Speech is impaired when it deviates so far from the speech of other people that it (1) calls attention to itself, (2) interferes with communication, or (3) provokes distress in the speaker or the listener." The advantage of this kind of definition is that it focuses our attention on what might be called the keys of communication abnormality. Van Riper and Erickson suggest, in fact, that their definition can be reduced to three key adjectives: *conspicuous, unintelligible,* and *unpleasant* (1996, p. 111). The disadvantage of this definition, in either the long or short form, is that it is very subjective. Nevertheless, it provides an appropriate foundation for understanding what is meant by disordered or defective communication.

Most communication disorders, in their most severe forms, are **conspicuous.** You have perhaps observed a severe stutterer whose face becomes distorted as he struggles to get out a single word. Maybe you have listened to a cleft palate individual who is so excessively nasal that you pay more attention to the quality of his voice than to the content of his words. Whenever speech is so far removed from normal that listeners' attentions are more drawn to the manner of speech than to the message being conveyed, it may be considered defective. Keep in mind, however, that a manner of speech conspicuous to one person might be ignored or considered perfectly normal by someone else. The nasal quality of a Texas dialect might be very conspicuous in Iowa but would be unnoticed in Dallas.

When speech differences reduce **intelligibility,** that is, when they interfere with the ability of listeners to understand what is being said, there is probably a communication disorder. We have all listened to youngsters who do not have complete sound systems. They leave out so many sounds, or substitute for them, that we can understand little of what they are trying to say. A speaker's voice might be so hoarse, or nasal, or breathy that we literally cannot understand the words he is trying to speak. Fluency problems can sometimes occur with such frequency and severity that intelligibility is reduced. One might conclude that reduced intelligibility is a fairly exact parameter of defective speech, but such a conclusion would not be entirely justified. When a child is 24 months old, we would not expect his speech to be completely intelligible, and if we could understand only half of what he was trying to say, we would probably not consider his speech defective, but if the same child, at the age of six years, was still only 50 percent intelligible, we would undoubtedly agree that his speech was defective. In addition, reduced intelligibility might be the consequence of regional or cultural dialects, and as we established in the preceding chapter, dialectal differences are not considered defects.

Deciding what is **unpleasant** to the speaker or his listeners might be the most troubling aspect of understanding disordered speech. We have grown up hearing the expression, "Beauty is in the eye of the beholder." "Unpleasant" is also the product of individual perception. The range of tolerance for speech differences is as wide as the range of tolerance for all other human differences. In the speech-language pathology business, we sometimes talk about colleagues with "long ears," which means these people hear problems most of us would ignore. They have little tolerance for speech differences. Other people can and do accept almost all kinds of speech differences as normal unless the differences reduce intelligibility. It would probably be fair to say that we would not call speech defective, on the basis of listeners' perceptions, unless *many* people find the difference unpleasant.

The only single perception that really matters is that of the speaker. If he considers his speech difference to be unpleasant, it really does not matter if anyone else agrees or not, especially if the rest of us cannot persuade him that nothing is wrong with his speech. An episode from my own clinical past will help make this point. A young man came to our clinic as a self-referral because he was concerned about what he called his stuttering problem. Two graduate students, under my supervision, evaluated his speech for about two hours. During that time, he did not produce a single behavior the students or I considered abnormal. When the evaluation ended, I asked the students what they concluded. They looked at one another, obviously concerned I had noticed something they had missed. We all agreed, however, that this young man sounded very normal and was, in fact, more fluent than the majority of normal speakers we all knew. When we shared our conclusions with the client, he was terribly upset. How could we not have noticed a problem which had troubled him since high school? He was absolutely convinced he was a stutterer, and he would not leave until he convinced us. I asked him to demonstrate to us exactly what he did when he stuttered. He picked up a college-level chemistry textbook, read aloud, and stumbled on a few words with which he was not familiar. This, he claimed, was his stuttering. When we failed to convince him that it was normal for speakers to hesitate and struggle a little with unfamiliar or difficult words, we agreed to enroll him in therapy because his speech difference was causing him to be distressed.

And now for the rest of the story. We designed a therapy to deal specifically with his perception of unpleasantness. He believed his problem was limited to oral reading, especially the oral reading of technical material. We had him read aloud for two or three minutes and asked him to evaluate his performance. We accepted whatever he said, especially in the beginning. If he identified words on which he "stuttered," we had him say these words in isolation perhaps five times, and then we had him put the words back into context and read entire sentences aloud. This exercise always resulted in fluent productions. We praised his efforts and the results. As time passed, his self-evaluations became more positive, and he actually became more tolerant of his nonfluencies. Each time he said something positive about his speech, we concurred, and told him he was making excellent progress. At the end of six weeks, he pronounced himself well and asked to be dismissed. We agreed, with the stipulation that he call us on a regular basis to let us know how things were going. He not only kept us informed about his continuing success, but he sent me Christmas cards for about five years telling me how wonderful we had been in helping him overcome his problem. In this case, there was nothing conspicuous about his speech, and he certainly was not unintelligible, but he did experience unpleasantness. Once the unpleasantness was gone, the problem was solved. I wish all communication disorders could be handled so easily!

Before we proceed to some specific communication disorders, I want to add an important footnote to the definition of defective speech. Even if we can agree on the basic parameters included in the definition discussed above, who decides whether they apply in a specific case? Who makes the judgment about whether a speech difference is a defect or simply a difference? I want to offer the viewpoint of a widely respected expert in speech-language pathology, a viewpoint I happen to share. According to Oliver Bloodstein (1979, p. 5), "the speaker is the one most competent to decide whether a speech disorder exists." There are undoubtedly many speech-language pathologists who disagree with this view. After all, they might argue, the physician does not or should not allow his patients to make their own diagnoses. Why should the speech-language pathologist allow speakers to decide whether or not they have speech disorders? Perhaps the best answer to this question is that speech disorders are not life-threatening. The speech-language pathologist can and should advise the client about how his speech deviates from normal, but the client must decide if this deviation is sufficient to warrant therapy. The client who is not convinced he has a communication disorder is not motivated to modify his speech behaviors, and an unmotivated client is not likely to make progress in therapy.

Obviously if the client is a child, we must amend this view. Children are not sophisticated or mature enough to make decisions about the appropriateness of their speech and language behaviors. I raise the issue, however, to emphasize how difficult it is to define defective speech.

The Classification of Communication Disorders

Communication disorders are usually classified according to their symptoms or their causes. When we classify by **symptoms,** we identify four disorder categories: (1) **phonological** disorders, which are problems with the production of speech sounds; (2) **language** impairments, which include difficulties in understanding and/or using the symbols of speech; (3) **voice** disorders, including a wide range of abnormalities in the laryngeal tone from the vocal folds to the resonating cavities that modify that tone into what we recognize as the voice; and (4) **fluency** disorders, which are problems affecting the rhythm, rate, or forward flow of speech.

When we classify communication disorders by **causes** or **etiologies,** we must first differentiate between organic disorders and functional disorders, and this differentiation is not as simple as it may first appear. One might assume that these terms represent opposite ends of a continuum, that functional means nonorganic. It is not accurate to use these terms as though they represent a dichotomy.

An **organic** disorder is caused by a demonstrable pathology of an organ system. If, for example, a cleft palate child cannot produce a "p" sound because every time he puts his lips together to build up pressure for the production of "p," the air escapes through the opening in the roof of his mouth and out of his nose, this is clearly an organic articulation problem. Or, if a child's voice has been normal until his vocal folds become infected and swollen, and his voice becomes hoarse, this is an organic voice problem.

Now consider what functional means. A disorder is considered **functional** if, after using the best diagnostic procedures and technologies available, we fail to identify a pathology of an organ system. This does not necessarily mean that there is not a pathology. It simply means that if there is an organic etiology, we have not been able to identify it. We generally use the term functional to describe disorders we believe are the result of learning, psychological, or environmental factors, but we need to be careful that we do not think of functional and nonorganic as synonyms.

Not many years ago, depression was widely understood as a psychological problem. We now understand that depression can be the result of biochemical imbalances that can be treated with medications. Until recently, alcoholism was viewed as strictly an environmental problem. We now understand that some people are genetically predisposed to alcoholism. These and similar conditions afflicting human beings cannot be easily dismissed as nonorganic, although there are undoubtedly cases of depression and alcoholism that are psychological and environmental.

There are many children who have problems with phonology or language that are identified as functional communication disorders. In some cases, there may be organic etiologies we are not able to identify. In many other cases, children have speech and language problems for reasons that have nothing to do with the integrities of their organ systems. If, for example, a child is reared in an environment that provides little or no speech and language simulation, or if he is reared by parents who are physically or emotionally abusive, we will not be surprised if there are communication disorders, and if the child's speech and language patterns are consistent with environmental or psychological causative factors, we will feel comfortable referring to these patterns as functional communication disorders.

Against this broad introductory background, we now examine some of the common communication disorders we see in children. The main headings refer to symptomatic categories, but we also consider etiologies within each category.

Phonological Disorders

For the past 20 years, speech-language pathologists have been in something of a quandary about the terminology used to describe speech sound disorders. Prior to the quandary, we referred to these problems as *articulation* disorders, but over the past two decades we have come to understand that the production of speech sounds is not limited to the speech apparatus; that it is more directly connected to language than we once thought, and that it is a rule-governed process, not just a mechanical process. We needed another, more comprehensive, term. The term that has been widely adopted is *phonology. Articulation* has been retained, but it is more narrowly defined today than it was 20 years ago. Some people might regard this fussing about terms to be much ado about little, but the difference between *articulation* and *phonology* is important in reference to understanding the etiologies of speech sound production problems and treating these problems.

Fey (1992) noted that "the notion of phonology and its role in Speech Pathology is a source not just of debate, but of bewilderment." The problem, it seems, is that many people are convinced that if we adopt the term *phonology,* we are obligated to discontinue using the term *articulation.* The fact is, the two terms, when used properly, co-exist without difficulty. What we are obligated to do is to understand how these two terms are related to one another conceptually. Fey offers an excellent beginning point by defining articulation as "the processes involved in the planning and execution of smooth sequences of highly overlapping gestures of the speech organs." In short, articulation is concerned with the motor aspects of speech production. Conceptually, phonology is a much broader term. It subsumes articulation, but goes far beyond the physical production of speech sounds to include the perceptual and cognitive aspects of speech sound production and understanding, as well as the rule system that governs how sounds are combined. In acquiring his speech sound system, for example, the child must learn that some consonants can be sequenced and others cannot. He must learn that some consonants can be used to open and close syllables, whereas others can only be used to open syllables or only to close syllables.

Clarifying the terms *articulation* and *phonology* leads us to a better understanding about how speech sound problems are categorized. To say that a child has an **articulation problem** means that he cannot physically produce a given sound. It is not in his inventory of sounds. For example, the child who cannot produce an "s" because his cleft palate will not allow him to trap air in his mouth so that he can force air through the narrow constriction between his tongue and alveolar ridge, has an articulation problem. Another child might be able to produce "s" in isolation, and he might be able to produce it correctly in some contexts, but he does not produce it correctly in all contexts. Perhaps he deletes "s" in the postvocalic position because he deletes all sounds that, given a place and manner of articulation, can be either voiced or voiceless. Perhaps he produces "s" when it is a single sound, but he deletes "s" when it occurs in sequences. If the child has the physical ability to produce "s" and produces it correctly in some contexts but not in all contexts, he has a **phonological disorder** in the sense that he is having a problem with some aspect of his speech sound system, but he does not have an **articulation disorder** because he is physically capable of producing the target sound. Because it is not always possible to isolate the articulatory portion of speech sound production from all other aspects of the speech sound system, we will refer to all speech sound production problems as **phonological disorders.** We will note, however, that in many cases, the speech sound problems associated with either structural defects of the speech mechanism or with neuropathologies that affect the function of the speech mechanism are primarily **articulation disorders.**

Etiologies of Phonological Disorders

When we classify phonological disorders according to etiology, we can identify three broad categories: (1) phonological disorders resulting from structural abnormalities in or around the mouth; (2) phonological disorders resulting from neuropathologies; and (3) phonological disorders of a functional origin.

In the chapter on the development of phonology, we briefly examined three approaches to describing normal and nonstandard speech sounds: traditional phonetics, distinctive features, and phonological processes. No matter which descriptive approach we use, however, speech sound errors take four basic forms. A speech sound might be **deleted,** as when the child says "bu" for *bus.* He might **substitute** one sound for another as when he says "thoup" for *soup.* If he produces the target sound, but there is a slight deviation in his production, we describe his effort as a **distortion.** In some cases, the child will **add** a sound that should not be present as when he says "fʌrog" for *frog.*

The sounds affected and the specific nature of errors depend on the etiology of the disorder, and of course, there are individual variations among speakers who have what appears to be the same etiological condition. For the sake of this discussion, we assume a uniformity of errors within each etiological category so you can see how a given condition is most likely to affect phonological acquisition and production, but keep in mind that the greatest consistency among phonologically disordered speakers is tremendous inconsistency.

Phonological Disorders Associated with Structural Defects

A speaker, child or adult, sometimes has difficulty with speech sound production because there is a structural defect in or around the mouth. These are called **orofacial** defects. If a phonological problem is the consequence of an orofacial defect, it is an articulation disorder. That is, the individual *cannot physically produce* the affected speech sounds. It is possible, of course, for someone to have an orofacial defect that does not cause a phonological problem. A child might have a deviation in his dental occlusion or bite. This is an orofacial defect, but not every person with a malocclusion develops speech sound problems. We must keep in mind that a person who has a phonological problem that is directly connected to an orofacial defect might have other speech sound problems that are not related to the orofacial defect. It also happens that some individuals have obvious orofacial defects, but have no speech sound problems as a consequence, even though they do have speech sound problems for other reasons. The moral of this story is that you do not always get what seems obvious. The speech-language pathologist learns that one should not assume that a phonological disorder is related to an orofacial defect unless the error patterns are consistent with the orofacial defect. Does all this really matter? Of course it does. If a phonological disorder is the direct result of an orofacial defect, speech treatment will be of little or no value until we do whatever we can to correct or compensate for the orofacial defect.

Congenital Clefts

Among the most serious orofacial defects that almost always affect speech are congenital clefts of the lip and/or palate. We call these clefts congenital to indicate that they are present at birth. The face, including the lips and the palate, develops as the various parts fuse together during the first trimester of pregnancy. If something happens to interrupt the normal fusion of these parts, the child is born with splits in these structures where they should have been joined together. Depending on exactly when and how the growth is interrupted, the child will be born with a variety of clefts, ranging from a partial cleft of the upper lip to a complete bilateral cleft of the lip together with a complete cleft of the hard and soft palates. Obviously, the more extensive the cleft, the more extensive the speech problems are likely to be. Few of these children grow up without some speech difficulties.

Clefts occur for a variety of reasons, including heredity, oxygen deprivation, rubella, maternal diet, medications taken by the mother during pregnancy, or even because a body part of the developing fetus gets in the way of the parts that need to fuse.

The problems encountered by the cleft palate child and his parents can be extensive and overwhelming, and more of these children are surviving birth today than several generations ago because of advances in medical science. This child is typically treated by a team of specialists, which might include a **plastic surgeon, pediatrician, orthodontist** (teeth straightener), **prosthodontist** (specialist who creates devices to cover or compensate for clefts), **psychologist** to help the child and his parents with the emotional problems often associated with clefts, **audiologist** (evaluates hearing problems that are frequent in this population), and the **speech-language pathologist,** who not only administers speech therapy but advises other specialists about how to best prepare the speech mechanism for optimal results. With the help of these and other specialists, the outlook for the cleft palate child is not nearly as bleak as it might appear at birth.

The speech problems that result directly from clefts are related to inadequacy of the velopharyngeal mechanism, described in Appendix A. The child has difficulty with most consonants, but especially with plosives, fricatives, and affricates because these sounds require a great deal of intraoral breath pressure.

Because the child cannot effectively close the passageway between his mouth and his nasal cavities, he cannot trap air in his mouth. The air escapes through his nose. In addition, his speech is hypernasal because the nasal cavities are permanently coupled with the oral cavity. Until the treatment team is able to close the cleft surgically or with prosthetic devices, speech therapy will have limited success.

Defects of the Tongue

Since most speech sounds involve placement or movement of the tongue, if this structure is defective in some way, speech is likely to be affected. Sometimes the tongue is too large, a condition called **macroglossia.** Actually there are no absolute dimensions for a normal-sized tongue, so macroglossia means that a given tongue is too large for the mandible in which it lies. If we transplanted the tongue of a 7'4", 500-pound man into a 5'2", 120-pound man, we would almost certainly have a case of macroglossia, but in the mouth of the large man, the large tongue would be just right. The phonological problems associated with macroglossia are predictable. Since there is not enough room for normal movement, speech sounds are slurred and nondistinct.

A more common problem with the tongue is a condition called **ankyglossia,** known more commonly as tongue-tie. There are two forms of ankyglossia. Sometimes the lingual frenum, a thin connective tissue under the tongue, inserts too close to the tongue's tip. If the tongue's mobility is significantly restricted by the frenum, it can be surgically clipped. In the other form of ankyglossia, the muscular root of the tongue inserts at or near the tip. This is a much more serious condition that can be relieved by surgery, but when we begin to cut into muscle, we risk permanent neuromuscular impairment. It is most important to note that what looks like ankyglossia seldom is. If a child can place the tip of his tongue between his teeth and raise it to the alveolar ridge, he probably has adequate mobility for normal speech.

Dental Malocclusions

Dental malocclusions are the most common orofacial defects, but they are also the least significant, at least in terms of speech. The term malocclusion literally means bad closure, and that is a fairly apt description of what we see. When the dentist asks you to bite down normally, he looks to see how your upper and lower teeth line up, using the first molars as the fixed points of reference. In a normal bite, the upper teeth are aligned a little ahead of the lower teeth. If the molars line up as they should, but the teeth in the front of the mouth are crooked, the condition is called **neutrocclusion,** a common problem frequently corrected by the orthodontist and miles and miles of wire. When the upper teeth bite too far ahead of the lower teeth, the deviation is called **distocclusion,** or more commonly overbite. **Mesiocclusion,** or underbite, refers to a bite in which the lower teeth are too far forward. Neutrocclusion and distocclusion usually have little effect on speech, but mesiocclusion can cause some phonological problems because when the lower jaw protrudes, the relationships of the oral structures are significantly disturbed. Try speaking with your lower jaw protruded, and you will quickly see that it is difficult to produce many of the consonants, especially labial sounds like "p," "b," "w," "f," and "v" and tongue-tip consonants like, "t," "d," "s," "n," and "l." In the case of any malocclusion, appropriate dental treatment before and during speech therapy is important, but parents need to understand that orthodontia alone will rarely correct the phonological disorders associated with malocclusions because the articulatory habits established before orthodontia are often firmly established and can be corrected only through speech therapy.

Dysarthria

The term **dysarthria** properly refers to a range of neurogenic motor speech disorders, including communication problems associated with neuromuscular impairments in respiration, phonation, resonation, prosody, and articulation. To understand the range of articulation problems in dysarthria, it is important to remember that the nervous system begins in the brain and includes the spinal cord and the countless nervous pathways that course throughout the body. A dysarthria can result from a problem in any speech-associated part of this pervasive and complex system.

If the damage occurs to the cranial nerves originating in the brain stem or in other segments of the peripheral nervous system, the resulting speech disorder is called **lower motor neuron dysarthria.** The common symptoms of this form of dysarthria are muscular weakness or paralysis and reduction or loss of muscle tone. Articulatory efforts are weak, labored, and imprecise, and virtually every other component of the speech mechanism is similarly affected. In severe cases, there may be no speech at all.

If there is a communication disorder as the result of damage to the upper motor centers of the brain, the condition is called **upper motor neuron dysarthria.** This is often the major speech problem in the cerebral palsied person. Although there may be weakness or loss of motion and reduced or abolished muscle tone in these patients, the most dominant characteristic is incorrect execution of movement and faulty coordination. Imagine what it would be like to have no control over how much the muscles of speech contract, or to have movements superimposed on speech over which you have no control, or to have the processes of speech out of synchronization. These are some of the problems encountered by cerebral palsied individuals when they try to speak. As with lower motor neuron dysarthria, every component of speech from respiration to articulation is likely to be adversely affected.

Therapy for dysarthric clients focuses on helping them gain maximal control over the neuromuscular abilities they have. By helping these people learn to carefully monitor what they feel and hear as they speak, and by using repetitive drill work designed to achieve optimal articulatory accuracy, it may be possible to facilitate some improvement in overall communication performance.

Developmental Phonological Disorders

The majority of phonological disorders are considered functional. As noted earlier, this means that although many of these disorders have nonorganic causes, there may be others that have organic etiologies which we simply cannot identify because our diagnostic procedures and technologies are not sensitive or sophisticated enough.

One factor that plays a role in most, if not all, phonological disorders is **habit strength.** If a child uses inappropriate articulatory habits that are purposely or inadvertently reinforced by adult listeners, these habits may persist, and the longer they do persist, the stronger they become. Articulatory habits are particularly difficult to break for a couple of reasons. By definition, motor habits are automatic, but articulatory habits are more automatic than others because speech is natural and instinctive in humans. These habits are also more difficult to monitor than some other habits because when we talk, we pay little or no attention to the act of speaking. Our focus is on sending and receiving messages. Habit strength, therefore, is a factor in almost all phonological disorders, no matter what the original cause may have been.

Environmental influences can certainly affect speech in positive or negative ways. Although a child's biological drive to acquire speech is sufficiently strong to overcome a poor speech and language environment, we cannot ignore these influences. In the extreme, if a child is reared in isolation, his oral output will consist of undifferentiated vocalized noises, including emotional interjections. The child must be exposed to models of speech if he is to learn how to speak. These models, usually provided by his parents, are critical to what the child learns about speech and language in his early years and to how well and quickly he learns it. Why does a child born in Main Street City, USA, speak English? He speaks English, of course, because that is the language to which he is exposed. If the version of English to which he is exposed is in Texas dialect, he will speak like a Texan. It is true, of course, that one or two poor communication models will probably not have long-term negative effects on the speech of a child because they will be balanced by many other, more appropriate models, but it would be a mistake to assume that what the child hears as he is learning speech and language will have no effect on his communication skills. There is no doubt that some communication disorders, including phonological disorders, are the direct result of poor speech and language models.

There is also a connection between **intelligence** and phonological disorders, although it is not as simple and direct as you might think. Phonological disorders are more common among mentally retarded children than among normally intelligent children, and there is a correlation between the severity of defectiveness and the degree of retardation. This correlation is far from perfect, however. Many children with normal or even superior intelligence have phonological disorders, and some mentally retarded children, even at low levels of intelligence, have very good articulation. Some severely retarded children, for example, will echo speech perfectly. They may not fully understand the language they are echoing, but what they imitate, they articulate without error.

Phonological problems sometimes result from **receptive deficits,** including sensory and perceptual problems. These phonological problems are considered functional because, even though there is a clear organic problem in the case of hearing loss, for example, the organic problem is not in the speech mechanism itself. The phonological disorders associated with hearing loss are consistent with the kind and severity of loss. For example, plosives, fricatives, and affricates are considered high-frequency sounds. If a child cannot hear in the range of frequencies characteristic of these phonemes, he will have problems acquiring these sounds. Common sense will also suggest that a child will have more problems with a severe hearing loss than with a mild loss, and that is certainly true. Whereas a mild hearing loss might simply slow up the acquisition of speech, congenital deafness makes the acquisition of speech extraordinarily difficult.

Sometimes a child can get sensory information into his brain because he has normal hearing, but he has trouble processing the information because he has a **perceptual deficit.** Perception is the process by which a person selects, sorts, organizes, interprets, and analyzes sensory information. If a child has a problem with this part of speech reception, he might not be able to figure out where words begin or end or which sounds or words are most important in strings of sounds and words. These and similar problems will affect speech output because we cannot separate how we speak from how we receive speech. Speech therapy for children with perceptual problems, therefore, begins with efforts to improve their processing abilities and does not immediately focus on how to produce speech sounds.

In many phonological cases, the speech-language pathologist is never able to figure out exactly why a given child is having a problem. There is not an obvious organic defect. The child is normally intelligent, has a typical family experience, and seems to be receiving and interpreting speech normally. In these cases, the clinician determines what the child knows about phonology and what he does not know, and then creates a program to fill in the gaps until the child's phonological system is intact.

Language Impairments

Terminology is a problem without end in all behavioral sciences, and that certainly includes the related disciplines of speech-language pathology and audiology. We had to deal with a terminology issue in the previous section on phonological disorders, and we revisit the tangled issue in this section. The word *language* did not appear in the name of the national professional association until 1979. Prior to that time, the national organization was called the American Speech and Hearing Association (ASHA). The association decided to add *language* to make it clear to all other disciplines that speech-language pathologists assess, diagnose, and treat language disorders. The national organization changed its name to the American Speech-Language-Hearing Association, but retained the ASHA acronym because it was the well-established short-form name of the professional organization and because there was concern that people might hurt themselves trying to say *ASLHA.* There is a point to this little story. For many years, the term *language disorders* seemed adequate to describe the broad category of problems people of all ages might have with language, but as is fashionable in the perception of some and necessary in the perception of others, some experts concluded that *disorders* in reference to language had outlived its semantic usefulness.

The argument about this particular term centers on the use of a single term to describe problems that are truly differentiated, or should be differentiated. Over the years, terms such as *language delay, language disorder,* and *language impairment* have been used to describe problems in language understanding and production grounded in limited skills, but the surface interpretation of these terms is not the same. Most people, whether or not they are expert in language matters, would understand *language delay* to mean that the language of a given child is immature for his age, that it fails to meet normative standards. A child with a language delay is acquiring language, but he is acquiring it more slowly than we expect he should. *Language disorder,* according to ASHA, is "impaired comprehension and/or use of spoken, written, and/or other symbol systems. This disorder may involve (1) the form of language (phonology, morphology, syntax), (2) the content of language (semantics), and/or (3) the function of language in communication (pragmatics) in any combination" (Ad Hoc Committee on Service Delivery in the Schools, 1993, p. 40). Clearly, *language disorder,* as defined by ASHA, goes well beyond *delay,* so how do we extricate ourselves from this little semantic quagmire?

Robert Owens (1995) advocates use of the term *language impairment.* It is his view that *impairment* is a broader, more inclusive term that accommodates both *delay* and *disorder,* and reason seems to be on his side. Not only does the term nicely accommodate delay and disorder, but it allows us to avoid the arguments that invariably occur about the kinds of language problems exhibited by certain communicative populations. Do individuals who are mentally retarded, for example, produce delayed language or disordered language? We can deftly avoid the potential discomfort of the question by describing the language as *impaired.* Reread the ASHA definition of *language disorder* and compare it to Owens' definition of *language impairment* as "a heterogeneous group of developmental and/or acquired disorders and/or delays principally characterized by deficits and/or immaturities in the use of spoken or written language for comprehension and/or production purposes that may involve the form, content, and/or function of language in any combination" (Owens, 1995, p. 22). This definition is certainly broad enough and inclusive enough to cover everything that could possible go wrong with language. We can only hope that someday in a galaxy not too far away, automobile bumper-to-bumper warranties will be as comprehensive. In any case, for all the reasons we have identified here and for all the reasons implied in the plethora of *and/or's*, we shall use the term *language impairment*.

What follows is an introductory overview of the major diagnostic categories associated with various language impairments common to children. The reader must approach this information on the tiptoes of an important caution, however. We use categories in this discussion as an organizational convenience. In doing so, we will be making generalizations about a mythical typical child. Real children are rarely considerate enough to behave exactly as they are described in any category of any set of behaviors, and that includes language. We tried to make that point in reference to stages early and often in this book, and we are now making that same point about language impairment categories. It is highly unlikely that any child, even correctly deposited into a given category, will exhibit all of the characteristics associated with that category. It is quite likely that a given child will exhibit characteristics associated with two or more categories, as well as a few characteristics of his own idiosyncratic category. Human beings, even when they walk and talk in small packages, are very complex creatures who defy all attempts to place them into tidy, clearly differentiated, categorical boxes. Just as present-day physicians are taught in medical school to treat people and not just organs or diseases, speech-language pathologists are taught from day one, or late in day two, that we treat individual people. Even when several individual people appear to have the same communication problem with the same etiology, we should expect differences because differences are the rule, not the exception. It is easy to fall into the trap of describing the speech of a client as "cleft palate speech," for example, as though all people with cleft palates produce speech in exactly the same way. It may also seem appropriate to talk about "autistic language" or "mentally retarded language," but while such terms may have a certain face validity, they are worthless descriptions. In fact, they are worse than worthless because they perpetuate stereotypes that can be harmful to the people to whom they are attached. Within the following discussion, therefore, the reader is strongly encouraged to keep in mind that there is significant variability within categories and across categories.

Specific Language Impairment

It should come as little surprise, after considering the problems we have experienced trying to define the broader category of language impairment, that there would be disagreements about how to describe and understand specific subcategories of language impairment. Though we can perhaps come to agreement about etiological subcategories such as mental retardation or autism, there has been considerable debate about the descriptive and causal boundaries for what is called *specific language impairment* or *SLI*. Perhaps the most widely applied description has been offered by Leonard (1987, p. 1), who observed that children with SLI "exhibit significant limitations in language functioning that cannot be attributed to deficits in hearing, oral structure and function, or general intelligence." Consider what Leonard is suggesting in this description. The etiologies of specific language impairments are essentially unknown. As one might imagine without working up an intellectual sweat, this a pretty heterogeneous group of language-impaired children. In fact, research by Aram (1991), Stark and Tallal (1988) and others have led language experts to conclude that there are several identifiable subgroups within the larger SLI population.

Even though there seem to be few common denominators connecting the language impairments of SLI children, some generalizations about their language behaviors seem warranted. Craig (1993) noted, for example, that there are qualitative and quantitative differences between SLI children and children who have normal language when they are matched for mental age. SLI children seem to experience failure in the classroom more often than their peers. These failures are typically blamed on pragmatic problems. That is, SLI children have trouble initiating interactions with other children, and they have problems with conversational turn-taking. In general, SLI children use pragmatic functions we would expect of younger children. They have trouble adjusting their language to fit particular speaker–listener interactions, and they do not effectively repair conversations when failures occur.

SLI children do not acquire their first words as early as other children, and their vocabulary growth is slower than normal. They sometimes have difficulty naming things, probably not because they have word retrieval problems, but because they do not possess adequate mental dictionaries. SLI children, in comparison to younger children with comparable MLU's, have fewer grammatical morphemes, including auxiliary verbs, tense and number markers for verbs, and function words such as conjunctions, articles, and prepositions. Whereas younger children with comparable MLU's tend to make random pronoun errors, SLI children tend to use the same pronoun repeatedly, whether or not it is applicable.

Mental Retardation

In the case of mental retardation, we should begin with the common ground. There is no dispute about the fact that there is a connection between mental retardation and language impairment, and there is no dispute about the fact that the severity of language impairment is correlated with the degree of mental retardation. Please keep in mind, however, that "mentally retarded language" is a meaningless description. It is meaningless, in part, because the mentally retarded continuum stretches a considerable distance. Some individuals at the mild end of the continuum use language quite well. Individuals at the severe end are often noncommunicative, and we find a wide range of language abilities between the extremes.

Before we consider the generalizations we can make about the language abilities of mentally retarded individuals, we need to establish some form of definition of *mentally retarded*. The definition most often used today was established by the American Association on Mental Retardation (AAMR). Mental retardation, according to an AAMR committee, is "significantly subaverage general intellectual functioning existing concurrently with deficits in adaptive behavior and manifested during the developmental period" (Grossman, 1983, p. 1). I can almost hear some readers groaning that this sounds like a statement a committee would generate. This complaint duly noted, the definition has significant value if we consider its constituent parts. What does it mean, for example, to function at a "significantly subaverage intellectual" level? A person meets this criterion if he or she has an IQ of 68 or lower, an IQ cutoff determined by appropriate statistical manipulations. What is meant by "deficits in adaptive behavior?" A person demonstrates *adaptive behavior* by functioning in an independent and socially responsible manner. Conversely, a person exhibits *deficits* in adaptive behavior when he or she demonstrates an inability to function independently or behaves irresponsibly in common social situations. What is meant by the "developmental period?" As presently understood, the developmental period extends from the moment of conception to adulthood (Nelson, 1993, p. 98). Most importantly, how many of these three criteria must be met before a person is classified as mentally retarded? The answer is simple and quite clear. A person must meet all three criteria in order to meet the AAMR definition of mental retardation.

Keeping in mind that there are wide individual variations among mentally retarded individuals in terms of their speech and language abilities, Kamhi (1981) observed that mentally retarded children experience more language difficulties than normally developing children even when they are matched for mental age. That is, a typical mentally retarded child who is six years old, but who has a mental age of three years, will have more trouble with language than a normally developing child whose chronological and mental ages are three years. It is also noteworthy that even when mentally retarded children have other developmental problems, including neuromuscular difficulties or social skill deficits, language impairment is usually the most critical problem they face. Language impairment may, in fact, be the single most defining characteristic of this population.

Owens, after thoroughly reviewing the literature, provides an excellent summary of the language behaviors of mentally retarded children (1995, p. 26). Even though these children exhibit gestures and intentions that are similar to those used by normally developing children, they tend to be submissive conversational partners and are not as effective as their mental age-matched peers in clarifying their messages when misunderstandings occur. Children who are mentally retarded acquire morphemes in the same order as other children, and the sequence in which they produce varying types of sentences is similar to that of normal children, but they tend to use shorter and less complex sentences than their mental age-matched peers. Whereas all children begin with word meanings that are concrete, children who are mentally retarded do not make the change from concrete to abstract meanings as quickly and easily as other children, and their word meanings remain restrictive. They experience a slower vocabulary growth, and they have more trouble with figurative forms of language than their mental age-matched peers. Children who are mentally retarded tend to use phonological processes that are typical of younger children, and they are slower to suppress these processes than their peers who have normal intellectual abilities. Finally, these children produce more articulation, or motor production, errors than other children.

If we put all these pieces together, we understand that children who are mentally retarded acquire language forms more slowly but in the same order as normally developing children. In some cases, when we match mentally retarded and normally developing children for mental age, they perform about the same. In other cases, even when we account for mental age, mentally retarded children are less effective in their use of language and more restricted in their use of the language forms they do have than their mental age-matched peers.

Autism

The term *autism* typically conjures up images of children who are withdrawn into their own egocentric worlds, children who appear to have rejected reality in favor of a fantasy place outside people cannot reach, children who engage in a wide range of abnormal and socially unacceptable behaviors, children whose language is severely impaired. Autism was first named as a syndrome, or aggregate of symptoms that in combination describe a condition, by Leo Kanner, a child psychologist, in 1943. The American Psychiatric Association, in 1987, categorized autism as a *pervasive developmental disorder* and described autism as an impairment involving a stringent repertoire of activity, a limited range of behaviors, a severely reduced interest level, and little or no social interaction. According to the National Society of Autistic Children, autism develops in 4 out of 10,000 children, and it is more common in males than females by a ratio of 4:1. The onset of autism usually occurs before 30 months. Physical appearance is normal, but motor, social, and cognitive development tends to be erratic. Autistic children do not react to sensory stimuli the same way other children do. That is, they tend to be either hypoactive or hyperactive in response to visual and/or auditory stimuli. Sometimes their responses are ritualistic, and they are intolerant of any environmental changes. Autistic children may appear to be preoccupied with mechanical devices at the same time that they seem uninterested in establishing contacts with people. Their speech and language problems include echolalia, mutism, and failure to use abstract terms. They also experience cognitive difficulties, even when, on occasion, they seem to be gifted in one particular area such as math. They not only have trouble relating to people, but sometimes even to objects, and to events. Autistic children tend not to show affection. Their play behaviors are often unusual, ritualistic, and perseverative, and when they are interrupted while they are playing or manipulating objects, they often become agitated (Ritvo & Freeman, 1978). The cause of autism has not been established, but there is speculation that it may be a genetic disorder, that it may result from a degenerative neurological disease, or that it may be an autoimmune disease. Prognosis is uncertain in all cases, but is considered poor for autistic children who are not talking by the time they are five years old. At this time, there is no single established treatment, but most treatments stress educational and behavior modification principles with emphases on teaching small segments of information and on strictly controlling inappropriate and maladaptive behaviors.

The primary focus of concern for autistic children, as it is with mentally retarded children, is severe language impairment. According to Tager-Flusberg (1985), all autistic individuals have impairments that affect both their ability to understand language and to produce language. Paul (1987) noted that half of the autistic population fails to develop functional language and fails to develop more than a few communication skills of any kind. Beyond this general and not very positive view, there are a number of generalizations we can make about the language abilities of autistic children.

Autistic children have difficulty establishing the kind of mutual attention that is necessary for communicative exchanges. They have trouble initiating conversation and using language to inform, skills that are basic to social interactions (Wetherby, 1986). These children lack conversational turn-taking skills, and they utilize a very limited range of communication functions (Donnellan & Kilman, 1986; Mirenda & Donnellan, 1986). Considering our general description of autistic individuals, it is not surprising that autistic children have difficulty with abstract words. They struggle to retrieve words, and they have trouble expressing their emotions. Autistic children often refer to themselves with second-person (*you*) and third-person pronouns (*he, she*). They often construct sentences without regard to underlying meaning (Bartolucci, Pierce, Streiner, & Eppel, 1976). The least affected component of language is phonology, although phonological problems are common in this population. The sequence of phonological development is the same as for normal children, and development is not distinctly delayed (Fay & Schuler, 1980).

In summary, the language problems of autistic children are diverse because they are members of a diverse population. Some of these children eventually use functional language, but just as many never do. Some of the language problems associated with autism seem to be the result of developmental delay, but other problems seem to go beyond delay. When autistic children are matched for mental age with mentally retarded, SLI, and normally developing children, the syntactic abilities of the autistic children are equal to the syntactic abilities of the mentally retarded and SLI children. What does this mean? According to Swisher and Demetras (1985), it may mean that autistic children construct sentences differently than normally developing children, that they derive surface structures from incompletely understood deep structures. Taking into account research on the development of all components of language, Swisher and Demetras (1985) conclude that there is evidence of delay, but in some cases, there is also evidence that autistic children follow developmental patterns that are unique. And we will reiterate one more time that, given what we know about the characteristics of autism, it is not surprising that there would be evidence of unusual developmental patterns.

Brain Injury

The general category of brain injury includes *traumatic brain injury* (TBI) resulting from a blow to the head that might occur in a fall or automobile accident, as well as the kind of brain injury that occurs in a *cerebrovascular accident* (CVA), commonly called a *stroke*. In this section, however, brain injury will be limited to traumatic brain injuries affecting children. In the United States, there are about one million victims of TBI who are children and adolescents. Some of these young people will experience complete, or nearly complete, recoveries from their brain injuries. Sadly, others will remain in essentially vegetative states for the remainder of their lives.

This next sentence should be annoyingly familiar. Children with traumatic brain injury are members of an extraordinarily heterogeneous group. This means, as we should now be able to chant in unison, that they will exhibit widely varying behaviors over a wide range of severity, and in the case of TBI, for varying periods of time. In addition, we must note that the language impairments associated with TBI differ in some respects from the language impairments that have developmental etiologies. In their review of studies focusing on the effects of traumatic brain injury on children, Ewing-Cobbs, Fletcher, and Leven (1985) found that these injuries impact general intellectual functioning, memory, psychosocial skills, academic performance, and, of course, language. Depending on the severity of the injury and on the site and extent of the damage, problems in these areas might persist for weeks or months, or they might be permanent. Compounding the problems identified by Ewing-Cobbs et al., these children tend to be highly distractible. They tend to perseverate, and to have low thresholds for frustration. Imagine for a moment the combination of these behavioral characteristics and language impairment, academic problems, and the social challenges inherent in interpersonal relationships. To say that traumatic brain injuries, even those in the mild and moderate categories, can be life-altering is something of an understatement.

As with the other categories of language impairment we have already discussed, we must be careful to acknowledge that whatever generalizations we make about the language impairments of TBI children are just that, generalizations. Here then are a few generalizations. These children often make statements during conversations that are not topic-focused. They have problems organizing their thoughts into language forms, and they have difficulty expressing complex ideas. Language that is automatic, including the language we use when we greet one another, tends to be unaffected by TBI, but when language is intentional or purposive, and when it is important, communication becomes more difficult. Individuals with traumatic brain injuries often struggle to name things, and they have problems with word retrieval even if their vocabularies are relatively intact. The sentences they produce tend to be long, aimless, fragmented, and inappropriate. TBI children typically do not have phonological problems as a result of their brain injuries, but they might have some articulation difficulties associated with injury-induced dysarthria and/or apraxia. It is not unusual for children with traumatic brain injuries to experience some problems with language comprehension. They might, for example, have problems affixing meanings to the syntactic structures of sentences, but most of these children will be able to interpret the sentences included in ordinary conversational exchanges.

A Few Words About Other Categories

Learning disabilities may hinder language development. Many people believe that mental retardation and learning disability mean the same thing. They do not. A child with a learning disability may have a normal or superior intellectual capacity. You will best understand learning disability by taking the term literally. This is a child with a deficit that renders traditional learning strategies ineffective, perhaps useless. If, for example, a child sees visual stimuli backward or scrambled, he will have problems learning to read. If he is unable to group auditory sounds into appropriate segments, he will have problems organizing and interpreting spoken language, because he may have difficulty grouping sounds into words and words into sentences. Children with learning disabilities often have difficulty attending to, sorting, or organizing stimuli, and they may have deficits in memory. Try to imagine learning language with these problems. The normal child learning language attends, even if unconsciously, to thousands of language samples each day. He is eventually able to sort through all those samples to figure out how verbs and nouns differ, how to organize words into subjects and predicates, and everything he learns about language is stored in memory. A deficit in any of these or related areas can have a significant impact on language acquisition and may result in language impairment. Treatment focuses on helping the child compensate for his learning disability by teaching him to rely more heavily on learning skills not affected or by helping him discover alternative learning strategies.

It will surprise no one that **hearing loss** and **deafness** are related to language impairments, and it should be obvious that, all other factors being equal, the greater the hearing loss, the greater the language impairment is likely to be. The deaf child lives in a speech-impoverished environment, no matter how much speech is generated by his parents and siblings and no matter the quality of those models. If the deafness is congenital, it is unrealistic to hope for normal speech. If the child has had normal hearing during the speech and language learning period and then becomes deaf, the outlook for oral communication is much more promising, but it will still fall short of the language quality we expect from normally hearing children. Consider the fact that adults who have had normal speech and normal hearing throughout their lives and who become deaf in adulthood experience some deterioration in the quality of speech (Goehl and Kaufman, 1984). It should be emphasized that hearing losses, even deafness, do not preclude language. The congenitally deaf child has the same natural language abilities as the hearing child, but he will best receive and express language visually. For this reason, most experts today recommend that the deaf child be provided opportunities for acquiring a visual language communication system as early as possible.

In Conclusion

In this section, we have considered some of the factors that might be responsible for language impairment, but we have certainly not considered all the possibilities. A comprehensive analysis of the possible etiologies of language impairment goes beyond the scope of this book. What we have tried to emphasize in our limited treatment of this subject is that anything that affects the way language develops and anything that affects the way language is received, processed, understood, or produced can result in language impairment. We have also tried, to the point of near exhaustion, to sensitize the reader to the idea that no matter how narrowly we might define a category of language impairment, there will always be a great diversity of language behaviors produced by the people we drop into that category. That diversity exists, no matter how hard we try to arbitrarily limit the possibilities by establishing strict categorical criteria, serves to remind us that language is an extraordinarily complex phenomenon produced by incredibly complex human creatures. When language is acquired normally and used routinely, we take this uniquely human gift for granted. Only when there is failure do we begin to appreciate how awesome, complicated, and impossible language really is.

Voice Disorders

Most of us are impressed by the ability of some birds, like the mynah or the parrot, to imitate human speech. I would submit that even more impressive is the ability of humans to imitate the sounds produced by birds, other animals, musical instruments, machines, almost any kind of sound imaginable. This virtually unlimited imitative ability is made possible because of the extraordinary range and versatility of the human voice mechanism, including the larynx and the resonating cavities. Within this range, we must try to determine what is a so-called normal voice, an exceedingly difficult task. Although we can identify many voices as unusual, surveys conducted by experts in this disorder indicate that about 1 percent of adults and perhaps as many as 6 percent of children have voices that can be considered abnormal or disordered (Miller & Madison, 1984; Silverman & Zimmer, 1975). We can agree that when a voice is disordered, there is a problem with pitch, loudness, and/or quality. For the sake of convenience, we examine each of these possibilities separately, but it is very important to stress that on a practical level, we cannot separate pitch, loudness, and quality. Each affects and is affected by each of the others. For example, when we describe a voice as breathy, we are making a judgment about the quality of the voice, but a breathy voice is also weaker in volume and usually lower in pitch than it should be.

Pitch Disorders

Pitch can be atypical in three ways. It may be **too high, too low,** or it may be **monotonous.**

A voice may be higher pitched than expected for one's size and/or sex because the speaker's larynx is abnormally small or because the vocal folds are short and thin. As long as the pitch is consistent with the size and capabilities of the larynx, nothing can or should be done to lower it. Trying to force a small larynx to produce a low-pitched voice might cause damage to the larynx of much greater consequence than the high pitch. A higher than normal pitch might simply be one symptom of slow overall maturation, in which case time is the best treatment. Boys especially might be a little slow to mature physically, but the boy who looks and sounds like he is twelve when he is fifteen will probably look and sound his age by the time he is eighteen or nineteen. When the voice is high-pitched as a result of tension or stress or because the speaker is consciously or unconsciously imitating someone with a high-pitched voice, therapy can help the speaker find his normal pitch range.

It is less common to find someone with a lower than normal pitch, but when this occurs, it may be because the speaker has a larynx that is larger than normal for his/her size or sex or because the vocal folds are longer or thicker than usual. Some people, males and females, force their voices lower than they should because they are trying to match what they perceive as appropriate voices. A female in business, for example, might unconsciously force her voice too low in order to project an image she believes is important for success, or because she is trying to fit in with her male counterparts.

A voice that is monotonous in pitch is often produced by someone who is generally hypotense or low in self esteem. A monopitched voice may also be one of the consequences of a hearing loss. It is difficult to feel changes in pitch, so when a speaker can no longer monitor pitch changes by hearing, pitch variations tend to decrease. As with other voice differences, a monopitched voice can also be learned by imitation.

Loudness Disorders

There are three common loudness problems. A voice can be **too loud, too weak,** or there may be no voice at all, a condition known as **aphonia.**

People who have hearing losses as a result of problems in the inner ear or along the nerve pathway from the ear to the brain often talk too loudly because they have difficulty hearing themselves talk. You may experience something similar to this when you speak too loudly while listening to music through headphones. In some cases, a loud voice is a reflection of the speaker's personality. People who might be described as overbearing, obnoxious, or self-centered sometimes speak in loud voices. Others might habitually speak too loudly because they are accustomed to working in noisy environments or because they have occupations, like preaching or teaching, which require them to project beyond normal volume. Although a loud voice might be bothersome to listeners, it becomes a problem to the speaker only if the strain associated with excessive volume produces a pathology of the vocal folds like nodules, polyps, or contact ulcers.

Sometimes people speak too softly because they have hearing losses associated with problems in the middle or outer ears that cause them to judge their own voices to be louder than they really are. You can get some sense for this condition by covering your ears and listening to yourself talk. As is true with a loud voice, a too soft voice might provide some insight about the speaker's personality. Someone who is shy, withdrawn, or insecure, or feels inferior to others might speak in a weak voice. Of course, a too soft voice might also be symptomatic of a physical condition such as partial vocal fold paralysis.

The most serious loudness problem is aphonia. A speaker may have no voice at all if both vocal folds are paralyzed in the open position, and it is impossible for the folds to adduct. In many cases, however, aphonia is not physical but psychological or emotional. When aphonia exists as a result of emotional trauma, it is often called hysterical aphonia. In hysterical aphonia, there is nothing physically wrong with the larynx, but the speaker does not produce voice because he truly believes he is incapable of producing voice. Treatment of these patients can be quite complicated because the voice problem is symptomatic of a psychological problem. Should we treat it as a voice problem or a psychological problem? The answer is *Yes!* In some cases, the psychological problem is addressed first, and if the aphonia persists, the speech-language pathologist addresses the voice disorder. Others recommend voice therapy combined with an opportunity for general emotional catharsis, followed by psychotherapy as needed (Aronson, 1985).

Vocal Quality Disorders

We now come to the least tidy subsection of voice disorders. There is so much disagreement among the experts about quality disorders that it is difficult to find terms and impossible to compose definitions for these terms that are acceptable to all of them. We can perhaps agree that quality disorders are the result of problems with resonance and/or laryngeal tone. When resonance is disordered, it is because there is too much nasality, **hypernasality,** or not enough nasal resonance, **hypo-nasality.** Quality disorders associated with the laryngeal tone are **harshness, breath-iness,** and **hoarseness,** or combinations of these conditions.

Hypernasality is almost universal in cleft palate patients. If the soft palate is cleft, it is difficult or impossible to achieve adequate closure of the velopharyn-geal mechanism to stop the flow of air into the nasal cavities. As we have already noted, the nasal cavities should be coupled with the oral cavity for only three American English sounds: "m," "n," "ng." If a speaker cannot achieve adequate velopharyngeal closure, all sounds are produced with nasal resonance. Some speakers are hypernasal, not because of cleft palates, but because they have con-genitally short soft palates that do not provide enough tissue mass for effective closure. Still other speakers have structurally and functionally sound velopha-ryngeal mechanisms but have become hypernasal by habit. A child, for example, might imitate the hypernasal voice of a parent and retain that resonance quality into adulthood.

Less commonly, speakers are hyponasal. That is, they do not produce nasal quality on "m," "n," "ng." Consider what this means about the velopharyngeal mechanism . For some reason, it remains closed all the time. This may occur because of enlarged adenoids or as the result of allergies that cause swelling of the tissues in the pharynx. The velum may be in a lowered position, but because of the enlarged adenoids or swollen tissue, the opening into the nasal cavities is obstructed, and normal nasal resonance cannot be achieved. As is true with all other voice disor-ders, hyponasality may also be acquired by habit.

A voice may be described as breathy when too much air is being released dur-ing phonation. There may be excessive airflow as the result of a paralyzed vocal fold that will not allow the speaker to adduct the folds completely. Excessive air may escape because vocal nodules prevent the folds from closing completely. Some people learn to speak in a breathy voice by imitation or because they prefer the breathy quality, one of the characteristics of what some perceive as a sexy or seductive voice in women.

Harshness is the quality resulting from a hard glottal attack and sustained, tense closure of the vocal folds. That is, when the speaker initiates voice, he slaps the vocal folds together in a hard, forceful manner and continues this excessive muscular tension as he talks. The result is a voice that sounds strained and labored. There is often a harsh quality in the voice of someone who is using inappropriately high pitch levels. Speakers who have harsh voices often work in noisy environ-ments or have jobs that require them to speak at high volume levels. The danger, of course, is that this kind of vocal fold abuse can result in nodules, polyps, or con-tact ulcers.

A person who has a harsh voice may eventually develop a hoarse voice, which combines breathy and harsh qualities. There is the same sustained strain we hear in the harsh voice, but there is also an excessive release of air along with phonation, usually as the result of nodules or polyps that prevent the folds from achieving complete closure.

Voice therapy can be most simply described as vocal education or reeducation. The clinician helps the client identify a target voice that is appropriate for the client's sex, age, and physical status, and then guides the client toward producing that voice. Voice is so habitual, however, and so much a part of one's personality, that changing from an inappropriate voice to the target voice is very difficult. When the voice has been so badly misused or abused that polyps, nodules, or contact ulcers have developed, surgery may be necessary before voice therapy is initiated. It must be stressed, however, that surgery alone is not likely to solve the voice disorder. Unless the speaker learns how to produce a proper voice within the appropriate pitch range, with reasonable volume, and with normal muscular tensions, the vocal fold pathology will probably return.

Fluency Disorders

When most people think about fluency disorders, they think about **stuttering.** Stuttering is actually only one of a number of fluency disorders, but since it is the most common, it is the focus of our discussion. You should know, however, that any disorder characterized by hesitations, repetitions (of sounds, syllables, words, or phrases), or prolongations of sounds, which impedes the forward flow of speech, is a fluency disorder. Fluency problems often accompany neuropathologies. People with epilepsy or cerebral palsy, or people who have suffered strokes or head injuries often have fluency problems. Whether or not all of these problems should be called stuttering is subject to debate (Hulit, 1996). In the context of this presentation, the term stuttering is used in reference to people who are normal neurologically and without serious psychological problems. Even if we limit ourselves to this population, however, we have another problem. All speakers, on occasion, have fluency difficulties. All speakers repeat syllables and words, stumble, hesitate, revise, and produce all the other behaviors we associate with stuttering. Separating stutterers from nonstutterers is not as easy as it may appear, because it is not just a matter of frequency of fluency failure. As noted in the opening of this chapter, some people we would all agree are stutterers have fewer fluency breakdowns than some people we would all agree are normal speakers. Stutterers and nonstutterers actually have more similarities as communicators than they have differences (Hulit, 1989). They are separated as much by their perceptions of speech, speaking situations, words, and listeners as by the struggle we all associate with stuttering.

One of the most difficult problems in discussing stuttering, as indicated by the preceding paragraph, is defining it (Bloodstein, 1990; Perkins, 1990). Experts over the centuries have argued about what stuttering is, what causes it, why it seems to come and then disappear in young children, and how to treat it. Although more has been written about stuttering than any other speech disorder, there is still far more we do not know about it than we know. Experts have described stuttering as a mystery, an enigma, and a riddle.

For the purposes of this discussion, let's identify a few of the things we know—or think we know—about stuttering. Stuttering is a disorder that begins in childhood, usually between the ages of two and four years. Many children who begin to stutter, perhaps as many as 80 percent, spontaneously recover by the time they are six years old. Stuttering is much more common in boys than in girls. When children are young, the sex ratio is about 2:1, but by adulthood, the ratio is 4:1 or 5:1. When stuttering begins, it is relatively simple and uninvolved. The child repeats single-syllable words, without struggle or awareness, and the stuttering is cyclic. That is, there will be days, weeks, or months of normal fluency followed by days, weeks, or months of fairly noticeable stuttering. Sometimes these cycles will go on for several years until the child enters a normal period and does not have another stuttering period. As stuttering develops, the behaviors become more complicated and the stutterer becomes more aware of his difficulty until he begins to think of himself as a stutterer. As severity increases, we see facial grimaces, and the stutterer seems to have difficulty breathing and making his articulators move. The experts do not agree about the prognosis for adult stutterers. Some believe it is possible for adult stutterers to become normal speakers. Others believe adult stutterers can learn to control their speech but will never be normal again.

We do not know what causes stuttering, although many theories about its etiology have been developed over the centuries. Some believe stuttering is an organic disorder that can be blamed on neurological problems related to articulatory function or phonatory control. Others believe it is a symptom of a psychological disorder, and still others believe stuttering is learned behavior. In one form or another, these theoretical views have been around for centuries, and they will likely be recycled for many more years to come.

Why do more boys stutter than girls? There has been much speculation about this question, but the fact is we do not know. Some have argued that boys are subject to more pressure than girls. Although that may have been an attractive explanation in the 1940s and 1950s, it seems less viable today. Others believe that boys stutter more often than girls because they are slower to mature and do not have the neuromuscular abilities to respond to the communicative demands placed on all children.

Why do many stutterers become suddenly fluent when they sing, or speak in unison, or when they whisper, or when they speak in a very distinct rhythmic manner? Again there are many different explanations, but the important insight to be gained here is that stutterers can be fluent and may be fluent as often, or even more often, than they are nonfluent. Stuttering, therefore, is more than disrupted motor speech. There is a perceptual component that basically operates like this.

When the stutterer believes he will stutter, or when he thinks speaking will be difficult, or when he is saying something he believes is very important, he is likely to stutter. When he is concentrating on something other than the content of his speaking, or when he is saying something meaningless, or talking to someone or something he perceives as unimportant or nonthreatening, or when he thinks speaking will be easy, he is less likely to stutter. Stuttering is indeed a mystery, an enigma, a riddle, and it is a frustrating speech disorder for the stutterer, his family, and the speech clinician.

The treatment of stuttering is much too complex to discuss here. Suffice it to say that when stuttering is treated early, the prognosis is excellent. When there is any doubt, therefore, about whether a child is stuttering or producing normal nonfluency, an evaluation is in order. If the evaluation indicates there may be a problem, the problem should be addressed. In the case of stuttering, the old adage that an ounce of prevention is worth a pound of cure holds very true.

Final Thoughts

We have come to the end of our story. As you have progressed through the pages of this book, we hope you have developed a new appreciation for the miracle of speech and language. We may never fully understand how human beings can think, edit thoughts, pull language from their memory banks, transform language into speech, and combine speech with all the critical aspects of nonverbal communication. We should, however, appreciate that this communicative ability is one of the great gifts humans pass from generation to generation. Although there is a powerful innate drive to acquire language and to speak in all human children, parents should do all they can to encourage their children during the acquisition period. Parents and teachers are usually the first to notice when a child is having difficulty with speech and language. It is their responsibility to seek professional help from speech-language pathologists who are qualified to diagnose and treat communication problems. If there is any doubt about whether a child has a communication disorder or not, the child should be evaluated and treated, if necessary. It is far easier to treat communication disorders in their early stages than after inappropriate habits have become established. The child who can talk has one of the most important tools he or she needs to explore and understand the exciting world awaiting him or her.

Review Questions

1. Why is it difficult to determine what constitutes a communication defect?

2. In your own words, and taking into account our discussion of the inherent problems in differentiating between "normal" and "abnormal" speech and language, define *communication defect*.

3. How do categories of communication disorders differ when we classify them by symptoms as opposed to classifying them by causes?

4. What does the term *functional* mean, and why is it inappropriate to think of *functional* as a synonym for *nonorganic*?

5. What is the difference between *phonology* and *articulation?* What is the difference between a *phonological disorder* and an *articulation disorder?*

6. Identify the members we would expect to find on a cleft palate treatment team and explain the role of each team member in the treatment of the cleft palate patient.

7. Identify and briefly describe the three most common forms of malocclusion. Which form of malocclusion is most likely to adversely affect speech and why?

8. Compare and contrast the symptomotologies of lower motor neuron dysarthria and upper motor neuron dysarthria.

9. Identify the common causes of developmental phonological disorders.

10. Discuss the problems associated with terms such as *language disorder* and *language delay.* Why is *language impairment* a better term?

11. Why should we avoid using terms such as *autistic language* or *mentally retarded language?*

12. What is meant by *specific language impairment?* How do the language behaviors of SLI children compare to the language behaviors of normally developing children?

13. How do the language behaviors of mentally retarded children compare to the language behaviors of normally developing children?

14. What is *autism?* Identify some of the behaviors and problems commonly associated with autism.

15. Describe the language behaviors commonly associated with autism and explain how these behaviors are related to other problems typically experienced by autistic children.

16. What is a *traumatic brain injury?* What are some of the common effects of TBI on a child's behavior in general and on language behavior specifically?

17. In what major ways can the voice be disordered?

18. Define the terms *aphonia, hypernasal, harsh,* and *hoarse?*

19. What are some of the differences between normal nonfluency and stuttering?

20. What are some things we know about stuttering, and what are some questions we have yet to answer about this disorder?

References and Suggested Readings

Ad Hoc Committee on Service Delivery in the Schools, ASHA (1993). Definitions of communication disorders and variations. *Asha, 35*(3) (Suppl. 10), 40–41.

Ainsworth, S., & Fraser, J. (Eds.). (1988). *If your child stutters: A guide for parents* (3rd ed.). Memphis, TN: Speech Foundation of America.

Aram, D. M. (1991). Comments on specific language impairment as a clinical category. *Language, Speech, and Hearing Services in Schools, 22,* 84–87.

Aronson, A. (1985). *Clinical voice disorders* (2nd ed.). New York: Thieme-Stratton.

Bartolucci, G., Pierce, S., Streiner, D., & Eppel, P. T. (1976). Phonological investigation of verbal autistic and mentally retarded subjects. *Journal of Autism and Childhood Schizophrenia, 6,* 303–316.

Bernthal, J., & Bankson, N. (1988). *Articulation and phonological disorders* (2nd ed.). Englewood Cliffs, NJ: Prentice-Hall.

Bishop, D. V. M., & Adams, C. (1992). Comprehension problems in children with specific language impairment: Literal and inferential meaning. *Journal of Speech and Hearing Research, 35,* 119–129.

Bloodstein, O. (1979). *Speech pathology, an introduction.* Boston: Houghton Mifflin Company.

Bloodstein O. (1995). *A handbook on stuttering* (5th ed.). San Diego, CA: Singular Publishing Group.

Bloodstein, O. (1990). On pluttering, skivering, and floggering: A commentary. *Journal of Speech and Hearing Disorders, 55,* 392–393.

Bloodstein, O. (1993). *Stuttering, The Search for a Cause and Cure.* Allyn and Bacon: Needham Heights, MA.

Boone, D. R., & McFarlane, S. C. (1988). *The voice and voice therapy* (4th ed.). Englewood Cliffs, NJ: Prentice-Hall.

Byrne, M., & Shervanian (1977). *Introduction to communicative disorders.* New York: Harper and Row.

Coggins, T. (1979). Relational meaning encoded in two-word utterances of Stage I Down's syndrome children. *Journal of Speech and Hearing Research, 22,* 166–178.

Conture, E. G. (1990). *Stuttering* (2nd ed.). Englewood Cliffs, NJ: Prentice-Hall.

Conture, E. G., & Kelly, E. (1991). Young stutterers' nonspeech behaviors during stuttering. *Journal of Speech and Hearing Research, 34,* 1041–1056.

Craig, H. K. (1993). Social skills of children with specific language impairment: Peer relationships. *Language, Speech, and Hearing Services in Schools, 24,* 206–215.

Creaghead, N., Newman, P., & Secord, W. (Eds.) (1989). *Assessment and remediation of articulatory and phonological disorders* (2nd ed.). Columbus, OH: Merrill/Macmillan.

Crowe Hall, B. (1991). Attitudes of fourth and sixth graders toward peers with mild articulation disorders. *Language, Speech, Hearing Services in Schools, 22,* 334–340.

Curlee, R., & Perkins, W. (Eds.) (1984). *Nature and treatment of stuttering: New directions.* San Diego, CA: College-Hill Press.

Curtis, S., Katz, W., & Tallal, P. (1992). Delay versus deviance in the language acquisition of language-impaired children. *Journal of Speech and Hearing Research, 35,* 373–383.

Donnellan, A. M., & Kilman, B. A. (1986). Behavioral approaches to social skill development in autism. In E. Schopler & G. Mesibov (Eds.), *Social Behavior in Autism.* New York: Plenum Press.

Egland, G. (1970). *Speech and language problems: A guide for the classroom teacher.* Englewood Cliffs, NJ: Prentice-Hall.

Ewing-Cobbs, L., Fletcher, J. M., & Leven, H. S. (1985). In M. Ylvisaker (Ed.), *Head Injury Rehabilitation: Children and Adolescents.* Austin, TX: Pro-Ed.

Fay, W. H., & Schuler, A. L. (1980). *Emerging Language in Autistic Children.* Baltimore, MD: University Park Press.

Fein, D. (1983). The prevalence of speech and language impairments. *ASHA, 25,* 37.

Fey, M. (1992). Articulation and phonology: Inextricable constructs in speech pathology. *Language, Speech, and Hearing Services in Schools, 23,* 225–232.

Goehl, H., & Kaufman, P. (1984). Do the effects of adventitious deafness include disordered speech? *Journal of Speech and Hearing Disorders, 49,* 58–64.

Grossman, I. (1983). *Classification in Mental Retardation.* Washington, D.C.: American Association on Mental Deficiency.

Ham, R. E. (1990). *Therapy of stuttering, preschool through adolescence.* Englewood Cliffs, NJ: Prentice-Hall.

Hegde, M. N. (1995). *Introduction to Communicative Disorders* (2nd ed.). Austin, TX: Pro-Ed.

Hobbs, J. (Ed.) (1987). *Cleft lip and cleft palate from birth to three years.* Pittsburgh, PA: The American Cleft Palate Educational Foundation.

Hobbs, J. (Ed.) (1987). *Cleft lip and cleft palate: The child from three to twelve years.* Pittsburgh, PA: The American Cleft Palate Educational Foundation.

Hulit, L. M. (1985). *Stuttering: In perspective.* Springfield, IL: Charles C Thomas.

Hulit, L. M. (1985). *Stuttering therapy, a guide to the Charles Van Riper approach.* Springfield, IL: Charles C Thomas.

Hulit, L. M. (1989). A stutterer like me. *Journal of Fluency Disorders, 14,* 209–214.

Hulit, L. M. (1996). *Straight talk on stuttering.* Springfield, IL: Charles C Thomas.

Hulit, L., & Wirtz, L. (1994). The association of attitudes toward stuttering with selected variables. *Journal of Fluency Disorders, 19,* 247–267.

Ingram, D. (1991). *Phonological disability in children* (2nd ed.). San Diego, CA: Singular Publishing Group, Inc.

Johnson, B. (1996). *Language disorders in children: An introductory clinical perspective.* Albany, NY: Delmar Publishers.

Johnson, W., et al. (1967). *Speech-handicapped school children* (3rd ed.). New York: Harper & Row, Publishers.

Kamhi, A. G. (1981). Developmental vs. difference theories of mental retardation: A new look. *American Journal of Mental Deficiency, 86,* 1–7.

Larkins, P. (1985). *Speech-language pathology update.* Rockville, MD: American Speech-Language-Hearing Association.

Lass, N., Ruscello, D., Schmitt, J., Pannbacker, M., Orlando, M., Dean, K., Ruziska, J., & Bradshaw, K. (1992). Teachers perceptions of stutterers. *Language, Speech, Hearing Services in Schools, 23,* 78–81.

Leonard, L. B. (1987). Is specific language impairment a useful construct? In S. Rosenberg (Ed.), *Advances in Applied Psycholinguistics* (Vol. 1). Cambridge, UK: Cambridge University Press.

Leske, M. (1981a). Prevalence estimates of communicative disorders in the U.S.: Speech disorders. *Journal of the American Speech-Language-Hearing Association, 23,* 217–225.

Leske, M. (1981b). Prevalence estimates of communicative disorders in the U.S.: Language, hearing and vestibular disorders. *Journal of the American Speech-Language-Hearing Association, 23,* 229–237.

Martin, H., McConkey, R., & Martin, S. (1984). From acquisition theories to intervention strategies: An experiment with mentally handicapped children. *British Journal of Disorders of Communication, 19,* 3–14.

McTear, M., & Conti-Ramsden, G. (1991). *Pragmatic disability in children.* San Diego, CA: Singular Publishing Group, Inc.

Miller, S., & Madison, C. (1984). Public school voice clinics. I: A working model. *Language, Speech and Hearing Services in Schools, 15,* 51–57.

Mirenda, P., & Donnellan, A. (1986). Effects of adult interaction style on conversational behavior in students with severe communication problems. *Language, Speech, and Hearing Services in Schools, 17,* 126–141.

Mowrer, D. (1990). *Methods of modifying speech behaviors* (2nd ed.). Prospect Heights, IL: Waveland Press, Inc.

Nelson, N. W. (1993). *Childhood language disorders in context: Infancy through adolescence.* New York: Macmillan.

Nippold, M. (1990). Concomitant speech and language disorders in stuttering children: A critique of the literature. *Journal of Speech and Hearing Disorders, 55,* 51–60.

Owens, R. (1995). *Language Disorders: A Functional Approach to Assessment and Intervention* (2nd ed.). Needham Heights, MA: Allyn and Bacon.

Pannbacker, M. (1992). Some common myths about voice therapy. *Language, Speech, Hearing Services in Schools, 23,* 12–19.

Paul, R. (1987). Communication in autism. In D. J. Cohen & A. M. Donnellan (Eds.), *Handbook of Autism and Pervasive Developmental Disorders.* New York: Wiley and Sons.

Perkins, W. H. (1978). *Human perspectives in speech and language disorders.* St. Louis: C. V. Mosby.

Perkins, W. H. (1990). What is stuttering? *Journal of Speech and Hearing Disorders, 55,* 370–382.

Ritvo, E. R., & Freeman, B. J. (1978). National Society for Autistic Children definition of the syndrome of autism. *Journal of Autism and Childhood Schizophrenia, 8,* 162–167.

Ruscello, D., St. Louis, K., & Mason, N. (1991). School-aged children with phonologic disorders: Coexistence with other speech/language disorders. *Journal of Speech and Hearing Research, 34,* 236–242.

Scheerenberger, R. (1987). *A history of mental retardation.* Baltimore, MD: Brookes Publishing Company.

Shames, G. H., & Rubin, H. (Eds.) (1986). *Stuttering: Then and now.* Columbus, OH: Merrill/Macmillan.

Shewan, C. (1988). ASHA work force study: Final report. Rockville, MD: American Speech-Language-Hearing Association.

Shewan, C., & Malm, K. (1990). The prevalence of speech and language impairments. *ASHA, 32,* 108.

Silverman, E., & Zimmer, C. (1975). Incidence of chronic hoarseness among school-age children. *Journal of Speech and Hearing Disorders, 40,* 211–215.

Silverman, F. (1996). *Stuttering and other fluency disorders,* 2nd ed. Needham Heights, MA: Allyn and Bacon.

Skinner, P., & Shelton, R. (Eds.) (1985). *Speech, language and hearing.* New York: Wiley.

Stark, R. E., & Tallal, P. (1988). *Language, Speech, and Reading Disorders in Children: Neuropsychological Studies.* San Diego, CA: College-Hill.

Starkweather, C. W. (1987). *Fluency and stuttering.* Englewood Cliffs, NJ: Prentice-Hall.

Stoel-Gammon, C. (1990). Down syndrome: Effects on language development. *Asha, 32,* 42–44.

Swisher, L., & Demetras, M. J. (1985). The expressive language characteristics of autistic children compared with mentally retarded or specific language-impaired children. In E. Schopler & G. B. Mesibov (Eds.), *Communication Problems in Autism.* New York: Plenum.

Tager-Flusberg, H. (1985). The conceptual basis for referential word meaning in children with autism. *Child Development, 56,* 1167–1178.

Van Riper, C. (1973). *The treatment of stuttering.* Englewood Cliffs, NJ: Prentice-Hall.

Van Riper, C. (1992). *The Nature of Stuttering,* 2nd ed. Prospect Heights, IL: Waveland Press, Inc.

Van Riper, C., & Erickson, R. (1996). *Speech correction: An introduction to speech pathology and audiology* (9th ed.) Needham Heights, MA: Allyn and Bacon.

Wall, M. J., & Meyers, F. L. (1984). *Clinical management of childhood stuttering.* Baltimore, MD: University Park Press.

Weiss, C., Gordon, M., & Lillywhite, H. (1987). *Clinical management of articulatory and phonologic disorders* (2nd ed.). Baltimore, MD: Williams and Wilkins.

Wetherby, A. M. (1986). Ontogeny of communicative functions in autism. *Journal of Autism and Developmental Disorders, 16,* 295–316.

Wilson, D. K. (1979). *Voice problems in children* (2nd ed.). Baltimore, MD: Williams and Wilkins.

Winitz, H. (1988). *Human communication and its disorders: A review.* Norwood, NJ: Ablex Publishing Corporation.

The Anatomical and Physiological Bases of Speech, Language, and Hearing

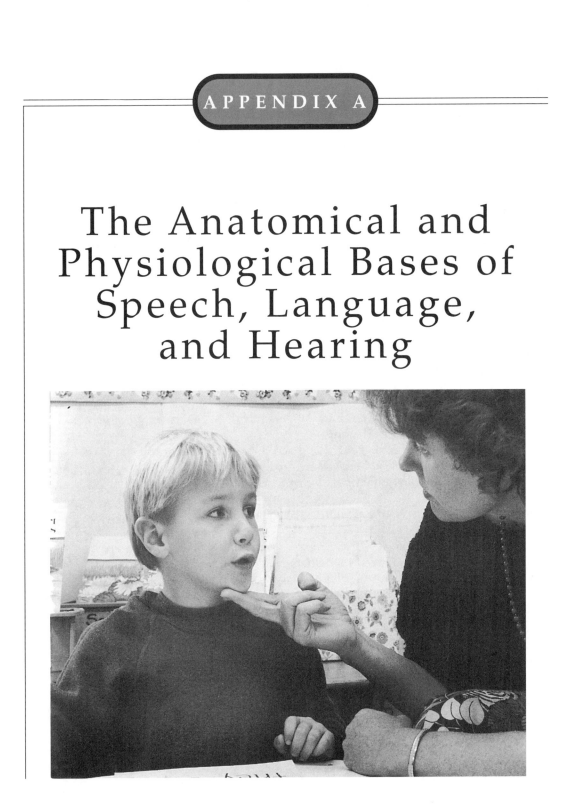

Chapter Objectives

Some of you will have a more thorough understanding of the anatomy and physiology of speech and hearing than others. Some will have no background in this area. All students of human communication development, regardless of knowledge level, need to be reminded that the speech portion of human communication is a physiological process. To fully understand how speech and language development occurs, therefore, one must have some appreciation for the anatomical equipment that makes the human communication system work. This chapter introduces the novice to basic information about the anatomy and physiology of speech and hearing and provides an adequate review if you already have a background. Specifically, this chapter is designed to facilitate understanding of the following topics:

- The integration of respiration, phonation, articulation, and resonation in the production of speech.
- *Respiration:* The power source for speech.
- *Phonation:* Using the larynx to generate voice.
- *Resonation:* Shaping the cavities of the speech mechanism to modify the tones of speech.
- *Articulation:* Using the structures of the mouth to produce the sounds of speech.
- The *human nervous system:* Linking the brain to the muscles of speech.
- The *ear:* Moving sound waves from the pinna to the brain.

Ⅰt is impossible to really understand human speech without examining the anatomic structures and physiological processes that produce speech. Speech is, after all, the direct result of muscle contractions innervated by the nervous system which move structures in ways that force air out of the lungs, vibrate that air, resonate it, and break it up into speech sounds. In this chapter, we look at the structures which together make up what we call the speech machine. We also examine the hearing mechanism, which is important to speech in two ways: (1) We receive the speech of others through the hearing mechanism. Unless there are ears to hear what is said, we cannot complete the **vocal-auditory channel,** one of the design-features of speech (Hockett, 1960). (2) The speaker depends on the ability to hear himself so that he can monitor the content of his speech as well as things like rate, pitch, stress, rhythm, and articulatory accuracy.

Speech as the Product of Borrowed Structures

It is important to note that all of the structures involved in producing speech are designed for other, more basic, biological purposes. Breathing, for example, is important for speech, but the primary reason a person breathes is to absorb oxygen into the bloodstream and to release waste in the form of carbon dioxide. The larynx, commonly called the voice box, is a valve in the throat that prevents the ingestion of foreign substances into the lungs. The tongue, which plays a major role in the production of speech sounds, exists primarily to facilitate eating. Every structure that is a part of the speech machine is, in a sense, borrowed from the body's life maintenance systems. Human beings have adapted certain bodily structures for the purpose of producing speech.

You should not interpret this to mean that speech is the product of an anatomy ill-suited for this purpose. On the contrary, every part of the body that plays a role in speech is ideally designed in structure and function for speech, but we should never forget that speech is an activity which is overlaid on biological functions which are more basic to our physical survival than is speech. This is one of the wonders of human oral communication, that we have been able to use structures intended for other purposes to create a communication system which is convenient and efficient and unmatched in power and sophistication by any other communication system in the animal kingdom. Other primates, for example, have anatomies remarkably similar to ours, but they have not been able to adapt their structures to produce oral communication systems even remotely comparable to speech. The structures themselves, while similar, are not capable of the intricate, controlled adjustments required for speech. The larynx of a chimpanzee, for example, resembles the human larynx, but the vocal folds in the chimpanzee's larynx do not allow the same range of length and tension adjustments as are possible in human vocal folds. Although it is true, therefore, that the structures humans use to produce speech have more fundamental vegetative responsibilities, they work so well for speech that they could have been specifically designed for that purpose.

The Four Processes of Speech

Speech can be most easily understood as the product of four separate but inextricably related processes: respiration, phonation, resonation, and articulation. As indicated in Figure A-1, each process makes a specific contribution to the end product. **Respiration** or breathing provides the power for speech. The speaker inhales to capture air in the lungs, and then in a controlled manner, exhales to force a column of air into the larynx. **Phonation** occurs when the vocal folds of the larynx are drawn together by contraction of specific muscles, and the exhaled air causes the folds to vibrate in a manner that disturbs or vibrates the air column. As the vibrating air column passes through the throat, mouth, and sometimes the nasal cavities, it is **resonated,** which means that the tone of the noise from the vocal folds is modified according to the size and shape of the resonating cavities. As the vibrating and resonated air column passes through the mouth, the tongue, teeth, and other structures in the mouth break up the airstream into the sounds of speech, a process called **articulation.**

As described here and depicted in Figure A-1, the reader might get the impression that there is a discrete order from one process to the next, beginning with respiration. It is more accurate to understand speech as the product of the successive and simultaneous interactions of these four processes. In other words, it is true that speech must begin with exhalation, and the air stream must be phonated before it can be resonated, and it is articulated as it passes out of the mouth, but in continuous speech, all four of these processes are occurring in a precisely integrated and synchronized manner. While one part of the vibrating air column is being articulated, another part of the air column is just beginning the journey from the lungs into the larynx.

For the sake of convenience, we will look at each process as a separate entity, but you should remember that, like any machine, each part of the speech machine depends on every other part, and the machine functions only as the parts work together. Many man-made machines have become so complicated in their structures and functions that they must be managed by internal computers. The human speech machine is also incredibly complex and also requires an internal computer to make sure all the parts function in proper synchrony. The speech machine's computer is the brain. It is the brain which coordinates the activities of all the processes of speech and insures that the product is speech, not jibberish. As indicated in Figure A-1, the brain sends out instructions along motor pathways to the structures involved in each process and constantly monitors how these structures are responding by analyzing the data sent back by the sensory pathways. Normal speech is maintained only if correct instructions are sent to the speech structures and reliable feedback is received from them.

FIGURE A-1 The Processes of Speech

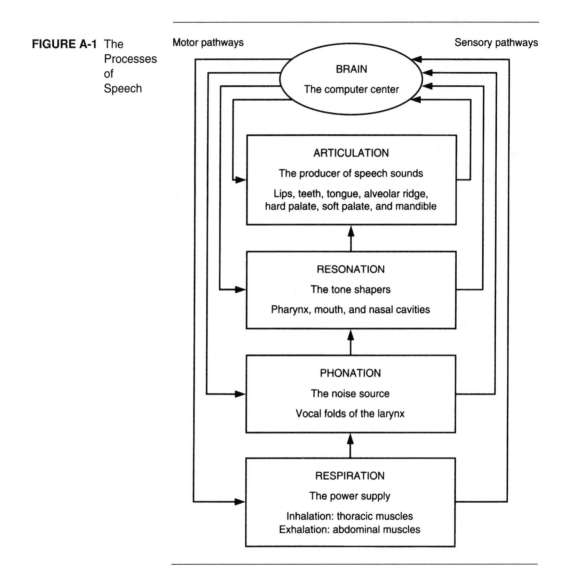

Motor pathways   Sensory pathways

BRAIN
The computer center

ARTICULATION
The producer of speech sounds
Lips, teeth, tongue, alveolar ridge,
hard palate, soft palate, and mandible

RESONATION
The tone shapers
Pharynx, mouth, and nasal cavities

PHONATION
The noise source
Vocal folds of the larynx

RESPIRATION
The power supply
Inhalation: thoracic muscles
Exhalation: abdominal muscles

Respiration

As has already been noted, the primary biological function of respiration is the exchange of life-sustaining oxygen for carbon dioxide. Breathing for life is involuntary and rhythmic. About 50 percent of each breathing cycle is spent on inhalation and about 50 percent on exhalation. Breathing for speech is very different. The speaker exercises voluntary control over the breathing cycle, especially exhalation, which forces air through the vocal tract. During speech, about 15 percent of the breathing cycle is devoted to inhalation and 85 percent to exhalation.

The Structures of Breathing

The primary muscle involved in inhalation is the **diaphragm,** which separates the trunk of the body into two sections. The section above the diaphragm is called the **thorax,** the cavity that houses the lungs, and the section below the diaphragm is called the **abdomen,** the cavity that houses internal organs like the kidneys, liver, and intestines.

The bony framework of the **thorax** (Figure A-2) is comprised of 12 **thoracic vertebrae** posteriorly, the **sternum** (breastbone) anteriorly, and 12 pairs of **ribs** laterally. The **lungs,** located inside the thorax, are the structures that exchange carbon dioxide and oxygen. The bases of the lungs rest on top of the diaphragm. Two moist membranes called **pleurae** surround the lungs. The lungs themselves consist of spongy tissue that is highly elastic, but there are very few muscle fibers in the lungs, which means they are passive structures. They receive air. They do not suck in air as some people think. The lungs receive air during inhalation when the thorax expands, creating a difference in air pressure in the lungs compared to the air pressure outside the body. Breathing depends on a very basic principle of physics known as Boyle's law.

The Application of Basic Physics to Breathing

According to Boyle's law, "If a gas is kept at a constant temperature, pressure and volume are inversely proportional to one another and have a constant product" (Zemlin, 1988, p. 33). This means that if we have a given number of gas molecules at a constant temperature, we can change the pressure exerted by those molecules by changing the volume of the container. If we double the volume of the container, the pressure is reduced by one-half. If we triple the volume of the container, the pressure is reduced to one-third of the original pressure, etc. On the other hand, if we cut the volume of the container in half, the pressure exerted by the gas molecules doubles, and if we reduce the volume to one-third of the original volume, the pressure triples, etc.

Consider how this law is applied to breathing. The lungs are housed inside the thorax, an airtight cavity connected to the outside air through the **trachea** or windpipe and the mouth and nose. If the volume of the thorax is increased, the air pressure inside the lungs decreases proportionately, and what will happen if the pressure inside is less than the pressure outside when there is a direct connection between the lungs and the outside air? Air will rush into the lungs to make the pressures equal, of course. Therefore, **inhalation** occurs when the volume of the thorax is increased, creating pressure in the lungs that is less than the outside pressure. In **exhalation,** the volume of the thorax is reduced, creating pressure inside the lungs that is greater than the outside pressure, and what happens? Air rushes

FIGURE A-2 The
           Thorax:
           Front and
           Rear
           Views

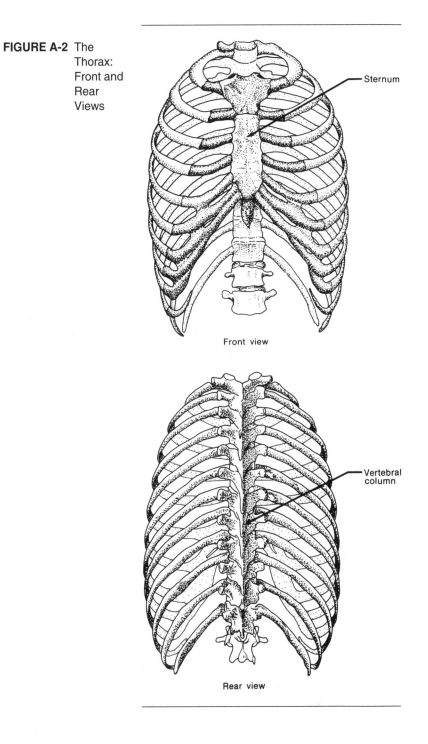

Sternum

Front view

Vertebral
column

Rear view

out of the lungs until the pressures are equal again. Breathing then depends on the very practical application of Boyle's law and the simple principle of equilibrium. What remains to be understood is how the volume of the thorax is increased in inhalation and decreased in exhalation.

Inhalation and Exhalation During Quiet Breathing

During normal quiet breathing, the amount of oxygen inhaled is approximately equal to the volume of carbon dioxide exhaled, and a complete inhalation-exhalation cycle occurs about twelve to fifteen times per minute.

The diaphragm is dome-shaped in its resting configuration. Inhalation begins when the diaphragm contracts or flattens, resulting in an increase in the vertical dimension of the thorax (Figure A-3). At the same time, muscles attached to the ribs contract, lifting the ribs and swinging them upward and outward in much the same way the handle on a bucket moves away from the side of a bucket when it is lifted (Figure A-4). This action also causes the sternum to be moved up and out. The muscles of inhalation, therefore, cause the thorax to be increased from side to side, front to back, and in the vertical dimension. The lungs, which are effectively attached to the sides of the thorax by the pleurae that surround them, expand when the thorax expands. This action creates reduced air pressure in the lungs relative to the outside air pressure, and air rushes into the lungs until the pressures are equal, completing the inhalation portion of the respiratory cycle.

Exhalation in quiet breathing is a passive process, not involving muscle activity. After the lungs fill with air, the muscles of inhalation relax, reducing the volume of the thorax and creating another imbalance of inside and outside pressures. Air now flows out of the lungs until the pressures are equal again. This completes exhalation and one complete cycle of respiration. We do this automatically and rhythmically about twelve to fifteen times per minute, whether asleep or awake (Zemlin, 1988, p. 94). There are obviously more cycles per minute when we are active than when we are relaxed, and when we sleep soundly, the number of cycles per minute is further reduced.

Breathing for Speech

Breathing for speech differs radically from breathing for life. As mentioned earlier, speech is a muscular activity requiring the precise synchronization of all four processes of speech, including respiration. Breathing for speech necessitates delicate control of each respiratory cycle and particularly the exhalation portion of the cycle. When we breathe for speech, we extend and control exhalation for up to 15 seconds. If we were unable to do this, talking time would be restricted to 2.5 second spurts, the average duration of exhalation during quiet breathing (Zemlin, 1990, p. 80). We would be able to produce only a few words at a time instead of the lengthy sentences which characterize normal speech.

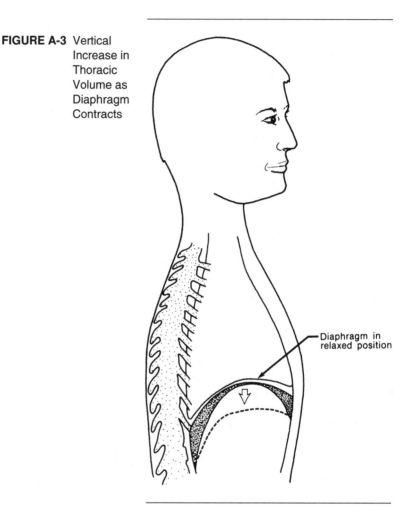

FIGURE A-3 Vertical Increase in Thoracic Volume as Diaphragm Contracts

Diaphragm in relaxed position

In addition to changing the nature of the respiratory cycle, speech affects breathing by introducing varying degrees of airflow resistance at a number of places in the speech mechanism. If the vocal folds are brought together, for example, and the lips or the tongue are positioned for the production of certain sounds, the power of exhalation must be great enough to force air through the constriction points. Instead of just relaxing the muscles of inhalation as we do during quiet breathing, we must partially contract these muscles and actively contract muscles of exhalation to maintain sufficient airflow force and control for speech production. Breathing for speech, therefore, requires a complex balance of the muscle activities involved in

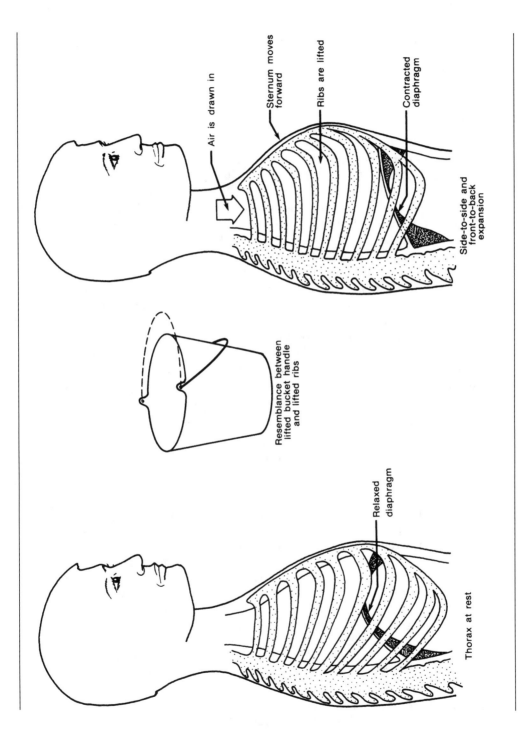

FIGURE A-4 Lateral and Antero-Posterior Expansions of the Thorax

Air is drawn in

Sternum moves forward

Ribs are lifted

Contracted diaphragm

Side-to-side and front-to-back expansion

Resemblance between lifted bucket handle and lifted ribs

Relaxed diaphragm

Thorax at rest

377

inhalation and exhalation, a balance that allows us to sustain exhalation for periods up to six times longer than exhalation during quiet breathing. The air we exhale for speech moves into the larynx, the tone-producing structure in the speech machine.

Phonation

The **larynx** is a structure in the anterior neck commonly known as the voice box. The **vocal folds** are the components in the larynx responsible for generating the noise upon which speech is superimposed. The larynx sits on top of the trachea and is suspended by means of muscles and ligaments from a U-shaped bone called the **hyoid.** Although the hyoid is not part of the larynx, it is important to laryngeal function because a number of laryngeal muscles are attached to it.

As mentioned earlier, the larynx acts as a valve to prevent foreign materials from entering the trachea and lungs. If something threatens to enter, the vocal folds close while exhalation continues until the force of the air below the folds literally blows them open. You may recognize this action as the cough.

The secondary function of the larynx is sound production, a purpose for which it is ideally constructed. The vocal folds are relatively long and are capable of the wide range of adjustments in length and tension that are essential for voice production. During normal quiet breathing, the vocal folds are relatively wide open, but during speech, they are drawn together to obstruct the flow of air from the lungs, setting up the conditions necessary for vocal fold vibration. We will take a closer look at the mechanics of voice production after we examine the structure of the larynx.

The Parts of the Voice Generator

The larynx is comprised of nine cartilages (Figure A-5) bound together by a complex network of membranes. The inside of the larynx is lined with a membrane that is continuous with the membrane lining the trachea below and the pharynx above. There are three single cartilages in the larynx and three pairs of smaller cartilages. We are concerned with only the most important of these cartilages: thyroid, cricoid, epiglottis, and the arytenoids.

The **thyroid** is the largest of the laryngeal cartilages. It is the part of the larynx that tends to protrude in the neck and is often referred to as the Adam's apple. This unpaired cartilage is made up of two plates joined in front in a V-shape whose open portion faces toward the back. Each plate has two projections called **horns.** The **superior horn** extends upward toward the hyoid bone, and the **inferior horn** extends downward to connect with the cricoid cartilage. This pivotal connection allows the thyroid cartilage to be tilted downward and forward, an action that lengthens the vocal folds.

The lowermost portion of the larynx is the **cricoid** cartilage, which sits on the top of the trachea. The cricoid is in the shape of a ring, with a plate on the posterior side and a narrower band forming the front and sides.

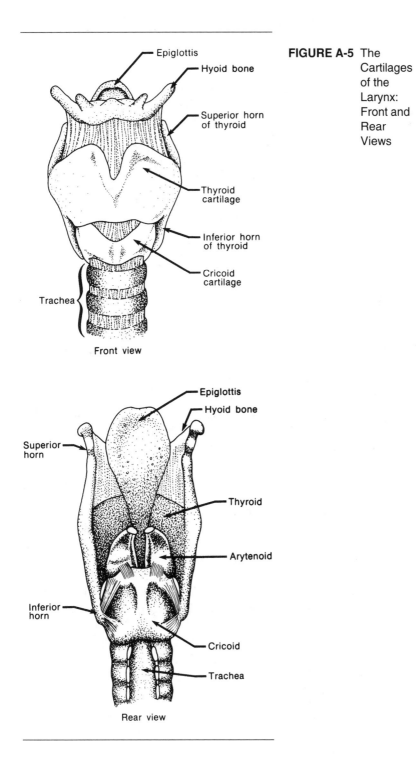

Epiglottis

Hyoid bone

Superior horn
of thyroid

Thyroid
cartilage

Inferior horn
of thyroid

Cricoid
cartilage

Trachea

Front view

FIGURE A-5 The
Cartilages
of the
Larynx:
Front and
Rear
Views

Epiglottis

Hyoid bone

Superior
horn

Thyroid

Arytenoid

Inferior
horn

Cricoid

Trachea

Rear view

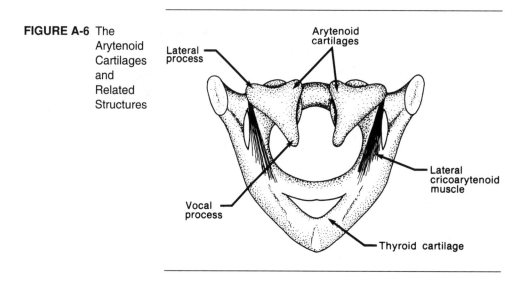

FIGURE A-6 The Arytenoid Cartilages and Related Structures

Attached to the angle of the thyroid is the third single cartilage called the **epiglottis,** which is shaped something like a narrow leaf. It is attached at its top margin to the hyoid bone by a ligament. Even though the epiglottis is an interesting-looking structure, it makes little, if any, contribution to speech.

The only paired cartilages that are important to laryngeal function are the roughly pyramid-shaped **arytenoids** (Figure A-6), which are situated on top of the posterior plate of the cricoid. Each arytenoid has a **vocal process** and a **lateral** or **muscular** process. The vocal processes extend anteriorly and have the vocal folds attached to them. The lateral processes have muscles attached to them that act to move the vocal folds together or apart.

As has already been mentioned, the **vocal folds** (Figure A-7) are the vibrating elements of the larynx and consist of muscles and ligaments. They originate at the angle of the thyroid, extend posteriorly along the inner sides of the thyroid, and attach to the vocal processes of the arytenoids. As indicated in Figure A-7, each vocal fold extends into the opening of the larynx like a shelf. The space between the folds is called the **glottis.** The glottis varies in width, depending on which laryngeal muscles contract and how much they contract. During normal breathing, the glottis is relatively wide open. When the speaker whispers, the front part of the glottis closes, but the posterior portion remains open. During full voice, the folds are closed along their entire length, and the glottis disappears.

Making the Voice Generator Work

Muscles in the larynx allow the speaker to open and close the vocal folds, and the muscles making up the vocal folds allow the speaker to make the folds tense or lax.

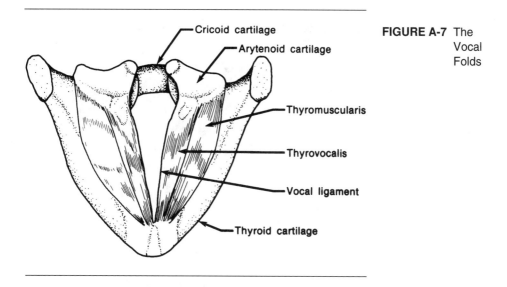

FIGURE A-7 The Vocal Folds

These adjustments are basic to producing the voice. Muscles that have both of their attachments within the larynx itself are **intrinsic muscles** of the larynx. These are the muscles primarily responsible for the adjustments necessary for voice production. The extrinsic muscles, with one attachment in the larynx and the other attachment outside the larynx, move the entire structure up and down, but these adjustments have little to do with generating voice. This section, therefore, focuses on those intrinsic muscles most directly involved in opening and closing the vocal folds.

The muscles whose primary responsibility is to open the vocal folds are called **abductors.** To **abduct** means to move or pull away from the middle. In the case of laryngeal function, the abductors pull the vocal folds away from one another, opening the glottis between them. Those muscles primarily responsible for closing the vocal folds are called **adductors,** which means that they move the vocal folds toward the middle, effectively closing the glottis.

The muscles of abduction are the **posterior cricoarytenoid** muscles (Figure A-8). As is true of most muscles of the body, the name itself identifies the points of attachment. These muscles originate on both sides of the posterior plate of the cricoid cartilage and attach to the lateral or muscular processes of the arytenoid cartilages. When these muscles contract, they pull the arytenoids in a manner that causes them to rotate, opening the folds attached to their vocal processes.

Adduction of the vocal folds is accomplished by contraction of the paired **lateral cricoarytenoid** muscles and the **interarytenoid** muscles (Figure A-9). The lateral cricoarytenoid muscles originate on the sides of the cricoid cartilage and insert into the lateral processes of the arytenoids. When they contract, they pull the vocal processes and the attached vocal folds toward the middle, partially closing the glottis. To achieve complete closure of the vocal folds, the interarytenoids must also be

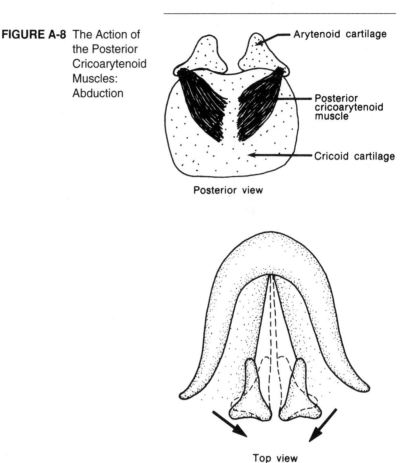

FIGURE A-8 The Action of the Posterior Cricoarytenoid Muscles: Abduction

Arytenoid cartilage

Posterior cricoarytenoid muscle

Cricoid cartilage

Posterior view

Top view

involved. There are actually several interarytenoid muscles which, as the name implies, run between the arytenoid cartilages. The **transverse interarytenoid,** an unpaired muscle, courses from the outside edge of one arytenoid to the outside edge of the other. Each of the two **oblique interarytenoid** muscles originates on the lower outside edge of one arytenoid and attaches to the top or apex of the other. When the interarytenoid muscles contract, they pull the arytenoid cartilages and the vocal folds together, and when they work together with the lateral cricoarytenoid muscles, they completely close the vocal folds.

We have now examined all of the laryngeal parts that are active in generating the tone upon which speech is produced. The laryngeal tone is the result of very rapid vocal fold vibrations. Consider what happens in a single cycle of vibration:

Transverse muscle

Arytenoid cartilage

Cricoid cartilage

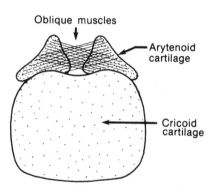

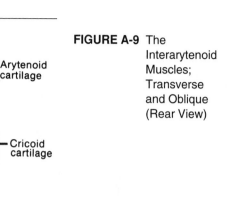

FIGURE A-9 The Interarytenoid Muscles; Transverse and Oblique (Rear View)

Oblique muscles

Arytenoid cartilage

Cricoid cartilage

(1) The vocal folds are adducted to restrict the flow of air from the lungs. (2) At the same time as the folds are being adducted, exhalation is producing increased air pressure beneath the folds. (3) When this pressure is sufficient, the folds are blown apart, releasing a small puff of air into the trachea above. (4) This release results in reduced pressure beneath the folds. (5) The reduction of air pressure combined with the elasticity of the folds forces the folds to snap back together, ready to be blown apart again when the pressure builds up. This five-step sequence is repeated 120 to 145 times per second in adult males and 200 to 260 times per second in adult females (Zemlin, 1990, p. 93). Pitch changes are accomplished by varying the length and mass of the folds. In general, pitch rises when there is an increase in length and a decrease in mass, adjustments that result in more rapid vocal fold vibrations. The tone produced by the larynx is most often called the **glottal** or **laryngeal tone.** It sounds like the combination of a hum and a buzz until it is shaped by the resonating cavities of the neck and head and eventually broken up by the articulators into the speech sounds we combine into words and sentences.

Resonation

The next speech process is **resonation.** Have you ever blown over the top of a partially filled bottle of pop? The sound you hear results from the size and shape of the resonating cavity, in this case the space in the bottle above the pop. If you drink more of the pop and blow over the top again, the tone will change. The change is the result of a larger and, depending upon bottle shape and the amount of pop remaining, differently shaped resonating cavity. In other words, if the tone fed into the bottle remains constant, but the size and shape of the resonating cavity within the bottle changes, the resulting tones will change. In general, the larger the resonating cavity, the lower the perceived pitch of the tone, because the larger cavity will reinforce the lower frequencies in the original tone. Resonance in speech, therefore, is the process whereby certain frequencies in the laryngeal tone are reinforced or emphasized depending upon the size and shape of the speech resonators, including the pharynx, mouth, and nasal cavities (Figure A-10). Although a bottle's resonating cavity has a fairly limited range of adjustments, the resonating cavities for speech are capable of seemingly limitless adjustments.

Although resonation is important for shaping all speech sounds, it is particularly important for vowels. The primary characteristic differentiating vowels from consonants is that they are open sounds, produced with a relatively free flow of air. There is very little constriction anywhere in the vocal tract when a vowel is produced. Say the following sounds aloud: *p, t, k.* Notice that the airflow is actually stopped and released on these sounds. Now say *s, f,* and *th.* Notice that the flow of air continues, but it is constricted. Now produce a few vowels aloud like *a, o,* and *e.* There is little restriction of air flow in the mouth. Now try producing a constant laryngeal tone and simply change the size and shape of your mouth by opening it wide and narrowing the opening, by lifting the tongue and lowering it without touching anything, and by moving the tongue forward and pulling it back. These are the kinds of adjustments we make to produce different vowels. When we produce a vowel like the *ee* in *feet,* we create a narrow, high, front-of-the-mouth resonating cavity. When we produce a vowel like the *a* in *father,* we shape a wide, low, back-of-the-mouth cavity, and notice that the *ee* sounds higher in pitch than the *a* even though the laryngeal tone remains the same. Keep in mind that we have considered changes only in the mouth. The pharynx, which connects the trachea and the mouth, is a muscular structure capable of many adjustments, and it is constantly changing its shape during speech, adding subtle resonated qualities to the laryngeal tone.

It is generally understood that the nasal cavities are opened for resonation only for the production of the consonants *m, n,* and *ng.* We actually experience some nasal resonance on vowels in words containing these consonants because we cannot close off the nasal cavities quickly enough to eliminate the nasal quality. You may also have noticed that there is a nasal quality in some dialects of American English, particularly in the southern and southwestern parts of the country.

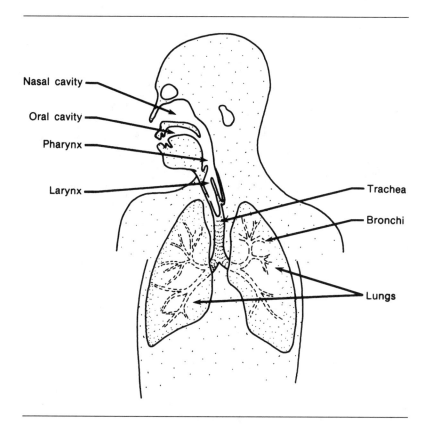

FIGURE A-10 The Resonating Cavities

Articulation

We now come to the final process of speech, **articulation,** which is most simply understood as the breaking up of the air stream into the sounds of speech by the structures of the mouth. It should be clear at this point, however, that it is not possible to separate articulation from the other processes of speech, particularly resonation, with which it is closely integrated. Although it is true, for example, that vowels are primary the products of resonation, they are also the products of articulatory adjustments, especially varying jaw openings and tongue manipulations. We most commonly associate articulation with consonants, but as has already been noted, the consonants *m, n,* and *ng* are very much the products of nasal resonance. Whatever separation we make between resonation and articulation, therefore, is somewhat arbitrary and must be understood as an effort to emphasize and

FIGURE A-11 The
Articulators

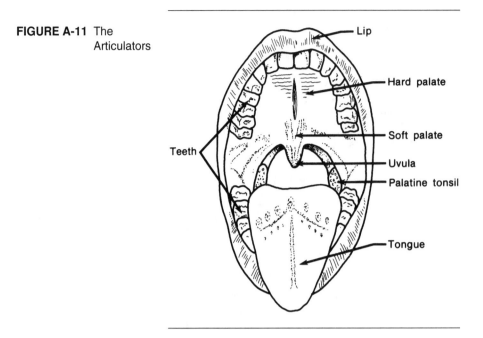

clarify the most important function of each process. With that purpose in mind, it is reasonable and accurate to note that resonation is primarily concerned with vowel production, and articulation is primarily concerned with consonant production, although each process is involved in the production of all speech sounds.

The articulators include the teeth, tongue, lips, alveolar ridge, hard palate, soft palate (velum), and the jaw (Figure A-11). Notice that some of these structures can move and others are fixed. The tongue, lips, soft palate, and the jaw can move, but not at the same speeds. The tongue is capable of relatively rapid movements, but the soft palate moves very slowly. The soft palate is the muscular tissue at the posterior end of the roof of the mouth. For all of the sounds of speech, except *m, n,* and *ng,* it lifts up and back to close off the opening between the mouth and the nasal cavities. The alveolar ridge is the bony shelf into which the upper teeth are set. The hard palate is the bony portion of the roof of the mouth. These structures and the teeth do not move. Another way to understand articulation, therefore, is that the mobile articulators move toward and away from, and sometimes make contact with, the fixed articulators. These adjustments account for how most, but not all, speech sounds are articulated, since the sounds *k, g,* and *ng* involve contacts between the back of the tongue and the soft palate, two mobile articulators.

The Four Processes in Review

Now that we have examined each process as a separate part of the anatomy and physiology of speech, we will consider how they work together in the simple production, *be*.

The speaker *inhales* by contracting the diaphragm and the muscles of the thorax, which has the effect of increasing the volume of the thorax in the vertical, side-to-side, and front-to-back dimensions. This increase in volume creates reduced pressure in the lungs, which expand along with the expanding thorax. Air comes into the lungs until the pressure in the lungs equals the pressure outside the body. The speaker then *exhales* by relaxing most of the muscles of inhalation and contracting the muscles of exhalation in a prolonged and controlled manner. These actions push a column of air out of the lungs, through the trachea, and into the larynx.

Since both sounds in the word *be* require vocal fold vibration, the speaker contracts the adductor muscles to bring the vocal folds together. As the column of air is pushed through the folds by the forces of exhalation, the folds vibrate, creating a disturbance in the particles of air we refer to as the *glottal* or *laryngeal tone*. The now vibrating column of air passes out of the larynx into the pharynx.

The speaker adjusts the *resonators,* including the pharynx, mouth, and nasal cavities, to shape the laryngeal tone according to the characteristics of the sounds being produced. In producing *be,* for example, the speaker will lift the soft palate to close off the nasal cavities because the sounds in the word do not receive nasal resonance. The speaker closes his lips to stop the flow of air and then quickly releases this closure to *articulate* the *b* sound, and at the same time, raises the tongue toward the front part of the hard palate to create the high, narrow resonating chamber for the *e*. The vocal folds vibrate throughout the entire production.

The reader should once again be impressed with the complexity of these adjustments and the speed at which they occur. The human anatomy has been ideally developed for the production of speech, and the physiology involved occurs so naturally and effortlessly that we make these rapid, intricate adjustments thousands upon thousands of times every day without giving them a conscious thought.

The Computer Center for Speech and Language: The Brain

The reason speech is produced with so little conscious effort is that the speech machine is directed by a central nervous system unmatched in any other animal on earth. Some physiological functions in humans and all animals are automatic, of course. Our hearts beat and we breathe without any conscious efforts on our parts, whether we are awake or asleep.

The behaviors of speech and language are voluntary and require more conscious control than breathing, but they require far less direct attention than, for example, putting thread through the eye of a needle. Remember too that people sometimes

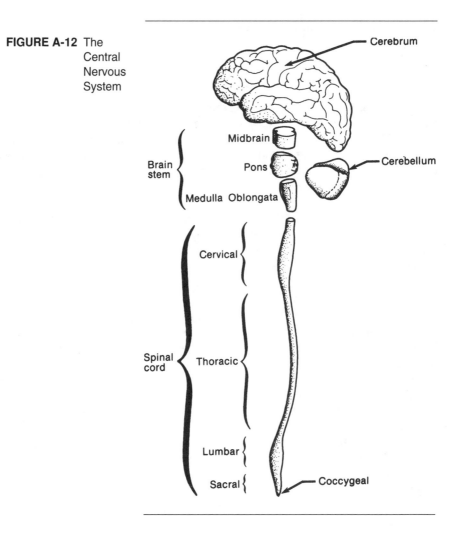

FIGURE A-12 The Central Nervous System

Cerebrum

Midbrain

Brain stem

Pons

Cerebellum

Medulla Oblongata

Cervical

Spinal cord

Thoracic

Lumbar

Sacral

Coccygeal

talk while they are asleep, so the behaviors of speech and language are voluntary, but they are so natural and instinctive and require so little effort that we can sometimes talk in our sleep. This would not be possible without the complex and highly reliable nervous system that serves as a kind of computer center for speech and language.

A detailed description of neuroanatomy and neurophysiology is beyond the scope of this book, but if you want to learn more about these subjects, see the list of readings at the end of this chapter. For the purposes of this book, we will focus on the major features of the human nervous system, and especially on those parts which are most directly related to speech, language, and hearing.

The nervous system can be arbitrarily divided into two major divisions: (1) central nervous system and (2) peripheral nervous system. The **central nervous system** (Figure A-12) includes the brain and the spinal cord. The brain is divided into halves called the right and left **cerebral hemispheres,** the **brain stem,** and the **cerebellum.** The brain is encased in the skull, and the spinal cord is surrounded by the bony **vertebral column,** sometimes called the **spinal column.**

The peripheral nervous system consists of all the cranial and spinal nerves that carry information to the brain in the form of sensations such as hearing, pain, or temperature, and information from the brain in the form of motor commands to the muscles of the body.

The most basic anatomic unit of the nervous system is the **neuron.** There are millions of neurons in the body, which are organized into complex networks or circuits. Any message carried anywhere in the nervous system is carried by the tiny neuron.

Speech and Language Functions of the Brain

Even though the speech and language functions of the brain are not fully understood, we have been able to identify certain areas of the cerebral hemispheres that have primary responsibilities for this uniquely human range of behaviors. What follows is a brief overview of the information researchers have gathered over the years about those structures they believe are most closely associated with speech and language functions. The reader should be forewarned that because this is only an overview and intentionally introductory in nature, we will focus only on the most obvious relevant structures. The reader who is interested in a more detailed description of all neural structures believed to be relevant to speech and language functions should consult the references and suggested readings included at the end of Appendix A.

The Cerebrum: Left and Right Cerebral Hemispheres

The **cerebrum,** the largest portion of the brain, is incompletely divided into two hemispheres. The two halves of the cerebrum are connected by a large band of neural fibers known as the **corpus callosum,** a structure that serves as a major communication pathway between the two hemispheres. Although we cannot generalize left and right hemispheric functions for all people, it is appropriate to indicate that in most people the left hemisphere has greater responsibilities for speech and language activities than the right. Three areas of the left hemisphere and a bundle of neural fibers (Figure A-13) are of particular interest: **Wernicke's area, Broca's area,** the **motor cortex,** and the **arcuate fasciculus.** Wernicke's area is primarily concerned with the comprehension and formulation of language. Language information is transmitted to Broca's area from Wernicke's area via a bundle of neural fibers called the arcuate fasciculus. The term *fasciculus* refers to a bundle of nerve fibers that share a common origin, termination, and function. In Broca's area, language information is organized into the appropriate articulatory motor sequences

FIGURE A-13 Left
Cerebral
Hemisphere

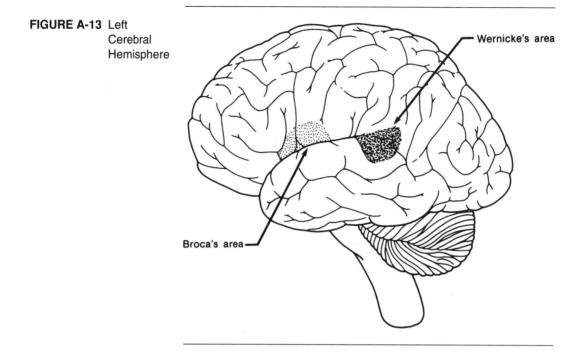

for speech. These motor commands are then transmitted to the motor cortex. The neural messages carrying speech and language information are eventually sent to the speech musculature along special pathways that will be described in the **Motor Speech Control** section.

The right hemisphere is less involved with speech and language than the left but it does contribute to the processing of emotional content that often underlies speech and language. There is also evidence that the melodic patterns we superimpose on speech when we sing are associated with right hemispheric functions (Blumstein and Cooper, 1974; Knox and Kimura, 1970).

There is the suggestion here that functions of the hemispheres are highly specialized, and although areas in each hemisphere do seem to have specific functions, it is important to understand that there is significant integration of the functions of the cerebrum. For example, we have noted that emotional processing is associated with the right hemisphere, and language and speech functions are associated with the left hemisphere. It should be immediately clear, however, that we can communicate emotional messages through speech and language only if the two hemispheres interact with one another in a manner that allows us to integrate emotional messages into language form, which are then expressed in meaningful speech.

Motor Speech Control

How do we get our speech and language messages from the cerebrum to the muscles of speech? Once thoughts are formulated and put into language form, the cerebrum sends the motor messages of speech along a complex neural network of special pathways within the central nervous system. The information contained in these pathways ultimately reaches the various motor portions of the cranial and spinal nerves that constitute the peripheral nervous system. The peripheral nerves are connected to the muscles of the body and are the final pathways over which the messages will be delivered.

It may help to think of this process of getting motor commands from the cerebrum to the structures of speech as being analogous to a relay race. The "runners" who will be the initial carriers of information in this complicated delivery system are the many neurons that make up specialized pathways in the central nervous system. Positioned at strategic locations within the nervous system are the other runners or neurons that make up the cranial and spinal nerves of the peripheral nervous system. Once the communication plan is developed, the runners of the central nervous system are given complex messages, which they carry to the runners of the peripheral nervous system by way of the special pathways. Upon reaching the stations where the peripheral nervous system runners are waiting, the messages are passed on and carried by those runners to the muscles of the body that must be activated to produce the message in its final form—speech.

Central Nervous System Pathways: The Beginning of the Race

One of the special pathways of the central nervous system is called **pyramidal** because the tiny neurons that give rise to this system have cell bodies shaped like pyramids. This part of the system has **direct** input into the motor cranial and spinal nerves which represent the second leg in the relay race to the structures of speech. The pyramidal pathway controls refined, intricate movements in structures like the lips and tongue. This kind of control is crucial to an activity like speech, which is the product of complex, precise, and delicately integrated motor adjustments.

The **extrapyramidal** system has a more **indirect** connection to the motor cranial and spinal nerves than the pyramidal, and it is responsible for providing commands for more gross and unskilled motor activities such as those involved in postural adjustment. We might refer to the act of writing to provide a simple example of the difference between pyramidal and extrapyramidal responsibilities. When you write, the extrapyramidal tract gets your hand to the paper, and the pyramidal tract controls the fine motor skills necessary for you to write on that paper. In the context of our relay race analogy, the runners in the extrapyramidal system stop at a number of locations within the central nervous system to gather additional information in order to make the necessary adjustments to provide a background against which the pyramidal system makes its more precise, finely tuned movements.

The **cerebellum** coordinates the activities controlled by the pyramidal and extrapyramidal systems. It is constantly receiving sensory information about the status of the muscles and limbs of the body and monitors the motor commands being sent along the pyramidal and extrapyramidal pathways. Using this steady flow of information to and from the central nervous system, the cerebellum makes crucial adjustments in commands to insure that the final motor products are performed as accurately as possible.

Peripheral Nervous System Pathways: The Relay Race Continues

The commands that have been formulated in the cerebral hemispheres, carried through the central nervous system along the pyramidal and extrapyramidal pathways, and fine tuned by the cerebellum are now passed to the message carrier who will run along the pathways of the cranial and spinal nerves that comprise the peripheral nervous system.

There are pairs of **cranial nerves.** Some of these nerves carry only sensory information, some only motor, and others are mixed and carry both sensory and motor information. Only six of the cranial nerves are concerned with motor speech (Figure A-14).

There are thirty-one pairs of **spinal nerves** and they are all mixed. That is, they carry both sensory and motor information. More than half of these nerves control the muscles of respiration. Since, as we observed earlier in this chapter, controlled and prolonged exhalation is crucial to speech production, these nerves make important contributions to the speech machine.

The Relay Race in Review: Instant Replay

There is much we do not understand about the nervous system in general and much we do not understand about those functions related to speech and language. We do know, however, that the nervous system is organized in a hierarchical manner. That is, there are levels in the system at which information is developed, refined, and integrated as it works its way to the speech musculature.

Using the relay race analogy, we can now summarize the process. At the highest level in the system, the cerebrum, thoughts are developed, and language to express those thoughts is formulated. The message is carried by runners along the pyramidal and extrapyramidal pathways of the central nervous system. These runners carry the message through the cerebellum, which fine tunes the motor commands, before they hand off the message to other runners who carry the message along the pathways of the cranial and spinal nerves involved in speech. The race ends when the commands reach the muscles of the speech structures, which contract in patterns producing strings of sounds that are a direct translation of the original thought.

In continuous speech, of course, the relay race is infinitely more complicated than this summary indicates because new thoughts, new language forms, and new

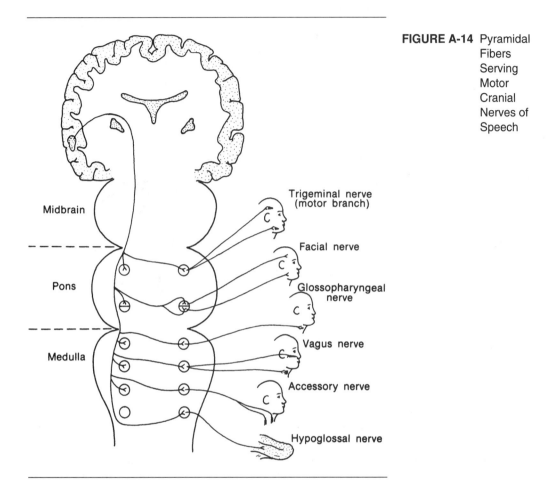

FIGURE A-14 Pyramidal Fibers Serving Motor Cranial Nerves of Speech

Midbrain

Pons

Medulla

Trigeminal nerve
(motor branch)

Facial nerve

Glossopharyngeal
nerve

Vagus nerve

Accessory nerve

Hypoglossal nerve

motor messages are being sent and monitored and fine tuned constantly. The nervous system carries so much information so quickly with such tremendous efficiency that it makes the most sophisticated telephone systems invented by man and hyped by Madison Avenue look like tin cans connected by kite string.

The Ear: An Energy Transformer

It is impossible to understand speech as a physiological process without considering the hearing mechanism that allows us to receive speech and monitor our own speech productions. You will quickly appreciate the importance of hearing if you consider how the child learns to talk. He does not buy a "How to Talk" manual,

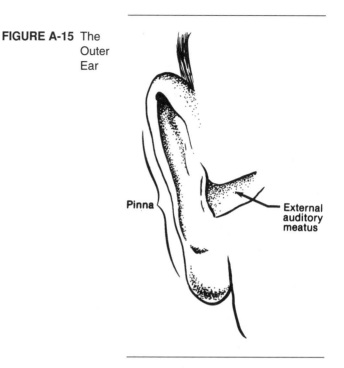

FIGURE A-15 The Outer Ear

Pinna

External auditory meatus

and he does not enroll in Human Speech 101 at his local university. He learns to talk by *listening* to the speech around him. If a child has any significant deficit in hearing, it is highly likely that the acquisition of speech will be impaired. At the other end of the age spectrum, a normally speaking adult who loses hearing later in life will not lose language but may experience some deterioration in speech because he cannot hear his own productions. Articulation may not be as precise as it once was, for example, and there may be some nasality on speech sounds that are not supposed to have nasal resonance. The point is simple but important. Hearing is as crucial to normal speech as any other part of the complete anatomical and physiological speech package.

The human hearing mechanism is an extraordinary energy transformer, and tracing the changes in energy forms is one of the best ways to understand the parts of the hearing system and how they are related to one another. For the sake of convenience we will consider the three traditional anatomic divisions of the ear, *outer, middle,* and *inner,* but it is important to note that the outer and middle ears function together to transform acoustic energy into mechanical energy.

The Outer Ear

Sound travels to the outer ear (see Figure A-15) in the form of sound waves which, as we noted in the first chapter, are disturbances of air particles characterized by

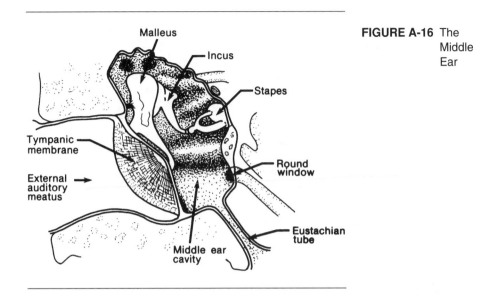

FIGURE A-16 The Middle Ear

compressions and rarefactions. These waves are caught by the pinna, the visible fleshy part of the ear attached to the side of the head. The pinna contributes minimally to our ability to hear, but it does serve to direct sound waves into the **external auditory meatus** or ear canal. This canal is slightly curved, about an inch long and a quarter of an inch across, dimensions that make it a resonator specifically tuned to the frequencies of speech sounds. At the end of the canal is the **tympanic membrane** or eardrum, which serves as the boundary between the outer and middle ears.

The Middle Ear

In the middle ear (see Figure A-16), the tympanic membrane is semitransparent and is usually pearl gray when it is healthy. The center of the membrane is pulled in because it is attached to one of the tiny bones in the middle ear. The tympanic membrane absorbs the acoustic energy of sound waves and transforms it into mechanical energy, which is the vibration of a solid material.

The tiny bones in the middle ear, called the **ossicles,** are the **malleus** (hammer), **incus** (anvil), and **stapes** (stirrup). The malleus is the largest ossicle and its "handle" is attached to the center of the tympanic membrane. The middle ossicle is the incus, which is attached to the innermost ossicle, the stapes. The bottom part of the stapes, known as the footplate because of its similarity to the footplate of the stirrup of a saddle, fits into an oval-shaped hole in the bony wall of the inner ear called the **oval window.**

The ossicles operate together in transferring energy from the tympanic membrane to the oval window, and for this reason, are often referred to as the ossicular chain. This chain is suspended in the air-filled cavity of the middle ear by ligaments

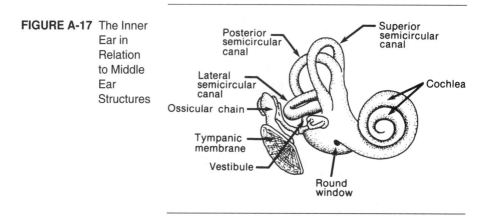

FIGURE A-17 The Inner Ear in Relation to Middle Ear Structures

Posterior semicircular canal

Superior semicircular canal

Lateral semicircular canal

Cochlea

Ossicular chain

Tympanic membrane

Vestibule

Round window

and muscles and spans the cavity like a bridge. The physics involved in how the ossicular chain and the eardrum function to transfer energy from the outer to inner ears is beyond the scope of this discussion. It is enough to consider that the ossicles take all the energy captured on the surface of the tympanic membrane and focus this energy onto the much smaller surface of the oval window. The surface area difference between the eardrum and the oval window, when coupled with a lever action of the ossicles, causes an increased concentration of energy at the oval window. Perkins and Kent (1986, p. 251) have likened this to a woman wearing spike heels trying to walk across a wet lawn. Regardless of how petite she is, her total body weight will be focused on the small heels, causing them to sink into the ground. In the same way, all of the sound energy captured on the tympanic membrane is focused onto the much smaller footplate of the stapes. The increased concentration of energy achieved by the tympanic membrane and the ossicular chain is necessary to set the dense fluids of the inner ear into motion.

The Inner Ear

Although the inner ear is very small, its anatomy is complex and its functions not fully understood. Before we continue to trace hearing through the inner ear, we need to examine its anatomy. The inner ear (Figure A-17) actually serves two functions. It contains structures important to hearing, of course, but it also contains a system we use to maintain balance or equilibrium. The structures of equilibrium are called the **semicircular canals.** Even though the inner ear has two functions, the divisions are connected, and they share the same fluid system.

The inner ear is encased in the temporal bone of the skull. The division containing the organs of hearing is called the *cochlea,* a structure that coils about two and a

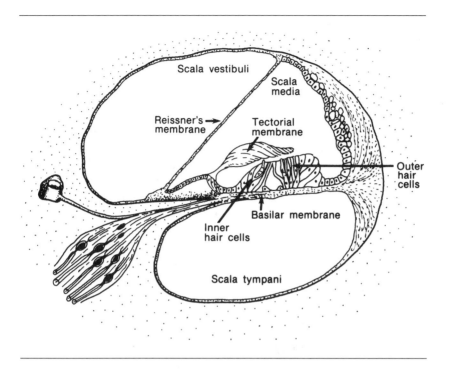

Scala vestibuli

Scala media

Reissner's membrane

Tectorial membrane

Outer hair cells

Basilar membrane

Inner hair cells

Scala tympani

FIGURE A-18 Cross Section of the Cochlea

half times around a cone-shaped bone called the **modiolus.** The nerve pathways from the cochlea feed into the modiolus where they merge into the **auditory nerve,** which carries hearing messages to the brain.

Figure A-18 shows a cross section of the cochlea. Imagine that we have uncoiled the cochlea, laid it lengthwise, and cut it. This figure shows what you would see if you looked through the cochlea as you might look through a pipe. Remember that everything you see here continues along the length of the structure. The cochlea is actually a bony tube containing two membranes that divide the tube into three sections: the **scala vestibule, scala media,** and **scala tympani.** The scala vestibule and scala media are separated by **Reissner's membrane,** and the scala media and scala tympani are separated by the **basilar membrane.** All three of these divisions are filled with fluid. The scala vestibule and scala tympani, which are connected at the top of the cochlea through a small opening called the **helicotrema,** are filled with fluid called **perilymph.** The fluid in the scala media is called **endolymph.**

The **organ of Corti,** sometimes called the essential or end organ of hearing is situated along the length of basilar membrane. It consists of thousands of tiny auditory nerve receptors that contain **hair cells** which are the delicate final endings of the auditory nerve. These receptors and their hair cells are arranged into one inner row and three outer rows along the basilar membrane. A jelly-like structure called the **tectorial membrane** hangs suspended over the tops of these highly sensitive hair cells. The tectorial membrane is a relatively free-floating membrane that responds to movements in the fluid of the scala media.

The **oval window,** which is occupied by the footplate of the stapes, serves as the communicating link between the middle ear and the scala vestibuli of the inner ear. The **round window** is located below the oval window and is adjacent to the scala tympani section of the inner ear. Sound vibrations enter the cochlea through the oval window. When the stapes pushes into the oval window, the mechanical energy of the ossicles is transformed into hydraulic energy in the form of fluid motion. The pressure of this motion is relieved by the round window, which moves toward the middle ear as the footplate of the stapes moves inward toward the inner ear.

There is some uncertainty about what happens next. We do know that motion of the fluids in the inner ear causes the tectorial membrane to move in a manner which somehow excites the hair cells, triggering neural impulses. The net result is that the hydraulic energy of the fluids is transformed into neural energy, which is carried by the peripheral pathways of the auditory nerve to the brain.

Tracing the Pathway of Hearing: A Brief Summary

By way of summarizing the hearing mechanism, we will follow a sound wave through the system and note the major structures of hearing along the way.

The sound wave is captured by the pinna, directed into the external auditory meatus, and strikes the surface of the tympanic membrane, setting it into vibration. This vibration is carried by the ossicles across the middle ear cavity and is focused onto the footplate of the stapes in the oval window. The inward movement of the stapes sets the perilymph of the scala vestibuli into motion, which causes Reissner's membrane to move, which then causes motion in the endolymph of the scala media. The motion of the endolymph causes movement of the tectorial membrane and movement along the basilar membrane. The motion finally makes its way along the scala tympani to the round window, which bulges slightly into the middle ear cavity. The motion of the tectorial membrane triggers neural responses in the hair cells, which are connected to the peripheral pathways of the auditory nerve. The auditory nerve carries the hearing information to the brain where it is processed.

Finally, notice the transformations of energy accomplished by the hearing mechanism. The acoustic energy of the sound wave is transformed into mechanical energy by the tympanic membrane and the ossicles. This mechanical energy is transformed into hydraulic energy by the fluids of the inner ear. The hydraulic energy is eventually transformed into neural energy by the action of the tectorial membrane and the hair cells.

The Complete Speech and Language Machine

We have now examined the anatomy and physiology, albeit briefly and superficially, of the structures that make up the speech machine. It is a complex system of systems, each part precisely and efficiently integrated with every other part, and directed by a reliable and constantly adapting central nervous system. Humans are born with all this equipment, and we quickly and easily adapt it for expressing language through speech.

Review Questions

1. Identify and define the four processes of speech. How are they integrated to produce speech?
2. How does quiet breathing differ from breathing for speech?
3. What happens in a single cycle of vocal fold vibration?
4. Describe the role of resonation in speech production.
5. What are the articulators? Which are mobile and which are fixed?
6. Trace the neurological relay race from the cerebrum to the muscles of speech.
7. Trace the journey of a sound wave from the pinna to the brain.

References and Suggested Readings

Abbs, J., Gracco, V., & Cole, K. (1984). Control of multimovement coordination: sensorimotor mechanisms in speech motor programming. *Journal of Motor Behaviors, 16,* 195.

Barlow, S., & Abbs, J. (1978, November). *Some evidence of auditory feedback contributing to the ongoing control of speech production.* Paper presented at American Speech and Hearing Association Convention, San Francisco, CA.

Bateman, H., & Mason, R. (1984). *Applied anatomy and physiology of the speech and hearing mechanism.* Springfield, IL: Charles C. Thomas.

Bell-Berti, F. (1975). Control of pharyngeal cavity size for English voiced and voiceless stops. *Journal of the Acoustical Society of America, 57,* 456–461.

Berti, F., & Hirose, H. (1975). Palatal activity in voicing distinctions: A simultaneous fiberoptic and electromyographic study. *Journal of Phonetics, 3,* 69–74.

Bless, D,, & Miller, J. (1972, November). *Influence of mechanical and linguistic factors on lung volume events during speech.* Paper presented at American Speech and Hearing Association Convention, San Francisco, CA.

Blumstein, S., & Cooper, W. (1974). Hemispheric processing of intonational contours. *Cortex, 10,* 146–158.

Borden, G. (1980). Use of feedback in established and developing speech. In N. Lass, (Ed.), *Speech and language advances in basic research and practice* (Vol. 3). New York: Academic Press.

Borden, G., & Harris, K. (1984). *Speech science primer* (2nd ed.). Baltimore: Williams & Wilkins Company.

Brown, J. (1975). On the neural organization of language: Thalamic and cortical relationships. *Brain and Language, 2*, 18–30.

Calvin, W., & Ojemann, G. (1980). *Inside the brain.* New York: New American Library.

Darley, F., Aronson, A., & Brown, J. (1975). *Motor speech disorders.* Philadelphia: W. B. Saunders.

Denes, P., & Pinson, E. (1993). *The speech chain* (2nd ed.). New York: W. H. Freeman and Co.

Dimond, S., & Beaumont, J. (1974). Experimental studies of hemispheric function in the human brain. In S. Dimond & J. Beaumont (Eds.), *Hemispheric function in the human brain.* New York: John Wiley.

Fritzel, B. (1969). The velopharyngeal muscles in speech: An electromyographic and cinefluorographic study. *Acta Otolaryngology.* (Stockholm) Suppl. 250.

Galaburda, A., & Sanides, F. (1980). Cytoarchitectonic organization of the human auditory cortex. *Journal of Comparative Neurology, 190,* 597–610.

Hixon, T. (1987). Respiratory function in speech. In T. Hixon, (Ed.), *Respiratory function in speech and song.* Boston: College-Hill Press.

Hockett, C. (1960). The origins of speech. *Scientific American, 203,* 89–97.

Hoit, J., Hixon, T., Watson, P., & Morgan, W. (1990). Speech breathing in children and adolescents. *Journal of Speech and Hearing Research, 33,* 51–69.

Hollien, H. (1960a). Some laryngeal correlated of vocal pitch. *Journal of Speech and Hearing Research, 3,* 52-58.

Hollien, H. (1960b). Vocal pitch variations related to changes in vocal fold length. *Journal of Speech and Hearing Research, 3,* 150–156.

Hutchinson, J., & Putnam, A. (1974). Aerodynamic aspects of sensory deprived speech. *Journal of the Acoustical Society of America, 56,* 1612–1617.

Isshiki, N. (1959). Regulatory mechanism of the pitch and volume of voice. *Otorhinolaryngology Clinic.* Kyoto, *52,* 1065.

Isshiki, N. (1964). Regulatory mechanisms of voice intensity variation. *Journal of Speech and Hearing Research, 7,* 17–29.

Isshiki, N., & Ringel, R. (1964). Air flow during the production of selected consonants. *Journal of Speech and Hearing Research, 7,* 233–244.

Kahane, J., & Folkins, J. (1984). *Atlas of speech and hearing anatomy.* Columbus, Ohio: Merrill.

Kelso, J., Tuller, B., & Harris, K. (1983). A dynamic pattern perspective on the control and coordination of movement. In P. MacNeilage (Ed.), *The production of speech.* New York: Springer-Verlag.

Kent, R. (1984). Brain mechanisms of speech and language with special reference to emotional interactions. In R. Naremore (Ed.), *Language science: Recent advances.* San Diego, CA: College-Hill Press.

Knox, C., & Kimura, D. (1970). Cerebral processing of nonverbal sounds in boys and girls. *Neuropsychologia, 8,* 227–237.

Kuehn, D., Lemme, M., & Baumgartner, J. (eds.). (1989). *Neural bases of speech, hearing, and language.* Boston: College-Hill Press.

Lieberman, P. (1975). *On the origins of language: An introduction to the evolution of human speech.* Series in physical anthropology. New York: Macmillan.

Liebman, M. (1991). *Neuroanatomy made easy and understandable* (4th ed.). Rockville, MD: Aspen.

Lubker, J. (1968). An electromyographic-cinefluorographic investigation of velar function during normal speech production. *Cleft Palate Journal, 5,* 1–18.

Marin, O., Schwartz, M., & Saffran, E. (1979). Origins and distribution of language. In M. Gazzaniga (Ed.), *Handbook of behavioral neurobiology.* New York: Plenum Press.

MacNeilage, P. (1970). Motor control of serial ordering of speech. *Psychological Review, 77,* 182–196.

McKeough, D. (1982). *The coloring review of neuroscience.* Boston: Little, Brown, and Company.

Millikan, C., & Darley, F. (1967). *Brain mechanisms underlying speech and language.* New York: Grune & Stratton.

Moll, K., & Daniloff, R. (1971). Investigation of the timing of velar movements during speech. *Journal of the Acoustical Society of America, 50,* 678–684.

Netsell, R., Kent, R., & Abbs, J. (1980). The organization and reorganization of speech movement. *Soc. Neurosci. Abstr., 6,* 462.

Negus, V. (1962). *The comparative anatomy and physiology of the larynx.* New York: Hafner.

Ornstein, R., & Thompson, R. (1984). *The amazing brain.* Boston: Houghton Mifflin.

Perkins, W., & Kent, R. (1986). *Functional anatomy of speech, language, and hearing: A primer.* Boston: College-Hill Press.

Putnam, A., & Ringel, R. (1979). Oral sensation and perception. In Williams, W., & D. Goulding (Eds.), *Articulation and learning,* Springfield, IL: Charles C. Thomas.

Scott, C., & Ringel, R. L. (1971). Articulation without oral sensory control. *Journal of Speech and Hearing Research, 14,* 804–818.

Subtelny, J., Oya, N., & Subtelny, J. (1972). Cineradiographic study of sibilants. *Folia Phoniatrics.* (Basel), *24,* 30–50.

Sussman, H. (1979). Evidence for left hemisphere superiority in processing movement-related tonal signals. *Journal of Speech and Hearing Research, 22,* 224–235.

Tucker, D. (1981). Lateral brain function, emotion and conceptualization. *Psychological Review, 89,* 19–46.

Zemlin, W. (1988). *Speech and hearing science, anatomy and physiology* (3rd ed.). Englewood Cliffs, NJ: Prentice-Hall.

Zemlin, W. (1990). Anatomy and physiology of speech. In G. Shames & E. Wiig (Eds.), *Human communication disorders* (3rd ed.). Columbus, OH: Merrill/Macmillan.

Name Index

Subject Index